YOU'RE NOT FAT

YOU'RE TOXIC

D1599831

Also by Stephanie Relfe

Perfect Health with Kinesiology and Muscle Testing
Training Manual

Perfect Health with Kinesiology and Muscle Testing
Practitioners Manual

Perfect Health with Kinesiology and Muscle Testing
DVD Training Course

Homeschool Natural Health & Biology Comprehension Curriculum
Workbook, for Grades 7 - 12. A companion to *You're Not Fat. You're Toxic*

YOU'RE NOT FAT

YOU'RE TOXIC

Stephanie Relfe B.Sc.

Sherrington House

Disclaimer

The information presented in this book has been obtained from authentic and reliable sources and is for educational and informational purposes. It is not intended as a diagnoses or treatment of any medical condition. The information given is not medical advice nor is it presented as a course of personalized treatment. Before changing any medical treatment or before discontinuing any course of medical treatment you may now be undergoing, you should consult your physician. The reader should not stop prescription medications without the advice and guidance of his or her personal physician. Although great care has been taken to ensure the accuracy of the information presented, the author and the publisher cannot assume responsibility for the validity of all the materials or the consequences of their use. Before starting any health regimen you should consult with your physician. Any application of the material set forth in the following pages is at the reader's discretion and sole responsibility.

FAIR USE NOTICE

This book may contain copyrighted material the use of which has not always been specifically authorized by the copyright owner. We are making such material available in our efforts to advance understanding of issues of health, ecological and humanitarian significance. We believe this constitutes a 'fair use' of any such copyrighted material as provided for in section 107 of the US Copyright Law.

Amazon Services Disclosure

Stephanie Relfe and Relfe.com is a participant in the Amazon Services LLC Associates Program, an affiliate advertising program designed to provide a means for websites to earn advertising fees by advertising and linking to Amazon.com. All publications referenced or reviewed in *You're Not Fat, You're Toxic™*, are available at Amazon.com and other major book retailers. Their inclusion in this book is unrelated to any affiliate payments due to their possible future purchase.

DEDICATION

I was travelling with my husband and son from Iowa to Florida. At one time, we stopped in a restaurant, and struck up a conversation with the young waitress who served us. Unfortunately, while she was very young and attractive, she had too much fat on her. I started to explain to her some of the simple ways that one could become slim, and stay slim, which are in this book.

She was amazed. In fact, she was so amazed that she brought five other waitresses over to hear what I had to say. They were shocked at what I had to say, and all of them eagerly soaked up every morsel of information that I gave them. My heart went out to these young girls who were trapped in bodies and a future where fat and toxins were bound to affect them in many different ways; from personal feelings of happiness, wellbeing and success to likely major health problems.

I was shocked that the mega-corporations had done such a good job of keeping simple truths from these young women and thereby ruining their lives. It was the thought of these young women, and the millions more like them, as well as all the poor little children that we see now who have fat where none should exist, that pushed me on when I did not want to keep writing and researching. I hope those young ladies get to see a copy of this book.

Stephanie Relfe

You're Not Fat. You're Toxic.

Contents

Foreword

Where the title for this book came from

My wife Stephanie had spent the better part of seven years planning, researching and writing *You're not fat, You're toxic*. So I was familiar with the poisons in our food, water and air and what they are doing to people everywhere. I will never forget how I created the name for her book. We were in Australia in 2004 visiting her family. One afternoon we were shopping at the grocery store. Stephanie went searching for things on her list and she sent me to the other side of the store to find our favorite tea tree oil toothpaste. The health and personal care products were in the same aisle and as I was searching for the toothpaste, a woman walked next to me and asked me a question about the protein supplements, thinking that I was an employee.

I asked her why she thought she needed a protein supplement and she replied "I want to speed up my metabolism because I am just *so fat*". She was so *sad*. She said it with downcast eyes, like she was embarrassed and like she was apologizing to me for somehow offending me. I could feel how sad she felt and so I could do only one thing:

"You're NOT fat, you're TOXIC", I told her. She just stared at me. She was stunned. I continued, "You are being poisoned to death by something. It could be food, or something in your house or parasites from your animals or some other thing. It's something you need to find out about."

We talked for a short time. I told her about food and chemicals in the food. I told her about parasites and how she needed to do a cleanse to get rid of them. I told her about not eating meat, coffee or soft drinks, including diet drinks. And I told her about how microwaved food slowly kills people while making them fat. When we were done she looked happy. And she looked like she had hope. She was not embarrassed. She kind of looked mad, like someone looks when they realize they have been conned.

And so after telling Stephanie what happened, she agreed that what I told that woman would be a great title for her book. We discussed other titles and approaches, but finally settled on *You're not fat, You're toxic.*

I think about that woman sometimes and hope that what I said helped her. No one should feel sad or embarrassed about being lied to, cheated or defrauded by a system that poisons them and tries to make them feel that they are the cause.

If you are beyond your normal weight, I hope that Stephanie's book will give you a blueprint for reducing your weight and regaining your health. And I hope you will get so angry about being victimized by the Food Mafia that you will tell your friends and help them stop eating poisoned food, just like you.

Best Regards,

Michael Relfe

CHAPTER 1

YOU'RE NOT FAT. YOU'RE TOXIC

Have you found that you are getting bigger and bigger? Even though you are eating the same food, in the same quantities, that used to keep you smaller? Are you getting larger, no matter what you do? Are you hungry a lot of the time? Are you depressed about having little control over your body? Have you given up? Do you believe that you are addicted to food? Are you like some people, whom I saw on a documentary[1], who amazingly said that they did not expect to live past 55, or even 50? Do you want to be slim, not just for looks, but also because you want to *feel good*? Do you have children who are too pudgy, and you don't know what to do about it?

If you said yes to any of these questions, then this book is for you. It's unique. With unique answers, not found in virtually any other weight loss book. In this book you will find reasons why you are not thin, even if you have been doing many things correctly.

There is a plague growing all over the world, and its name is obesity. One in three Americans are obese[2],[3]. But it's not just America. In Europe now, a majority of adults are overweight.[4] And the World Health Organization warned that a billion people are overweight and obese, and this number is rising[5].

An extensive country-by-country report in the 2011 *Lancet*, the world's leading medical journal, found that America was the 20th fattest country[6]. Number one was the United Arab Emirates with an average BMI (body-mass index of fat percentage) of 28.9. Anyone with a bodymass of 25 or higher is considered overweight. The average BMI in the United States is 28.4. Note that this is an average. Thin people help to keep the average from skyrocketing.

Just looking around will show you that people have grown enormously in just the last five years. It's becoming so common place for people to be larger than they should be, that many people in America now think that it's 'normal'.

Perhaps worst of all is what's happening to children, since children traditionally were always a healthy, slim size. Now in the USA, one in five four-year-olds are obese[7]! The frightening thing is that huge body size is becoming so 'normal', that some people now think that this is how it 'should' be, and look at children who are a healthy slim size as 'needing to put on weight'. It's quite a terrifying sight to me to see ten year old children with fat arms and legs and double chins, knowing that this is, for many, a life sentence of health & emotional problems.

In Europe, for example, the European Union is particularly concerned that it is children who are increasingly contributing to making Europe a fat continent. In 2007 the European Union reported that 21 million children are overweight, and this number is increasing by 400,000 children each year. This is a tragedy, because there is absolutely no reason why *any* child should be overweight.

It is a travesty when people get so much fat on their bodies that it even shows up around their faces. A fat face covers up the majesty and beauty of your character, of who you truly are. But in addition to personal appearance, this is a deadly serious question about health, about destroying people's lives. Try this: Right now, go and pick up four pounds of sugar or flour. Walk around the house with it. See how heavy it is? Imagine what an extra 50 lb. feels like, and how much work you have to do to do that. It's terrible that so many people have to carry so many extra pounds around with them, especially if they are children with growing bones.

In addition, one pound of fat has about 100 miles of blood vessels[8].

That's a lot of extra work your body has to do, just to maintain that extra weight! No wonder over-weight people get tired so easily.

Why are so many people so overweight, when this did not happen very often a few decades ago? This is a plague that's spreading – a super disease. Something is seriously wrong. People did not look like this in 1950. And yet, every year, many new books come out on dieting and weight loss. "Weight loss" is a $60 billion a year industry[9], and it's not working.

There is a saying, "It's no use running faster, if you are on the wrong road."

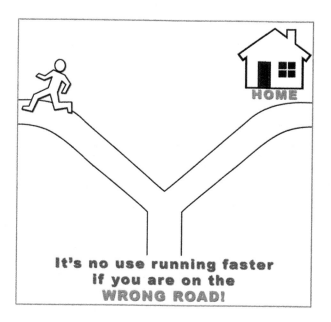

In fact, the commonly held causes of obesity, overeating and inactivity, do not explain the current obesity epidemic. While there is a perception that people are consuming more calories, studies in England show that overall levels of daily caloric consumption have actually declined substantially throughout the twentieth century[10]. And while understanding how the right kind of exercise is important, evidence does not show that levels of physical activity have plummeted sufficiently to totally cause such a high incidence of obesity during this time period[11]. In fact, a report by the British Sports Council on physical activity noted the opposite phenomenon, stating that "participation is increasing across all age bands and all social groupings"[12]. It's time we looked elsewhere for answers.

THE ANSWER IS THAT FAT GAIN IS CAUSED LARGELY BY TOXINS

A toxin is a substance that hurts the body. The more toxins, and the stronger they are, the more damage is done to the body.

Here's yet more evidence that body weight is not about calories or genes. See how France and the United Kingdom, which are genetically and geographically very similar, eat on average the *same number* of calories each day. And yet their average weight varies by 26 lb. / 12 Kg[13] !

Country	Average Weight	Daily Intake
United Kingdom	176 lb. / 80 kg	2,200
Italy	163 lb. / 74 kg	2,100
Germany	162 lb. / 73.5 kg	2,400
France	150 lb. / 68 kg	2,200

More and more evidence is mounting to show that it is toxins, and not calories or lack of exercise, that cause obesity. For example, in a recent study, rats given toxic chemicals gained weight and increased their fat storage, without increased calories or decreased exercise. In 6 months, the rats were 20% heavier and had 36% more body fat than rats that had not been exposed to those chemicals.[14]

TWO SOURCES OF TOXINS

Toxins come from two main sources:

1. Some toxins are from the environment around us[15]. The amount of toxins in our environment from pollution, cleaning chemicals and

chemicals on products such as toys, clothes and furniture, has grown at roughly the same rate as the rise in fat gain. We should do what we can to eliminate toxins from our home, but the toxins in the environment are much harder for one person to control. In this book you will learn ways to help your body detox environmental toxins.

2. The other, and main, source of toxins we *can* control. This source is the toxins in our food and drink, plus a few other sources I will discuss later. These affect us much more strongly than those in the environment, because they are right inside our body, in large amounts.

This book will give you information you need to get slim, and to stay slim, *without going hungry*. To understand this fully, you will need to develop a completely new way of thinking about your body from the way that the medical establishment has taught you. Start to question everything. First of all, let's look at calories.

WHAT IS A CALORIE?

I was shocked when watching the very good documentary, *Super Size Me,* to see how many people did not have a clue what a calorie is. A calorie is a measurement of how much energy is in food. To determine calories, scientists burn food to see how much heat the food gives off when it is burned. And, yes, calories are part of the picture. Generally, the more calories you eat, the larger you will get.

But if you focus on calories, instead of on toxins and on what is healthy, you very well may never get the results you want, especially long term. There is no comparison between a normal engine, like the one in your car, and your body. The car needs only one kind of fuel to make it go. Our bodies are living and infinitely complex, and changing every second in billions of different ways.

YOU NEED NUTRIENTS TO TURN FOOD INTO ENERGY

If calories give energy, then it should follow that people with high calorie diets have the most energy, right? That means that a person who lives off cookies and French fries should have the most energy. But, in fact, these are generally the people with the least energy. Here's the reason for this: An engine gets energy simply by *burning* fuel. But our bodies do not do this. Instead, our bodies get energy from complicated *chemical reactions*. These chemical reactions require a *good supply* of nutrients, such as vitamins, minerals, trace elements and many other nutrients that we don't know much about as yet.[16]

Toxic food usually has very few nutrients. Therefore, without enough nutrients, the body cannot *use* the chemical energy you eat. So it stores it as fat, until it can use the chemical energy at a later date, when you do give it enough nutrients (if ever).

Plus, if you don't get enough of the right nutrition, you will be hungry, and eat more. If you consume toxins, your body will require extra nutrition to remove the toxins, and so will tell your body that you need to eat more food.

TOXIC FOODS CAN BE AS ADDICTIVE AS DRUGS

Plus, toxins are highly addictive, as we shall see, so the addiction will urge you to eat more of the toxic food. This is often the crux of the problem for many people. It's not that people are addicted to food in general. It's that they eat foods which are chemically addictive. Once you understand this, and switch to foods that are not addictive, your brain chemistry will change, and you will have the willpower to kick your previous habits, because you will no longer be hungry and your brain will be working better.

Here's an example of this: The New York Daily News wrote:

"Fatty foods may be just as addictive as heroin and cocaine[17]."

In fact, some addiction researchers have argued that potato chips and foods similar to them like bacon, cheesecake and chocolate frosting, are as addictive as crack[18]! Rats that were given unrestricted access to processed high-fat and high-sugar foods like these not only got obese, but their reward threshold kept getting bigger and bigger. The rats found it harder and harder to register pleasure, so they ate more and more than before, "very similar to what we have seen with animals that use cocaine and heroin[19]." In fact, if rats are given full access to junk food from the supermarket for long enough, they will then voluntarily starve when offered only healthy food[20].

It got so bad that after 40 days of addiction, the rats were willing to put up with painful electric shocks to the feet, just so they could get hold of more junk food! That's *really* bad. One of the ways that I will show you how to gain the strength to give up these addictions, is by giving your brain a lot of real, natural nutrition, so that the brain and body can start to function correctly again.

Unfortunately, weight loss 'experts' usually think only in terms of calories. They seem to think that our bodies are the same as metal engines that just burn everything. Calories are just a part of the picture for long term fat management. Our bodies are not made of metal. They are living and organic, and have virtually *nothing* in common with an engine that does not think, has no life in it, and does not grow and repair itself.

KEY #1 TO GETTING THIN: AVOID TOXINS

The main key to weight loss is toxins, not calories. Understand this, and you will understand the reasons behind nearly every successful weight loss story, and every single story of someone who gained weight.

FOURTEEN WAYS THAT TOXINS MAKE YOU FAT:

Some, but not all, of the ways that toxins make you fat, are as follows:

1. Our bodies do not get energy from burning fuel like a car engine does, but from complicated chemical reactions, that require a good supply of nutrients[21]. The more toxins you eat, the less nutrients you have. Therefore, the body cannot use all the chemical energy you eat, and so it stores it as fat until it can use it later.

2. Toxins cause chemical stress. This raises cortisol levels. High cortisol

levels makes you fat, especially on the belly[22].

3. Toxins make you hungry, by raising cortisol. They also make you crave sugary, high-calorie foods.

4. Toxins are acidic. High acid content is fattening. Your body needs an alkaline environment to burn fat.

5. Your body uses up magnesium to burn fat. Most of us are already deficient in magnesium. The more toxins, the less magnesium you will have, and the less your body can get rid of fat.

6. If your body can't get rid of excess toxins, because the liver is over-loaded from too many toxins to deal with, it stores them in the nearest fat cell, to be dealt with at a later date. Think of fat cells as *garbage dumps*.

7. The more toxins you ingest, the more nutrients your body needs to break them down. The less nutrients you have, the hungrier you will be, and the more food you will eat.

8. Toxins put your body out of balance, making it less efficient, and harder for it to burn fat and build muscle.

9. Much of the food we eat has too much estrogen, or toxic substances that act as if they are estrogen. Excess estrogen causes an increase in fat tissue. To make matters worse, the more fat you have, the more estrogen you make, which makes even more fat[23]!

10. Toxins are often highly addictive, as addictive as drugs. For example, that's why people keep going back to fast food outlets, even though they know they are making them fat. Once you know that you are dealing with a real chemical addiction, you will get the extra will power needed to go long enough without the food, to heal the addiction, even to the extent that you forget about that particular food.

Plus, eating foods that are healthy, and not addictive, will prevent you from feeling hungry and make your brain work better, so that eventually you no longer want toxic foods.

11. Toxins induce insulin resistance[24]. That is, toxins cause diabetes.

12. Toxins cause allergic reactions, which include fat gain. The more toxic a food is, the more chance there is that it will cause an allergic reaction. Even healthy foods may have a little toxin in them, which a healthy body handles normally, as long you get enough variety and nutrition in your diet. But if you eat a food nearly every day, then that increases the chance of you becoming allergic to that food. Any food that you just can't bear the thought of giving up, is almost guaranteed to be allergic to you, and a major cause of your fat gain, even if it's a low-calorie food, such as tomatoes.

13. The majority of restaurant, fast food and processed foods have chemicals added to them called excitotoxins. MSG and Aspartame are examples of excitotoxins. Companies do this to fool your brain into thinking the food tastes delicious and *because* they are addictive, and make money for the companies. Excitotoxins are called "excito" toxins because they literally excite brain cells, which is why they make food taste great. Unfortunately, they also excite the brain cells to death, within a few hours. *Just one dose* kills brain cells in a critical area of the brain[25]. Food is meant to support your body. How can it do that if it is killing brain cells?

14. When your body is toxic, you will not feel happy. Unhappy people are more likely to reach for a donut or cheeseburger.

Others are beginning to realize that toxins are part of the picture. For example, the UK Daily Mail reported:

"Chemicals found in household products may be causing significant increase in cancers, diabetes, *obesity* and falling fertility, the European Environment Agency has warned[26]."

Further evidence that it's toxins that are making us fat is provided, I do believe, by the 2011 report by *Lancet*, of which country is the fattest world wide. While some of us have the perception that women are fatter than men, the truth is the opposite. U.S. men are the 10th fattest in the world, while U.S. women rank at 'only' 36th. Therefore, women brought the total US fatness down to 20th in the world.

Generally it's easier for men to reduce weight than women, because nature designed man as a "four cylinder engine", but women as a "three-cylinder engine". And yet, American men are fatter than American women. No wonder men die, on average, five years before women! I believe this difference in fat is because more women care more about what they eat, and focus more on health than men do. Part of this idea comes from years of observing what people put in their shopping trolleys. I have seen that women are more likely to add some healthy foods, but men tend to throw in only what they like the taste of, with more processed goods and alcohol, a lot less variety, and hardly ever any vegetables.

But it's not just toxins from household products or pollution. The main toxins that are making us fat are the ones we put into our bodies. We will be looking at the major fat-causing toxins in this book. The good news is that when you remove toxins, and eat more nutritious foods, you will get healthier and happier, as well as thinner.

Much of the advice in this book is backed up by scientific research, and many references are included. Where I refer to another author, I have used only authors who had an extensive list of scientific research references. However, the general message in this book is not favored by the medical establishment. Why? Because we spend $2.2 trillion a year on so-called 'health' care in the United States of America. That's five times more than the defense budget[27]!

That's why some people in the government, and lobbyists, work for the drug companies, not for you and me. They fuel massive profits for the Medical Mafia by taking taxpayers money, and using it to give billions of dollars in subsidies to farmers to grow cheap corn, wheat, soy, meat and dairy[28]. You will learn how these foods easily cause obesity, heart attacks, diabetes and cancer, the main things that the Medical Mafia need in order to receive that $2.2 trillion each year. The government is not interested in subsidizing healthy, organic vegetables and fruit which prevent the drug companies from making their trillions of dollars.

This is why you can't look to most doctors or scientists for advice. Because the same advice that will get you permanently thin without being hungry, is the same advice that will get you *healthy*. And that will reduce their profits. There's no money in healthy people, and no money in dead people. They want to keep you somewhere in between.

Don't think the government is going to care about you either. That $2.2 trillion sure greases a lot of wheels, even if it isn't all profit. Plus, the more people who die early, the less the government has to worry about paying social security.

Unfortunately, most people still think that people with medical training are the ones to turn to. However, here's just one example of what's in the heart of many doctors and the companies that trained them: In 2012 just one drug company, Glaxo Smith Kline, was found guilty of bribing with financial kickbacks a massive network of 49,000 doctors to sell their products. That's right - forty nine *thousand* doctors. The company admitted to this and paid the federal government $3 billion in fines[29]. The company won't mind that though. That's just the cost of doing business.

If you think you can turn to doctors for advice on fat loss, consider what Dr. Wallach, the author of *Dead Doctors Don't Lie* says about doctors[30]:

"This profession tells you to follow their instructions to stay healthy and live a long life. I wondered just how good a job they did. So I went to the medical school library at the University of California in San Diego and pulled out the Journal of the American Medical Association. The average age of the 40 M.D. obituaries was 58 years old! Could this statistic possibly be accurate? Be nice to know about this, wouldn't it? Our average life span is 75.5. You can gain 17 years of life simply by not going to medical school!"

Doctors don't study health. They study sickness. ``Health insurance" should be called ``sickness insurance", just like we have ``fire insurance" and ``flood insurance". Having health insurance won't make you healthy, or thin.

However, not all doctors are evil or clueless. It's the system that's evil. Five brave doctors published a report "Death by Medicine" that analyzed all published data, and found that conventional medicine causes the death of more than 780,000 people in the USA each year[31]! I bet you did not see that statistic in the mainstream media.

You will find scientific evidence to back up my claim that it is toxins that are making people fat, as you read on. For starters, *Woman's World* magazine reported when a panel of nutrition experts from top universities, including Harvard, Yale and Cornell, was asked to pick the very best diet for Americans to try, they picked a plan that most people have never heard of. It's called the DASH diet. DASH stand for "Dietary Approach to Stop Hypertension". It's based on fruit and vegetables, plus low-fat dairy and small amounts of lean protein, nuts, whole grains and good fat[32].

If you look at the DASH diet, you will see that processed food and many toxins are removed, while a lot of unprocessed, raw plant foods are added. As you read on, you will learn why this plan works so much better than more famous diets. And you will also learn how to *vastly improve* on even the DASH diet.

Here's an example of how very different this book is from other weight loss books. I researched 43 books and documentaries for this book, among other sources, culling the gems of wisdom from them, and one of the books was *Crack the Fat-loss Code* by Wendy Chant. The book is pretty much your standard weight loss book, with a few good tips. I decided to look on the internet to see what Wendy Chant looked like. I was totally shocked and horrified to learn that she died at 44 years old of cancer! This is a woman who taught about health and fitness! What use is being thin if one dies of cancer?

It is a tragedy that this woman died of such a terrible disease, and at such a young age. Please, learn from her experience. Do not let this happen to you. Have you noticed how few people seem to die like they did in the old days, when they used to pass away peacefully in their sleep, or on the couch?

One thing that people don't mention much about cancer is how incredibly *painful* it is. A friend of my family died of cancer, and even with painkillers, she died screaming in her husband's arms. I do not want this to happen to you. I want to scare you into taking action now.

I want you to have the same goal that I do: when it is time to leave my body and travel to Heaven, I intend to leave my body with peace and grace, and free of pain and drugs, in my own home. While this book is about fat loss, many of the habits which you need to reduce fat are the same ones that are needed to stay free of cancer, stroke and other dreadful diseases.

Obviously, there were things about health that Wendy Chant did not know about. Her book says much the same as many other diet books, by talking about grams of fat, protein and carbohydrate. But there is very little discernment between what is toxic and what is not. For example, pepperoni pizza is on one of her menu plans. You will learn why pepperoni is a major no-no, for both fat loss and for health, because it's loaded in toxins. That's why it doesn't rot very much. Food is meant to rot. If it doesn't rot, that means it's so toxic that not even bacteria will touch it. Bacteria are needed to digest food in your intestines.

Here's an interesting thought; during all the time people have been getting fatter, *wild* animals have not gained a pound. Hmmm... Can wild animals give us some clues? I believe that they can. You see, while you are an immortal spirit, your body is separate from you. That's why we say "MY" body. The body is not "you".

While you are an advanced Spiritual Being, the body that you own and live in to play the game of life with, is biologically just an animal. One of the clues to finding the answers we seek in getting thin is to see what wild animals are doing right that we aren't. And if you think it's about exercise, think again. While many animals do more exercise than we do, it's not as much as you might think.

Wild animals generally maintain an ideal weight with high muscle and low fat throughout their life. The few exceptions are hibernating animals. For example, a bear may look fat in the summer, but that's not fat, it's muscle. Watch a video of a bear running down a dear and you will realize this. Eating natural, raw food keeps a bear at its correct weight. But as winter starts approaching, bears get a change in their brain chemistry so that they can eat past their normal satiation amounts, so that they can put on fat for winter. Somehow, the toxins and lack of nutrition in our food has done the same to us. We eat as though we are getting ready to hibernate!

In fact, wild animals prove to us that obesity has nothing to do with our genes. It's in our genes to be thin! Just like wild animals are! Even if the last few generations of your family were overweight, if you go back far enough, your ancestors did not have problems with fat. However, fat can run in families, not because we share the same genes, but because we 'inherit' the eating, lifestyle and child-rearing *habits of our parents.*

I am going to tell you information that others dare not, because it threatens trillions of dollars of profits of multinational companies. If you are desperate for a thin body and a thin face, and a new life, then this book is for you. It's not about your genes. It's about the things we do, which are very divorced from nature.

Some of the information that I am going to give will not be welcome to many readers, because you will learn that substances that you have grown to love and have been brainwashed into thinking are slimming, are actually making you fat, such as meat and dairy (even if it is low-fat), and even coffee. And you will realize how you have been victimized.

KEY #2 TO GETTING THIN: COMPLETE NUTRITION FROM RAW PLANTS

You will be reading about new scientific evidence that shows that eating meat and dairy causes many bad effects including:

- Damaged blood vessels.
- Damaged pancreas cells, so that they can't produce insulin.
- Cancer cells to grow.
- Fat.

Most people think they need lots of animal protein, because the meat industry has trained us to think that, so that we buy their products. Remember that meat is just a product that someone wants you to buy. But protein does not make protein. Amino acids make protein. Any protein that is eaten has to be broken down into amino acids before it can be used to make the particular proteins that your body needs. Our body builds 50,000 different proteins[33], as well as 5,000 enzymes, from just 22 amino acids[34],[35].

All plants have *more than enough* amino acids to do this, even the essential amino acids. You will see a graph in the chapter on meat which verifies this.

You will see how all of the above symptoms, including fat, can be reversed by changing to a whole foods diet of vegetables, fruit, seeds, nuts and legumes, plus a few extras such as organic eggs. That leaves a *long* list of foods which you can eat, which are given in the "Shopping list" chapter.

But if you want to be really thin, then you will take this one step further. There is one thing that wild animals eat that we don't, and that is the second key to getting and staying thin: That is *raw* plant food, just like gorillas do. If you think you need lots of cooked protein, realize that gorillas and chimpanzees, who are anatomically very close to us, don't eat cooked meat, but they still have plenty of muscle. By eating *raw* plant food, animals have what most of us don't – enzymes, plus thousands of other nutrients, which are destroyed by cooking. These are the nutrients that your body needs to get thin naturally.

Raw plants contain all the amino acids your body needs to build protein. *But cooking destroys 50% of protein.* Don't be threatened by the idea of eating raw plants. I am going to show you ways to eat raw food that make it easy, tasty and interesting. This may be hard to believe, but the more you do this, the more you will actually *forget* about the junk food of the past.

NUTRITION IS KEY TO GETTING THIN

You are going to learn how nutrition is key to getting thin. For example, abdominal obesity is associated with low levels of magnesium, zinc, and Vitamins C & E[36]. (One day, studies will find that obesity is associated with low levels of many other nutrients as well). A fat belly is associated with low nutrition levels, partly because the more toxins you ingest, the better your nutrition needs to be to remove them.

The only thing that works for life, is life-style changes to *what* you eat and drink, and when you eat and drink. It has less to do with quantity. Although, you will find, that once you eat a diet of vegetables, fruits, nuts, seeds and legumes with a lot of raw food, that you naturally eat less than before.

But, the question is, what life-style changes work? It was only when I discovered certain teachings of natural health that I finally found the answers I was looking for. I am sorry to say, there is no magic bullet, no pill or 5 minute program that will work for life. Do not believe all the hype that tells you that is possible, so that the people selling the hype can get rich.

It takes a wholistic approach, meaning that you have to look at *everything* that affects your body. If you have bought into the concept of a magic pill to cure every ill, including fat gain, I am sorry that you have fallen for a marketing gimmick.

This book is going to do a very good job of showing you all the important parts of your lifestyle that you need to improve to get and stay slim. Once I used this knowledge, I was able to reverse my body's trend of increasing weight (scary!) and to keep my weight down, year after year, without being hungry, or missing what I gave up, and while still being happy and energetic.

This book will explain why people are growing fatter and fatter, and what to do about it, with a completely new way of thinking about food and your body. Some of the time you won't even have to change what you are eating. You will just do things differently to reduce the toxins in your body, such as change the way you prepare food or when you eat it.

You are not fat. You are toxic. We need to shift the focus from calories to toxins. This is a revolutionary concept, but please read on to learn more.

I am not the only one to make this realization, although I do take it further than others. For example, a study entitled *"Chemical toxins: a hypothesis to explain the global obesity epidemic"* concluded that:

> "The commonly held causes of obesity - overeating and inactivity - do not explain the current obesity epidemic[37]."

The study suggests that because "the obesity epidemic occurred relatively quickly", that the cause is toxins in the environment. While this is part of the problem, the toxins you eat and drink are a much bigger cause of the problem. After all, wild animals aren't obese, and they share our environment. You will learn in this book unique concepts, such as that a person can get fat by consuming food or drinks that have no calories, and get thin by eating food with high calories.

Your body is not a car, that simply needs one form of energy poured into it. It is fabulously complex beyond our imaginations, and needs thousands of different nutrients to keep it working at optimum. When you don't give it the right nutrients, you will get hungrier, and eat more. And because the body is not getting what it needs, its ability to function as God intended is messed up, and it is much more likely that you will gain fat.

YOUR BODY USES FAT CELLS AS GARBAGE DUMPS

I first learned this secret key to weight loss from my teacher in natural health, Australian Naturopath and Kinesiologist, David Bridgman. David explained how the liver is an amazing organ of the body, which has the job of breaking down thousands of different toxins, so that they can be removed from the body. A toxin is like the exhaust of a car - it's the parts which didn't get used. Even food which is good for you will produce some toxins. But our current society has added a whole host of new toxins to the body, which is challenging our livers like never before.

In order to break down the toxins, the liver needs the right materials to do the job, and enough energy to do the job. If it doesn't have enough of the right materials, or energy, to do the job, it dumps the toxins in a fat cell!

That is why you have fat which hasn't budged. It's nothing to do with calories. It's because the body is using those fat cells as garbage dumps. In order to solve this problem, you need to stop taking in extra toxins, and give the body the right raw materials and energy to remove the toxins.

In addition, toxins are acidic. The more toxic, the more acidic. Non-toxic foods are alkaline in the body. A lot of people eat only acidic foods most of the time, which is why we now see so many growing people.

Added to this, people are eating much more processed food, rather than food they prepare fresh at home. The more something is processed, rather than prepared at home, even if you bought it from a health food store, the more toxins it has.

For example, sugar is a problem. But *raw* sugar cane is not a problem. If you eat something that is raw and untouched, as a wild animal does, the food has thousands of nutrients which work together to nourish your body, the way God intended. But each time we process something, the substances and energy are changed. Each step along the way, sugar becomes more and more toxic, because it loses nutrients that are needed, and concentrates substances which are never meant to be concentrated. Does raw, white sugar look anything like raw sugar cane? No. You see, no one has ever seen a sugar molecule, and until we have, we won't really know what processing does to natural food.

Another example of how processing food makes it worse and worse. Heroin is made from a flower, the poppy. When the poppy is processed it makes a dangerous drug, opium. When it is processed more, it becomes an even more dangerous drug, morphine. And ultimately it is processed into deadly, highly addictive heroin. Heroin bears no resemblance to the original poppy, but processing made it hugely more dangerous. And toxic.

In addition, the more processed a food is, the more addictive it may become, making you want to eat more. On the other hand, a meal prepared fresh at home will leave you satisfied with a smaller amount.

To make matters even worse, restaurants and fast food outlets *deliberately* add toxins, called excitotoxins, which make the food addictive, but which also kill brain cells. They drug the food so that you will buy more of it.

I had an argument with a family member about this once. No matter what I said, he just didn't get what I was saying. Like most people, he believed that getting thin was *only* about eating less calories. So I began to get clearer on what my argument was. We are not a furnace that burns everything that is put into it equally. Hey, even most machines aren't! If you put diesel in a car that wants regular gasoline, the car won't run.

It's the same with our bodies, except that because our bodies are alive, it's much, much more complicated than that. To get thin, we have to get back to eating as God intended. Did you ever see a fat wild animal? (Other than one that is getting ready to hibernate). No. Wild animals of the same species have similar body sizes mostly all the time. We are meant to do that as well. But because we have broken away from God, we have had to pay the cost with bodies that don't work properly, and hence put on pounds and more pounds.

Going back to my discussion with a member of my family, he finally got what I was saying. "Are you saying that if you eat 5,000 calories of apples that you won't get fat, but if you eat 5,000 calories of fast food that you will get fat?" (His wife correctly pointed out that it would probably be impossible to eat 5,000 calories worth of apples). While that was greatly oversimplifying things, basically, yes, that was the idea. Especially when this is applied over a long period of time. It's not that simple, because too much food, even healthy food, becomes toxic. So quantity still does play a part. But you will find that when you eat the right kind of food, you naturally end up eating less. Maybe a lot less.

As you give up toxins at every opportunity, you will find your body will have the ability to burn fat, build muscle and reduce your appetite. And at the same time, you will start to feel happier naturally. This will replace the chemical high that you used to get from junk food.

This book is unlike any other weight-loss book. While everybody is different, once you have read this book, you will understand why all those hundreds of other weight loss books and articles work for some people, and why they don't work for others. You will learn why we have the terrible situation in which even very young children are obese. And you will understand why the $60 billion a year weight loss industry will not reveal to you the secrets in this book.

Even if you are close to your ideal weight, somewhere in this book there is at least one answer to getting the body size you want. If you are very overweight, there are many answers that you have been looking for. Once you learn the common sense concepts that this book teaches – that you are toxic, not fat – you can change the habits which got you where you are today. Then you can have a thin body, and the power to know that your body size is finally within your control *permanently*.

This information is important for everyone to learn. Why? Because if you put on just four pounds every year, that is 40 pounds every 10 years. There are plenty of overweight people who were once thin. They are overweight because they did not know about the importance of toxins.

WEIGHT ALONE IS MISLEADING

As you remove toxins from your body and give it more nutrients, it is very important to keep in mind that while you will lose weight, that is not the only important thing. The important thing is how small and well-proportioned your body becomes. Two weeks after my husband and I started having 2-3 fresh-squeezed juices a day, we weighed only about 2 pounds less. But we looked thinner, and this was verified by a relative who told us, unprompted, that we both looked thinner. I will talk more about this in the chapter "Weight is deceptive". Therefore, on this program it is crucial that you regularly *feel* your body for changes. Plus once a week, try on a pair of pants that are one size smaller than you are now, until you get to your ideal size. Please go and buy a smaller pair of pants right now!

When I was 21 years old I got a job looking after racehorses in Sydney, Australia. I walked about 10 miles a day leading racehorses around and did a lot of other manual work, like mucking out horse boxes. After a while, people started giving me *huge* compliments on my new body. The problem was, during this time I did not lose one single solitary pound, and so I found it hard to believe the people complimenting me, although I dropped at least one whole size in jeans. It may have been more - I just did not even think to see if I could get into anything smaller, because the scales appeared to be saying that I was the same size.

There have been other times when I changed my eating habits and, while I did not change my weight greatly, I was able to get into smaller and smaller clothes. And just looked better. This is partly because weight for weight, muscle takes up less volume than fat. In addition, muscle is spread all over our body, whereas fat tends to go in just a few places, which makes the proportions wrong. But I suspect there is even more to this. Somehow, in many ways, our bodies get more dense when we switch from a standard western toxic-filled diet, to a natural, nutrient-filled one, especially one that has a lot more raw food in it.

THE PROBLEMS WITH SCIENTIFIC RESEARCH

We will look at the trillions of dollars which are made from keeping people fat and unhealthy. Many corporations profit from this scam through such avenues as:

- Drugs.
- Hospital stays (why does a hospital room have to cost $2,000 a day, when the food is so terrible?).
- Operations.
- Research which goes nowhere, and is sometimes fraudulent.
- Junk food which is addictive. Dr. Mark Hyman M.D. says, "Our immune response makes us crave foods we're allergic to."[38]

This causes a problem with finding scientific evidence to back up any theory that someone has, which does not make huge profits for giant corporations. A story from my university days illustrates this beautifully:

I was sitting in my first lecture of zoology, in third year science at Sydney University. The beginning of this lecture became my clearest memory from my university days. Professor Tony Underwood came in, and strode up and down the bottom of the lecture theatre, telling us to get out our textbook, and to tell him what the researcher of a particular chapter had proved. Like good little robots, we gave the expected answer. He then declared very forthrightly something to the effect of-

"NO! You can prove anything you want with a scientific test, you just have to design it in such a way as to make it do what you want. The truth is that the scientist who designed the test did not look at all the many different alternatives which could also give the same results."

In this book, I will give scientific evidence to back up my arguments wherever possible. Where I quote from a book, I have used only books that had a lot of scientific papers for references. But if you are the kind of person who always demands scientific research to support every single statement that goes against your beliefs, I ask you to please find out who paid for all of the research that gave you your beliefs in the first place. And who paid for the marketing that promoted that idea.

One major problem with health research is that it always zeroes in on one tiny aspect of the picture. But everything in the body affects everything else. As I say, "If you step on a cat's tail, it's the other end that screams". You need to know the whole picture, not just isolated facts, to get permanently thin.

One of the most powerful forms of proof is "social proof", which means that if enough people believe something, it must be true. Which, of course, is ridiculous. Some of what you are going to read goes against social proof.

However, if we are to get off the road of getting fatter and fatter, we need to do things very differently. Instead of looking to "social proof", I suggest that you look to another form of "proof" which can be much more powerful – the proof of your own personal experience.

Try the techniques in this book for three months, and see if they don't make a radical improvement to your body. Then, if I'm right, and these techniques are working, keep them going for the rest of your life.

THE LAW OF THE MINIMUM

There is a natural health law called the "law of the minimum". That is, if you do everything perfectly, but there is just one thing that you leave out totally, then you won't benefit much, if at all, from the perfect things you were doing. For example, you will learn why you may still have fat even though you eat healthily and eat little, but you aren't getting any sun or enough sleep. Please do your very best to do something of everything in this book.

THE CHALLENGE

While it's a horrible thought to contemplate, no matter how large you are now, you can still get larger, if you don't change what you are doing right now, and change for life. If you put on just four pounds every year, that's an extra forty pounds after ten years. Change your mind to change your behavior.

Removing fat is not the only thing you need to do. You also need to change the *habits* that got you where you are in the first place. If you don't do that, there is no reason why you could not put on another 50 or more pounds in the coming decades. So:

Do you live to eat? Or do you eat to live? If you are ready to eat to live, and to have the body shape that you never thought was possible, then this book is for you. You're not fat. You're toxic. So let's get started and change that.

REFERENCES
1. *Fat, Sick and Nearly Dead.* Documentary by Joe Cross
2. *Forks Over Knives* documentary
3. www.rt.com/usa/news/force-obese-counseling-us-799/
4. Yahoo News, 5/30/07.
5. Breitbart.com. 7/1/05.
6. *Lancet* 2011 Feb 12;377(9765):557-67. Epub 2011 Feb 3.
7. *Forks Over Knives* documentary
8. Ramzi Cotran (former Chairman of Pathology at the Brigham and Women's. Hospital. www.mblwhoilibrary.org/services/lecture_series/folkman/transcript1.html
9. www.prweb.com/releases/2011/5/prweb8393658.htm
10. Department for Environment, Food and Rural Affairs. *The National Food Survey2000*: Annual Report on Food Expenditure, Consumptions and Nutrient Intakes. London: Her Majesty's Stationary Office, 2001.
11. Morris JN. Obesity in Britain: Lifestyle data do not support sloth hypothesis (letter). BMJ 1995;311:1568-1569. Also Rasvussin E. Obesity in Britain: Rising trend may be due to "Pathoenvironment" (letter) BMJ 1995;311:1569
12. Trends in sports participation: Facilities factfile 2. Planning and provision

for sport. London: Sports Council, 1993.

13. Freeman, Sarah (14 December 2010). "Obesity still eating away at health of the nation". *Yorkshire Post*. Retrieved 18 December 2010.

14. Chen JQ, Brown TR, Russo J. Regulation of energy metabolism pathways by estrogens and estrogenic chemicals and potential implications in obesity associated with increased exposure to endocrine disruptors. *Biochim Biophys Acta*. 2009;1793(7):1128-1143.

15. "Chemical Toxins: A Hypothesis to explain the Global Obesity Epidemic", Paula F. Baillie-Hamilton, *The Journal of Alternative & Complementary Medicine*, Vol 8, No. 2, 2001, pp 185-192

16. *Excitotoxins*, by Dr. Russell Blaylock M.D., 1997, page 23

17. *New York Daily News*, 3/29/12

18. www.time.com/time/health/article/0,8599,1977604,00.html

19. *Nature Neuroscience*, 3/28/12.

20. www.cbsnews.com/2100-204_162-6343889.html

21. *Excitotoxins* by Dr. Russell Blaylock M.D., 1997, page 23

22. *First for Women* magazine, 2/12/12, quoting a Yale study discussed in Cracking the Metabolic Code, by James LaValle NC

23. *The Anti-estrogenic Diet*, by Ori Hofmekler, 2007, page 6

24. Remillard RB, Bunce NJ. Linking dioxins to diabetes: epidemiology and biologic plausibility. Environ Health Perspect. 2002;110(9):853-858. Review.

25. *Excitotoxins*, by Dr. Russell Blaylock M.D., 1997

26. *Daily Mail* May 11, 2012. www.dailymail.co.uk/health/article-2142953/Chemicals-household-items-causing-huge-increase-cancer-obesity-falling-fertility.html

27. *Forks Over Knives* documentary

28. articles.mercola.com/sites/articles/archive/2011/08/03/the-9-foods-the-us-government-is-paying-you-to-eat.aspx

29. www.naturalnews.com/036416_GlaxoSmithKline_fraud_criminal_charges.html

30. www.american-longevity.com/walet.htm

31. www.relfe.com/2011-2012/deathbymedicine.pdf

32. *Woman's World* magazine, 4/2/12

33. www.innovateus.net/health/how-many-proteins-exist-human-body

34. en.wikipedia.org/wiki/Amino_acid

35. www.libertyzone.com/hz-Amino-Acid.html

36. *The Magnesium Factor* by Mildred Seelig, M.D., 2003, page 91
37. J. Altern Complement Med. 2002 Apr;8(2):185-92. Occupational and Environmental Health Research Group at Stirling, Stirling University, Scotland.
38. *Woman's World* magazine, 7/9/12, page 18

CHAPTER 2

BEFORE YOU BEGIN

You are about to embark on a journey. This journey will give you a new body, and new health and happiness that you might never have dreamed was possible.

However, I have found from experience with my kinesiology clients that most people have very poor awareness of their bodies. It is not uncommon for clients to turn up for a second session of kinesiology, and when questioned say that they are no different from when I first saw them. When that happens, I say something like, "Well, you had an 8/10 back pain last week, that you felt for months. How is the back pain now?" And they will say something like, "Oh, that. Now that you mention it, my back is not hurting anymore." And so on and so forth for other symptoms.

That is, we tend to only notice what is happening NOW, and forget about how bad or good things were in the past. Corporations and governments know that most of us have no more than a 90 day attention span, at best, and they use that against us.

Therefore, *please*, right now, get out a piece of paper or write in a journal, all of the facts of how you are now, so that at the end of your journey, you have something to compare yourself to. Keep it forever. If you back slide in five years time, you might just come across it again and use it as motivation to get going again. Write a new list out in one month, and again in three and six months and twelve months, and compare them. You might be surprised at the changes.

This is a book about fat loss. But you will quite likely find that in the process of getting thin, that a whole host of other health symptoms improve at the same time. So include those on the list.

Write on the page:
- Date.
- Your weight.
- Your pants size.
- Which hole of which belt you wear with which clothes.
- Waist measurement.

List of symptoms including:
- Pain: Give location in body.
- For each location of pain in the body, give a rating from zero to ten of how severe the pain is (zero is no pain).
- With each location of pain, say how often you get it.
- Health problems.
- Skin problems.
- How often you do a poo. And how easy it is.
- If you are a woman, how painful and heavy your periods are.
- Emotional problems. Give your overall level of happiness a rating from zero to ten.
- Energy. Give your overall energy levels a rating from zero to ten.

Even better, please see a medical practitioner and get a full printout of your current physical condition, including blood tests. Do this again after you have been on the plan in this book for three months. I am betting that if you do that, you will be in for a pleasant surprise.

It might also be a good idea to take some full body photos (front and side), in case you later want "before and after" photos.

Well done! Now, please read on...

CHAPTER 3

WHY ARE SO MANY FOODS TOXIC?

When people start to learn about what food is toxic and what is healthy, they often get a shock, since *so much* of what most people eat is toxic. But please do not let fear of knowing the truth stop you from reading on and deciding for yourself. You have nothing to lose but fat and health problems.

There are a number of reasons for this. First of all, the longer something lasts on the shelf, the easier it is to produce. Manufacturers and store owners don't have to worry about food being spoiled and thrown out. The trouble with this is, that there is a general rule in natural health; the quicker that something rots, the better it is for you. You see, if it rots, it's bacteria doing the rotting. And it's bacteria that will digest it in your body.

There is one exception to this rule, and that is raw, *live* food. The better that a plant such as fruit and vegetables has been raised, the longer it will stay fresh on the shelf. There are special methods of growing food that are not used by commercial farmers that can extend the shelf-life of fresh fruit and vegetables for weeks. These methods, such as biodynamic farming, work with energy in ways that are not understood by science.

But back to making processed food last longer. The very thing that makes the food last longer, is the very thing that makes it toxic, and hence eventually fattening. The manufacturers add toxins to keep the bacteria from digesting the food. Your body has to work out what to do with these toxins so that *its* bacteria can digest the food. The liver has to do most of this, but if the liver doesn't have enough of the two things it needs to detox the toxins – the right nutrients and enough life energy – then it dumps the toxins in the nearest fat cell, which is like a rubbish dump, until it can deal with them later on.

Why don't processed meats like salami rot? Think of them as embalmed meat – like Egyptian mummies. So-called 'preservatives' (read 'toxins') are put in to stop it rotting. I was told by my kinesiology / naturopathic teacher, who is a mine of natural health information, that bodies in morgues are now lasting three to four times longer than they used to, because of all the preservatives in their fat cells. So think of all those preservatives as something that is *preserving* your fat in place.

Here's another reason why most food these days is toxic. Think of yourself as a detective. The crime is people getting hugely fatter. Now you need to find:

- The perpetrator of the crime.
- The motive.
- The evidence.

Could the following be a motive? Much food is made by giant multi-national companies that are partly owned by other multi-national companies.

Currently, about one in three people in the U.K. and U.S.A., will get cancer[1,2]. Although this statistic will likely get worse, since cell phones cause brain cancer (By the way, dying of cancer really, really hurts, even with drugs. Have you noticed how people are no longer 'passing away' gently in their sleep like they used to? Toxins are a major cause of cancer. You owe it to yourself to set a goal to do whatever it takes to keep toxins out of your life). I digress. According to the excellent website www.CancerTutor.org, the average cancer patient spends over $300,000 on treatment. Other people set the figure a lot higher at $1.3 million[3]. If we take the lesser figure and multiply one third of the USA by $300,000, we get about **$27,000,000,000,000** ($27 trillion) over the next 70 years to the medical industry. That's for cancer alone. There are plenty of other profitable diseases, like heart disease (operations start at $100,000) and diabetes (costs have risen 41% in just 5 years), and lots of other less well-known ones.

This figure fits in roughly with another estimate: We spend a total $2.2 trillion a year on so-called 'health' care in the United States of America. That's five times more than the defense budget[4]!

THE USA SPENDS $2.2 TRILLION EACH YEAR ON HEALTH CARE

Most of us can't imagine how big a million is, let alone a billion. And with the massive size of a trillion, it is mind numbing to even think of something that size. But we will try anyway. We'll start with a $100 dollar bill. Currently the largest U.S. denomination in general circulation. It makes friends wherever it goes.

A packet of one hundred, $100 bills is less than 1/2" thick and contains $10,000. Fits in your pocket easily and is more than enough for a nice vacation.

If we then take 100 of those packets of $100 bills, we now have one million dollars ($10,000 X 100). You could easily carry this around in a briefcase. And now you are a millionaire.

We could then take the contents of 100 of those briefcases and stack them on a standard pallet. We now have 100 million dollars and feel like one of those oil barrons we see in the movies.

If we then had 10 of those pallets, each containing 100 million dollars, we would become a billionaire like Donald Trump. But by government standards we are still at the bottom of the pile.

So what is a trillion dollars? It is a one followed by 12 zeros. If we then replicated our pallets until we had 10,000 of them, we would have a trillion dollars. Or if you wanted it in a giant building to keep your money dry, it would be a building encompassing abut 400,000 cubic feet (this is 4 1/2 olympic sized swimming pools filled with $100 bills).

So the next time you hear someone toss around the phrase "trillion dollars"... that's what they're talking about. Maybe you begin to get an idea why there could be a motive to do things to people which cause them to be more toxic, even if that means that they will also get fatter.

If you wonder why you have not heard about what I am going to tell you about food from the medical establishment, please consider this. In five years of medical training, how much time do you think the average doctor gets on training about food? Only zero to twelve hours!

How about the government? Does it benefit them in any way? Don't 'they' care for us? Well, they have this problem with social security. If adding a few toxins here and there to the food supply can reduce social security payment by billions (trillions?) of dollars by reducing the number of old people, well then ....

In fact, I talked with an author once at a natural health expo in Australia. She told me that a doctor told her that whenever the old peoples' homes get too full, they give everyone a vaccination. This kills off a certain percentage of the old people who receive it. The doctor said that he would totally deny having ever said that if she said that he had said this. You see, it's hard for normal people to imagine such evil. But then again, think of the amazingly enormous sums of money we are talking about. Is it possible that not everyone on the planet is as nice as you and me?

Whenever you decide what food is good for you, or what marketing or scientific research you can believe, remember that we spend $2.2 trillion a year on so-called 'health' care in the United States of America, and that's five times more than the defense budget[5]. So, why would they want you to know about how to get thin, since the same methods will also *make you healthy?*

When it comes to your health and the health of those you love, be like one of those private detectives in the books and the movies. Just follow the money.

REFERENCES
1. www.cancerresearchuk.org/cancer-info/cancerstats/keyfacts/ Allcancerscombined
2. www.cancure.org/statistics.htm
3. www.beating-cancer-gently.com/index.html
4. *Forks Over Knives* Documentary
5. *Forks Over Knives* Documentary

CHAPTER 4

DIETS DON'T WORK.
THE 60 BILLION DOLLAR A YEAR FRAUD

More people are waking up to the fact that diets don't work. Just look at Oprah Winfrey for example. Here is a great lady who is super motivated, and can have what ever she wants with regard to advice and access to diets, food and even personal cooks. And yet, we have all seen her ups and downs. It's just that when Oprah does it, it's a lot more public than for the rest of us.

If you've been on a bunch of diets by now, you probably know from experience that they don't work. Here are some reasons why[1]. When you use will power to deny yourself food, the body thinks you are starving it of nutrition and energy, which you are. So it makes sure that it survives the next 'famine' by the following:

- Your body adapts to less food, by slowing down your metabolism[2].

- When you finally do eat, your body stores up fat for what it considers the next famine.

- Exercising at the same time you restrict food intake results in an even more sluggish metabolism!

Instead of dieting, we need a totally different way of living. This book will show you how to do that.

In my early years I always seemed to be about ten pounds heavier than I wanted to be. Actually, looking back at my teenage years, I know now that there was a time when I thought I needed to reduce weight when I really didn't. That's the unfortunate power of the media to make young girls focus on their body size. So, like lots of people, I went on a bunch of diets. And like most people, the weight came back on, plus extra.

I have heard this quite a lot from people. Does this sound like you? "I've put on 10 pounds. What I can't understand, is that I am eating the same food that I always used to eat, when I didn't put on any weight."

There are a number of reasons for this, including:

1. As we get older, we tend to get more and more out of balance, because of all the different stresses on our body. These stresses are not just emotional. They are also chemical, nutritional, physical (like lack of sleep) and electrical (like from using an electric blanket).

2. Toxins build up because you are having too many of them, and not enough nutrition and good water to get rid of them. Eventually something has to give.

3. Eating the same food often, eventually can cause you to become allergic to that food. This can affect your body in many different ways, including how your brain operates, but also by causing fat gain.

I will talk more about this in the chapter "Health is like a bank account".

I read a story once about a man who ran a health farm. He got tired of the way that his clients would come to his farm, be put on a healthy diet and lose all kinds of weight, go home and then turn up months later with the weight back on. He got so exasperated with this situation, that he decided to prove that his diets worked. He went on one of his health farm diets. As expected, he lost weight. But it came as a shock to him to realize that within a few months after that, not only had he gained the weight back, he had put on *extra* weight. So he went on his diet again. The same thing happened again - he gained the weight back, plus some extra.

I have experienced this for myself. When I was young I thought I was overweight. The truth was, I probably wasn't much overweight at all. Years later, I would have done a lot to get back to being as thin as I was then. I would grab a bunch of skin and say "see, that's fat". I believe that too many young people obsess over their weight, thanks to the media and fashion industry.

If young people would just focus on eating and doing what's healthy and natural and not toxic, they would not have to think about their weight at all in later life.

I would go on a diet, lose eight pounds or more, be happy, and then go back to eating how I did before. The trouble was, the weight came back, plus more. And each time I went back on a diet, it got harder and harder to lose that eight pounds. Sound familiar?

Here is the way that dieting works. *You* may think it's a diet, but *your body* thinks it's a famine. Your body thinks we are back in the dark ages, and the crops have died, and it's winter, and it does not know when the next decent meal is coming. So it starts to store up food as soon as there is plenty again.

I believe this goes for people who go on a water fast, as well. I do not recommend water fasting. If one wants a total cleanse, one can drink water and do fresh squeezed juices, especially vegetable juices. A juice fast where you drink fresh-squeezed juice when ever you get hungry is not a real fast. That way, the body still gets all the nutrients, vitamins, minerals and amino acids for protein that it needs to run its factories.

It's easier to burn up muscle than fat, so if you don't eat enough food, the body burns up muscle rather than fat. But it takes a lot more energy to maintain muscles than it does to maintain fat cells. So, gradually your body needs less and less energy to stay alive. So, your metabolism goes down. You now need less energy each day, but you will also feel less energetic.

Worst of all, you have not changed the *habits* which caused you to put on the weight in the *first place*.

I only got my body back the way I wanted it when I gave up thoughts of dieting. Instead I focused on doing what was good for my health and wellbeing.

If you want to be thin and stay thin, you will have to face the hard fact of life. You have to change the habits that made you fat in the first place. You have to let your body know that there is no shortage of nutritious food, so it does not need to store it. And you have to remove the toxic food that made you bigger. You will have to learn about natural health and apply it to yourself.

You may think this is a hard thing to do, but my experience and the experience of many others is that once you do this, you will feel so much better, that you will eventually not even want to go back to the toxic food you used to enjoy.

By the way, I don't like to use the words "lose weight." If you lose something, then that means you can later find it again. I prefer "reduce fat" rather than "lose weight". It's more permanent. Words have power. And your body is listening to what you say. Plus you will learn in another chapter about how you can reduce fat, and get a thinner body, without losing any weight at all.

Here is a testimonial that a lady sent me about the advantages of giving up dieting:

> "I've had weight problems my whole life - been on every diet. Several years ago I decided that this was stupid and stopped dieting - I just couldn't afford to gain any more weight! Now after starting on a supplement program and adjusting my diet to include more protein and less carbohydrates I've lost 50 pounds. Pretty interesting…. Took over a year and I still could lose another 30 pounds".

DON'T FALL FOR THE "DIET" SCAM

Dieting does not work. If you don't know that yet, you are either too young or haven't been on enough diets yet. Don't bother. You may lose weight initially on a diet, but if you don't change the way you look after your body *all the time*, later on you will probably gain the weight back, plus some extra pounds. And then the weight will likely be more fat, and less muscle.

Keep reading and learn ways to reduce fat without dieting, by eating three meals a day, without ever going hungry, at the same time you remove toxins from your body and feel *wonderful*.

REFERENCES

1. *Outside* magazine, Jan 2002
2. *Mastering Leptin*, by Byron Richards CCN, 2002, 3rd edition 2009 pg. 52

CHAPTER 5

THE LAW OF THE MINIMUM

Do you believe that you do pretty much everything that is right for your body, but still have excess weight? In that case, you need to know about a natural health law called "The Law of the Minimum".

To be thin and healthy our body wants a *balance* of the right:

- Food (including a balance of the right minerals, vitamins etc.).
- Water.
- Exercise.
- Sleep.
- Rest (different from sleep).
- Air.
- Sun.
- Positive Emotions.
- Electromagnetics.

Unfortunately, because of the "law of the minimum", if you are very low in just one area, it can affect all the others. This means that if you are doing everything perfectly, but missing out on one of the necessary things your body needs, then your results could be very bad. For example, if you eat the right food in the right quantity, but don't get enough sleep or sunlight, then you could very well have fat that has nothing to do with your diet. The same applies if you eat healthily, but are missing out on an important mineral or essential fatty acid.

Yes, there are some people who get away with this – for now. They quite possibly have hidden health problems, but so far fat gain is not one of them. But give them enough time and some of these people may just start to get pudgy later on in life, just as a high percentage of the whole world is doing right now. Or, they just might have major health problems later on. The thing is, everyone is different. I assume you are not one of these people, or you would not be reading this book. If you are looking for the unique answers that will work for you, please read all the way to the end of this book, as you will likely find the answers you are looking for.

One piece of scientific evidence that backs up the theory of the "Law of the Minimum" is that it has been found that there are seventeen minerals that are essential for our bodies, and if there is a shortage of just *one* of these, the balance of the entire system gets upset.[1]

REFERENCES
1. *Transdermal Magnesium Therapy*, Mark Sircus, 2007

CHAPTER 6

TOXIC FOODS PRODUCE ACID

Toxins are acidic. The more toxic, the more acidic. And, conversely, the more acidic, the more toxic. Non-toxic foods are alkaline in the body. Acid makes you fat.

You have 75 *trillion* cells in your body[1]. A healthy and thin body is determined by the health of each of its single cells. All disease originates at the cellular level and not at the organ level. Healthy cells create healthy tissues. Healthy tissues create healthy muscles and organs, like the heart. Healthy organs create healthy systems like the endocrine system or the immune system, and healthy systems make up a slim and healthy body.

To be healthy and slim, all 75 trillion body cells must work together. A picture metaphor of how the cells in the body communicate would be to envision all seven billion people on this planet picking up a phone simultaneously and having a phone conversation. Now picture everyone clicking three-way and having a three-way conversation. Then picture everyone in the world clicking on conference call with total conversation capability of 1,000 different people simultaneously.

The question is, does your phone have good reception to transmit and receive messages? Your intestinal phone talks to the skin. Your spleen phone talks to the thymus. Your heart phone talks to the liver. All organs and systems work in unison. No organ or system works alone, just as no nutrient works alone. So what controls cell processes? The answer is pH, the measure of how acid or alkaline your body is. The lower the pH, the more acidic you are.

The pH of your tissues and body fluids affects the state of your inner cleanliness or filth. The closer the pH is to 7.35 - 7.45 or greater, the higher your level of health and well being, and your ability to resist fat gain and states of disease. From *The pH Miracle for Weight Loss*[2]:

> "Too much acid in the body robs the blood of oxygen, and without oxygen, the *metabolism slows*. Food digests more slowly, *inducing weight gain* and sluggishness, and, worse still, causing the food to ferment (rot!). Fermentation creates yeast, fungus, and mold throughout the body. These are all living organisms, so they need to "eat", and when they overgrow in an acidic body they feed on *your* nutrients, reducing the chemical and mechanical absorption of everything you eat by as much as 50%.

> Without enough nutrients, your body cannot build tissue (like muscle) or produce hormones, or hundreds of other chemical components necessary for cell energy and organ activity... And the result is *unwanted weight gain* as well as fatigue and illness".

As acid wastes back up, a chronically over-acidic body pH corrodes body tissue, slowly eating into the 60,000 miles of veins and arteries, like acid eating into marble. This is what science calls hemorrhage. If left unchecked, it will interrupt all cellular activities and functions from the beating of your heart to the correct firing of the brain.

Over acidification interferes with life itself, leading to all sickness and "dis-ease." Fundamentally, all regulatory mechanisms, including weight loss, circulation and hormone production, serve the purpose of balancing pH.

When you eat food, it ferments, just the way a banana on your counter ferments from green, to yellow, to brown, to black. The banana rots from the inside out, not from the outside in. That is why humans can look healthy from the outside, but are rotting and decaying from the inside.

PRIMITIVE PEOPLE WHO ATE PLANTS HAD ALKALINE URINE

Dr. Davis tells us in *Wheat Belly* that the alkalinity of early human diets has been estimated to be 6 to 9 times greater than that of modern diets[3]! This was due to the very high plant content of their food, with low grains and no processing other than a little cooking. Their urine pH was a very alkaline 7.5 - 9.0. Most people today have acidic urine that measures a shocking 4.4 – 7.0. No wonder people are so fat and so sick!

The following create an alkaline body, particularly if they are raw or as little cooked as possible[4]:

- Fruits.
- Vegetables.
- Nuts.
- Seeds.
- Legumes (lentils & chickpeas are better than beans. Soak for 8 hours before using, to sprout them and make them less toxic).
- Organic yogurt.
- Water (reverse osmosis).

ACID CAUSING FOODS

To maintain an alkaline body, all you have to remember is that virtually everything else that is not listed above is acidic, including:

- Meat & all foods that come from animals.
- Dairy.
- Eggs.
- Sugar.
- Grains, especially wheat[5].
- Processed Foods.
- Nicotine.
- Sodas.
- Fruit juice that is not fresh-squeezed.
- Drugs.
- Caffeine (coffee, tea, energy drinks), because it's a drug.

- Alcohol, because it's a drug.

Raw foods contain enzymes and life energy that cooked food does not. In addition, cooking creates toxins which are unknown in nature, which are acidic. This doesn't mean you have to go 100% raw, but the less cooked your food is, the better. Whenever possible, choose raw over cooked. (When I talk about eating raw food, I am talking about fruit, vegetables, nuts and seeds. I am not talking about foods which must be cooked to kill bacteria and parasites, such as eggs and meat). Drugs, including caffeine and alcohol, are particularly acidic.

One of the very best food groups for alkalizing the body is green plants, and especially leafy, green vegetables. Add to every meal something from the following:

- Superfoods like spirulina or chlorella.
- Salad greens.
- Kale.
- Spinach.
- Collard greens, turnip greens.
- Parsley / Italian parsley.
- Cilantro / Coriander (this has also been reported to help with removing heavy metals).
- Cucumbers.
- Different greens such as different choys, available from Asian stores.

What pharmaceutical drug neutralizes acids and increases pH? *Nothing*! What pharmaceutical drug addresses nutritional deficiencies, especially alkaline minerals? Nothing! What pharmaceutical drug boosts or enhances the immune system? Nothing! And how could they? They're poisonous and destructive, not nutritive and constructive. Pharmaceuticals are acid. How can you treat an acid condition with acid? That's like trying to cure someone who accidentally drank poison with another poison.

On the other hand, an acid-causing diet is a bone-breaking diet which helps the drug companies make at least $10 billion a year selling osteopororis drugs[6].

Dr. William Davis tells how one young man got his life back simply by totally giving up one toxic, ultra-acid-causing food – wheat. (I will talk more about wheat in a chapter on its own). Jason was a smart 26 year old who was getting ready to have a heart transplant. He had been told that he had a "congenital heart defect" since he was an infant. He was also in so much pain that he could barely walk. (If you can't walk, it's a lot harder to get thin). After just five days of zero wheat, he was shocked – his *pain was gone*! Plus, after three months of no wheat, his *heart failure was healed*! It looked like a miracle – and yet the solution was so simple.

The body *must* maintain pH. So if you eat acid-causing foods, the body draws on calcium from the bones to balance out what you ate. As Dr. Davis says in *Wheat Belly*:

"An excessively acidified diet will eventually show itself as bone fractures[7]."

It is now understood that decline in bone density affects both men and women, and it starts *years* before people are told they have osteoporosis.

The fact is that all doctors are drugging the symptoms of acidity and drugging the symptoms of nutritional deficiencies. Weight gain, pain, headaches, skin rashes, brain fog, severe tiredness and gastric bloating are some of the body's warning signals of a problem due to an acidic pH. Suppressing a symptom with an "anti" medication is analogous to snipping the wire to a blinking oil light on your car's dashboard and thinking that you fixed your engine, instead of lifting up the hood and putting oil in your engine so the light goes off.

I believe that our understanding of natural foods and alkaline foods is only in its infancy. Science has not seen the full truth of what really goes on in a body when it digests food. Can we really hope, at this stage, to fully understand how 75 trillion cells all work together to do all the things they do? Our understanding of God's design has only just begun.

There are articles that recommend that you add various chemicals to your water to make it more alkaline. I believe this is a dangerous mistake. It is unnatural, and only by studying the laws of nature can we get our proper natural looking bodies, as all wild animals do naturally. Alkaline chemicals can do as much damage as acidic chemicals. In the book, *The pH Miracle for Weight Loss*, Dr. Young writes:

> "Fat is used primarily as a way to store ... acids. Ask any plastic surgeon: The fat they liposuction out of their patients is brown and black because of all the acids it contains. (One of our associates, who is a plastic surgeon, put this to the test by sending samples of liposuctioned fat in for analysis: the lab reports concluded it was indeed full of acid)."

However, I believe the author is not seeing the picture fully. Excess fat that is liposuctioned is brown and black because of toxins, which just happen to be acidic. If you put the focus on toxins, and not just on acids, you will have more effective results.

Aerobic exercise, which is easy exercise with oxygen, the kind you can do for long periods of time without creating pain, also creates an alkaline body, because oxygen is alkalizing. Note that many so-called 'aerobic' exercises are really anaerobic. That is, they work without oxygen, because they are too fast and strenuous, and therefore create lactic acid, which is what causes pain and tiredness.

I realize that most people reading this book will have to learn new ways to prepare food. You can do it! There are tasty recipes and a shopping list in this book that will help you to get started. Remember, as long as you have the ingredients, if ever you don't know what to do with them, you can always go to a search engine on the internet and search for a recipe with those ingredients. For example, put in "vegetarian recipe cabbage lentils".

You're not fat. You're toxic. Toxins are acidic. A body full of toxins will be acidic. This causes fat gain. This is one reason why diets don't work. We need to change our whole lifestyle and focus on eating more alkalizing foods, and as few acidifying foods as possible. Please read on, to learn more about how removing toxins from your life will give you the body and happiness you deserve.

REFERENCES
1. www.britannica.com/EBchecked/topic/275485/human-body/3361/ Organization-of-the-body
2. *The pH Miracle for Weight Loss*, by Dr. Robert Young Ph.D., page 14
3. *Wheat Belly*, by William Davis M.D., 2011, page 122
4. *Wheat Belly*, by William Davis M.D., 2011, page 118
5. *Wheat Belly*, by William Davis M.D., 2011, pages 116-129
6. *Wheat Belly*, by William Davis M.D., 2011, pages 123
7. *Wheat Belly*, by William Davis M.D., 2011, page 119

CHAPTER 7

TOP SECRET
HOW WATER MAKES YOU THIN

Lots of diet books tell you to drink water to "fill you up" with something that has no calories. In fact, water does not fill you up! But it is one of the *most important* keys to weight loss, for other reasons.

The very best book to learn about the secrets of water is *Your Body's Many Cries for Water*, by Dr. Batmanghelidj[1]. Published in 1992, this is one of the most famous books among natural health circles. The book says:

"It has been shown experimentally that, when we drink one glass of water, it *immediately* passes into the intestine and is absorbed[2]."

That is, it doesn't stay in your stomach. It does not 'fill you up'.

Water is needed to flush the toxins out of your system. Note that I said 'water' and not 'fluids'. Fluids are not water.

- Fruit juice is food or toxins, depending on what is done to it.
- Soda, Gatorade, tea and coffee are toxins.

Would you wash your windows with Gatorade? Or your hair? No. Just like a wild animal, your body wants pure water. Not 'fluids'.

WATER GIVES YOU ENERGY

There is another amazing quality of water that helps in weight loss. We have been taught that anything which has no calories cannot give us energy. And that only glucose will give energy to the brain. But the amazing truth is that *water gives the brain energy!*

"Recently is has been discovered that the human body has the ability to generate *hydroelectric energy* when water, by itself, goes through the cell membrane and turns some very special energy generating pumps; very much like the hydroelectric power generation when a dam is built on a river[3]....This creates a voltage which is converted and stored in the form of ATP and GTP. These two chemicals are vital cell battery systems. Thus we see that water is turned into a *chemical* source of energy in the body![4].

Note: Salt is also needed to produce this hydroelectric energy. You will learn more about salt in the chapter on salt. Therefore, the brain gets energy from two sources:

- Glucose.

- 'Hydroelectricity' from water.

"It now seems that the brain depends *very extensively* on energy formation from 'hydroelectricity." Now, isn't that amazing? Something that has zero calories gives you energy. Which is evidence of what I said at the beginning – What *kind* of substances you ingest is much more important than counting calories.

Also note what else this means – dehydration makes a person less intelligent. I believe that dehydration due to drinking soda and other drinks, instead of water, is a contributing factor to declining abilities in schools and in life.

The brain is the most important organ in the body to keep functioning properly. Brain cells are 85% water.

"The front of the brain gets energy either from 'hydroelectricity' or from sugar in blood circulation. Its functional needs for hydroelectricity are *more urgent* – not only for the energy formation from water, but also its transport system ... depends on water.

Thus, the sensations of thirst and hunger are generated simultaneously to indicate the brain's needs. We don't recognize the sensation of thirst and *assume both indicators to be the urge to eat.* We eat food even when the body should receive water[5]

"We eat to supply the brain with energy for its constant round-the-clock activity. However, when food is eaten, only about 20% of it reaches the brain. The rest will gradually become stored if muscle activity does not use up its allocated portion. With water as a source of energy, this storage does not happen."[6]

WATER REGULATES ALL FUNCTIONS OF THE BODY, INCLUDING FAT METABOLISM

"Proteins and the enzymes of the body function more efficiently in solutions of lower viscosity. A body that is dehydrated has a higher viscosity. Therefore, it is water itself that regulates all functions of the body"[7]. Since burning fat is a function of the body, it follows that if you are not sufficiently hydrated, this function will not be working at full efficiency, if at all.

MANY HEALTH PROBLEMS CAN BE HEALED WITH CORRECT WATER AND SALT INTAKE, ALONE

Dr. Batmanghelidj explains how just drinking enough water at the right times, plus a little salt, can heal a huge range of symptoms. I will talk more about salt later. Chapter by chapter, with testimonials, he shows how this can heal, for example:

1. Allergies.
2. Alzheimer's disease (because brain cells shrink and then lose their functions, from prolonged dehydration. Imagine a plum turning into a prune. That is what the brain does without sufficient water).
3. Anginal pain (that is, chest pain).
4. Arthritis (because the joints contain much water as lubricant).
5. Asthma (the lungs are a main site of evaporation. If there is not enough water, the airways constrict to save water. Plus the lungs need to be moist to work properly. Dr. Batmanghelidj has numerous testimonials of people who completely healed their asthma after a month or more purely by increasing water (not fluid) intake, plus having a little salt.
6. Chronic pain – Including Rheumatoid pain, back pain, headaches, leg pain.
7. Depression.
8. Dyspeptic pain (indigestion) - Dr. Batmanghelidj treated with only water 30 minutes before meals, over 3,000 persons with dyspeptic pain. All of these people had their pains disappear. Symptoms included: Colitis, Duodenitis, Gastritis, Heartburn, Hiatal Hernia.
9. Headaches & migraines.
10. High blood pressure.
11. Morning / Pregnancy sickness.
12. Pain – such as in the neck (because there must be fluid in the spaces between the discs).
13. Sleeping difficulties.
14. Weight, excess.

Why haven't you heard about this? Could the fact that nearly half of all Americans are on prescription drugs have anything to do with it?[8] And do you think it could have anything to do with the huge markup on drugs? Here are a few examples: [9]

Celebrex: 100 mg, Consumer price (100 tablets): $130.27, Cost of general active ingredients: $0.60, Percent markup: 21,712%.

Claritin: 10 mg, Consumer Price (100 tablets): $215.17, Cost of general active ingredients: $0.71, Percent markup: 30,306%.

Lipitor: 20 mg, Consumer Price (100 tablets): $272.37, Cost of general active ingredients: $5.80, Percent markup: 4,696%.

Norvasc: 10 mg, Consumer price (100 tablets): $188.29, Cost of general active ingredients: $0.14, Percent markup: 134,493%.

Paxil: 20 mg, Consumer price (100 tablets): $220.27, Cost of general active ingredients: $7.60, Percent markup: 2,898%.

Prevacid: 30 mg, Consumer price (100 tablets): $44.77, Cost of general active ingredients: $1.01, Percent markup: 34,136%.

Prilosec: 20 mg, Consumer price (100 tablets): $360.97, Cost of general active ingredients $0.52, Percent markup: 69,417%.

Prozac: 20 mg, Consumer price (100 tablets) : $247.47, Cost of general active ingredients: $0.11, Percent markup: 224,973%.

Tenormin: 50 mg Consumer price (100 tablets): $104.47, Cost of general active ingredients: $0.13, Percent markup: 80,362%.

Vasotec: 10 mg, Consumer price (100 tablets): $102.37, Cost of general active ingredients: $0.20, Percent markup: 51,185%.

Xanax: 1 mg, Consumer price (100 tablets) : $136.79, Cost of general active ingredients: $0.024, Percent markup: 569,958%.

Zithromax: 600 mg, Consumer price (100 tablets): $1,482.19, Cost of general active ingredients: $18.78, Percent markup: 7,892%.

Zoloft: 50 mg, Consumer price: $206.87, Cost of general active ingredients: $1.75, Percent markup: 11,821%.

On the other hand, water is free (or almost free). So who is going to tell you about the healing and weight loss properties of water in a world that unfortunately, so far, is run more on greed than on love and caring?

Your Body's Many Cries for Water includes six testimonials (about half of the testimonials in the book), where people reduced their weight by an amazing 35-45 pounds! They did this purely by increasing their water intake, and stopping drinking other drinks, plus having a pinch of salt. (Your body needs salt – that's why your tears and sweat are salty. But it should be sundried sea salt, not sodium chloride. See the chapter on salt).

One of the problems with recognizing that almost all of us are chronically dehydrated is because we think that we can't be dehydrated, because water is so readily available. But unless you *actually drink* enough water, all that water won't do you any good. Your body can be greatly dehydrated. It is hard for most people to realize that the answer to so many problems can be so simple. And so they ignore this most basic of need of the body.

Water regulates *all* functions of the body. This naturally includes weight loss. Water is essential for the body to live, and especially to move toxins around the body. It has to be very careful to regulate what parts of the body receive how much water, because it may be a long time before it receives more water, especially if you don't drink enough.

The most important organ is the brain, so if there is limited water, the brain will receive the water and the other organs will go without. The brain is 2% of the total body weight, but it receives about 20% of blood circulation.

WATER IS NOT THE SAME AS 'FLUIDS'

In advanced societies, thinking that 'fluids' (tea, coffee, juices, sodas, beer etc) are desirable substitutes for water, is a "catastrophic mistake"[10]. While these do contain water, they also contain other substances which are dehydrating. They are dehydrating because they are toxic to the body, so the body requires *more water* to flush them out. It is a miracle and testimony of the power of the body to adapt to negative situations, that there are people who have never drunk plain water who are still alive.

"Currently, practitioners of medicine are unaware of the many chemical roles of water in the body." (This is largely because there's no money in it). "Because dehydration eventually causes loss of some functions" (which can affect weight loss), "the various sophisticated signals given by the operators of the body's water rationing program during severe and lasting dehydration have been translated as indicators of unknown disease conditions of the body. This is the most basic mistake that has deviated clinical medicine."[11]

Medical practitioners have been taught to silence the signals of dehydration with chemical products, instead of with water[12].

"The mistaken assumption that all fluids are equivalent to water for the water needs of the human body is the main cause of many of the ills of the human body, and it is frequently associated with the initial excessive *gain in weight.*"[13]

YOU CAN BE DEHYDRATED WHEN YOU ARE NOT THIRSTY

"At the moment, the "dry mouth" is the only accepted sign of dehydration of the body... This signal is the *last* outward sign of *extreme dehydration.*"[14] "The body can suffer from dehydration even when the mouth may be fairly moist."[15].

How can we be dehydrated if we don't feel thirsty? It's because we did not learn to drink water from childhood. Gradually, the body became less and less able to tell us when we are thirsty. The body can suffer from dehydration even when the mouth may be fairly moist.

"Proteins and the enzymes of the body function more efficiently in solutions of lower viscosity". This means that if a person doesn't have enough water in their body, the body will not work as well. When toxins come in, the body will be less able to handle them efficiently and will be more likely to dump them in the fat cells, to deal with later. That is, the person will be more likely to store fat. And naturally they will be less likely to burn excess fat that is already present.

DRINK A MINIMUM of 6-8, 8 OUNCE GLASSES OF WATER BEFORE MEALS, EVERY DAY

Adult humans should drink six to eight, 8 oz. glasses of water everyday (8 oz. is one cup or half pint). This should not be drunk all at once, as that can cause problems for the kidneys. It should be drunk throughout the day and especially before eating any food. The best time to drink is thirty minutes before a meal. To reduce fat, one of the most important things you can do is to drink two, 8 oz. glasses of water 30 minutes *before eating any breakfast.*

The order of the digestive system is:

+ Mouth.
+ Esophagus.
+ Stomach.
+ Small intestine.
+ Large intestine.
+ Colon.

The reason that water should be drunk 30 minutes before a meal is this: It has been shown experimentally that water passes immediately into the intestines after drinking. It doesn't stay in the stomach and make you feel 'full'. But, within 30 minutes, almost the same amount of water is secreted into the stomach. Also, the pancreas empties a lot of a watery solution containing bicarbonates into the duodenum (the first part of the small intestine), when the stomach empties into there, to neutralize the acids from the stomach. (Without this watery substance, one can get all kinds of digestive pains).

All of this is needed for efficient food breakdown. The body needs lots of water to digest food properly, and to prevent pains related to digestion. The better you digest your food, the better your body will operate, and the easier it will be for you to reduce fat.

The reason why drinking water makes people feel 'full' is partly because most bodies are so out of balance that the person can no longer distinguish the difference between a thirst signal and a hunger signal. When the body signals a desire for water, it feels as though the desire is a desire for food. Drinking water solves the dehydration, and so the feeling of being 'hungry' evaporates – because it never was a cry for food in the first place.

LACK OF WATER CAUSES DEPRESSION, WHICH CAUSES EX-CESS EATING

You are not fat. You are toxic. This one truth manifests in many, many ways, because the body is infinitely complicated. For example, what is one reason why a lot of people eat more than they need, and eat unhealthy food into the bargain? Because they are 'depressed'. A toxic body is more likely to be dehydrated, because the body needs extra water to move toxins out of the body. Why could they be depressed in the first place? -

"The brain uses electrical energy that is generated by the water drive of the energy-generating pumps. With dehydration, the level of energy generation in the brain is decreased. Many functions of the brain that depend on this type of energy become inefficient. We ... call (this) depression"[16].

That is, drink enough water, before meals, and eat and drink less toxins, and you might very well feel less depressed. Which will end up with you eating less food, and being less likely to eat unhealthy food.

In my kinesiology practice where I have helped many people to heal many health and emotional problems, I was not focusing primarily on weight loss. But just by doing kinesiology on them, and having them make some life-style changes that required them to heal their pain and health problems, a number people lost 8-20 pounds within a few weeks after seeing me.

One of the first things that is looked at in a proper kinesiology session is a muscle test that tests whether or not someone is dehydrated. It is so important to do, that it's called a "pretest", because if the person is dehydrated, any muscle tests will not give an accurate result. This is one of the reasons why so many people who claim that they do muscle testing do not get accurate results.

It's very simple to do, once you know how to muscle test properly. You give a gentle tug on a person's hair or skin, and immediately afterwards, do a muscle test on the person. Generally, an arm is tested. The person holds their arm out straight in front, at about 45 degrees to the body. If the person is dehydrated, the person will not be able to hold up their arm, no matter how strong they are, when the tester applies a pressure to it. It has nothing to do with strength. When you muscle test you are communicating with the brain, which is far, far smarter than most people realize.

If the person is hydrated, there will be an electrical signal going from the brain to the muscle and back again, all the time. But if the person is dehydrated, this signal will not be working as efficiently as possible. Therefore, when we muscle test, the muscle goes weak.

The correction is simple. The person drinks a glass of water. Once they do that, generally the next dehydration test you do will test strong, although there are exceptions to this. I worked on a lady once who had terrible health problems. She was only in her 30's and yet she had already had three operations. No matter what I did, she kept becoming dehydrated during the session, so I had to keep giving her more and more water. This was such an unusual situation that finally I asked her how much water she normally drank. It turned out that she never drank water! In fact, her mother had put coca cola in her bottle as a baby. No wonder she had such terrible health problems!

I have found in my own kinesiology practice that about half of the people who come to me are dehydrated. Now, these are the people who are already interested in natural health, so I suspect that if I muscle tested the general population for dehydration, the percentage of people who are dehydrated would be even higher.

I believe that many sports injuries occur because the person is dehydrated, because they are drinking so-called 'sports drinks' instead of water. I believe this because muscle testing shows that when a person is dehydrated they have weak muscles. So when the person falls over,, the muscles do not hold the bones together strongly, the way they were designed to do. And a body that is drinking water plus chemicals plus sugar will not be properly hydrated, the way that a body that drinks plain water will be. But how many people will believe this when their favorite sports star endorses the drink? The sales in 1997 of one sports drink were close to $2 billion. Is a sports star going to give up all those million dollar endorsements and tell you that water is better for you?

I believe that the best way for people to see through the propaganda and to know the truth is to learn muscle testing and to see, and feel, this for themselves.

I had often wondered how wild animals manage to stay healthy without drinking as much water as we need to. I believe that I had my answer when I went on a completely raw diet for three weeks. During this time, I ate as much as I wanted so long as it was raw fruit, vegetables, nuts and seeds. No dairy, and of course, no meat (since raw meat contains parasites). There are 'cook' books that tell you how to prepare raw food so that you don't feel you are missing out on normal meals. By the end of the three weeks, I had reduced my weight by ten pounds and was close to my desired body size. I looked five years younger and felt fantastic. An interesting discovery during this time was that I, who normally experienced a low level of thirst most of the time, lost the feeling of being thirsty. Muscle testing showed that I wasn't dehydrated. I believe this is because just the process of heating food, which does not occur in nature, produces toxins, which have to be processed by the body. Animal bodies, like the human body, are designed for digesting *raw* plant food.

I believe that babies should be given some water from the moment they stop 100% breast feeding and start eating solid foods. Water intake should increase with solid food intake. Good habits such as drinking a glass of water (not juice) before meals, and throughout the day, should be instilled in children. Put the money you would spend on juice and soda away towards more fruit and vegetables. If they have bottled juice, consider it as candy, not as a drink. Fresh-squeezed juice is food. Sodas are just toxins.

So, right now, please stop drinking any fluids except for water. Do your best to drink the water before meals, especially before breakfast. If you are working on a computer or driving a car, or anything else where your body is subjected to electromagnetic stress, sipping water periodically can help your body to withstand the electromagnetic stress.

THE BEST KINDS OF WATER

Dr. Batmanghelidj believes that drinking tap water is good enough. And, if that is the only water you have, then he is correct. Even tap water will do more to help your weight and health than no water.

But the trouble is that most tap water has a lot of toxins in it, which will make it harder for your body to do what it wants to do, namely, keep you trim and healthy. These toxins include the poisons chlorine, fluoride and now many places are even finding a huge range of *pharmaceutical drugs* in the water!

Of these poisons, fluoride is possibly the worst. On the global scale of poisons where five is the worst, fluoride rates 4 out of 5. There have been many cases reported of people having health problems who removed all fluoride from their lives, mostly in water and toothpaste, and their health problems went away.

However, it gets worse. The following notes are from a New York times article[17]:

"The 35 year old federal law regulating tap water is so out of date that it can pose serious health risks, and still be legal. Only 91 contaminants are regulated by the Safe Drinking Water Act, yet more than 60,000 chemicals are used within the United States...

Millions of Americans are drinking water that does not meet at least one commonly used government health guideline intended to help protect people from cancer or serious disease, according to an analysis by *The Times* of more than 19 million drinking-water test results...

Dr. Parekh says "People don't understand that just because water is technically legal, it can still present health risks".

Government scientists have evaluated 830 of the contaminants most often found in water supplies, according to a review of records from the EPA (Environmental Protection Agency) and the USGS (United States Geological Survey). They have determined that many of them are associated with cancer or other diseases, even at small concentrations...And in some places, tap water contains not just one contaminant, *but dozens*".

It gets even worse, if that's possible. The Associated Press reported[18]:

"A vast array of pharmaceuticals — including antibiotics, anti-convulsants, mood stabilizers and sex hormones — have been found in the drinking water supplies of at least 41 million Americans."

If your body can't detoxify all of these toxins, which is quite possible, it will deposit them in the nearest fat cell, to hopefully deal with at a later time. The more toxins you have, the more fat your body will need to store them.

Therefore it is important to remove toxins from your drinking water because:

- Your body won't have to store toxins in fat cells.
- Your body will work better.
- When the water tastes better, you will naturally drink more of it.

DISTILLED WATER IS WORSE THAN TAP WATER

You need a really good filter to get rid of all those chemicals and drugs. Some people believe that distilled water is the best to drink, but it is toxic. Distilled water is made by boiling water and then condensing it, which supposedly leaves all the toxins behind. Unfortunately, while distilling does leave behind some dangerous toxins such as heavy metals, it actually concentrates some other dangerous chemicals that cause cancer and other health problems, called DPBs. DPB stands for disinfection byproduct. DPBs are chemicals that form when chemicals that are used for disinfecting, such as chlorine, react with organic matter which is also in the water.

Scientists have found that DPBs are over 10,000 times more poisonous than chlorine, which is very poisonous to start with[19].

DPBs form a gas at a temperature lower than water. Therefore, when the water is boiled, they go along with the water vapor into the distilled water, but in an even more concentrated form!

In addition, distilled water has been super heated, which never happens in nature. Heating water changes the energy of the water. There is a whole science to the properties of water that scientists are only just now staring to understand. If you want to know more, I highly recommend studying the work of genius Viktor Schauberger.

DRINK REVERSE OSMOSIS WATER

Good spring or well water that has been fully tested and shown to be free of toxins is good for you. The other water that is good is water filtered by reverse osmosis. Reverse osmosis is a process in which dissolved toxins are removed from tap water, by pushing tap water through a semi permeable membrane, under pressure. Reverse osmosis filters are the only filters which remove fluoride. Reverse osmosis water tastes great!

Some people sell water 'purifiers' which are said to 'improve the energy' of the water (alkalizers, magnetic, far infra red etc). Never buy an ultra violet water purifier, because it kills the energy of the water, and makes it unhealthy. I believe that some of these purifiers may be good, but only when they are *combined* with a reverse osmosis filter. Changing the energy of water is not going to remove the effects of dozens of dangerous chemicals and drugs.

You can get a portable reverse osmosis filter which is reasonably cheap from hardware stores or www.ebay.com. The filters should be changed about *every six months*. We always buy ours cheaply from ebay.com.

Some people will say that reverse osmosis water is not good because it makes the water a tiny bit more acidic. If you are worried about this, just add a mineral cartridge to your machine. We added a magnesium cartridge to our machine and it works fine.

DRINK WATER BEFORE MEALS

Drink water before meals, preferably 30 minutes before. Yes, it's kind of boring, but if you will especially drink 2, 8 oz. glasses before breakfast, you may be surprised at how much less hungry you get. Anne Fletcher M.S., R.D., registered dietician, surveyed 208 people who reduced weight by an average of 64 pounds! And best of all, *kept it off,* for at least three years[20]. The number one thing they did was to drink a glass of water *before* (not during) eating. That is what I suggest you do now, and for the rest of your life.

REFERENCES

1. *Your Body's Many Cries for Water,* by Dr. F. Batmanghelidj, M.D.,.
2. *Your Body's Many Cries for Water,* by Dr. F. Batmanghelidj, M.D., Page 29
3. *Your Body's Many Cries for Water,* by Dr. F. Batmanghelidj, M.D., Page 101
4. *Your Body's Many Cries for Water,* by Dr. F. Batmanghelidj, M.D., Page 18
5. *Your Body's Many Cries for Water,* by Dr. F. Batmanghelidj, M.D., Page 99
6. *Your Body's Many Cries for Water,* by Dr. F. Batmanghelidj, M.D., Page 103
7. *Your Body's Many Cries for Water,* by Dr. F. Batmanghelidj, M.D., Page 19
8. Department of Health and Human Services report 2004.
9. pharmatruth.blogspot.com/2010/01/unbelievable-mark-ups-of-pharma-ceutical.html. Sharon L. Davis, Budget Analyst, U.S. Department of Commerce, Room 6839, Office Ph: 202-482-4458
10. *Your Body's Many Cries for Water,* by Dr. F. Batmanghelidj, M.D., Page 6
11. *Your Body's Many Cries for Water,* by Dr. F. Batmanghelidj, M.D., Page 6
12. *Your Body's Many Cries for Water,* by Dr. F. Batmanghelidj, M.D., Page 7
13. *Your Body's Many Cries for Water,* by Dr. F. Batmanghelidj, M.D., Page 105
14. *Your Body's Many Cries for Water,* by Dr. F.Batmanghelidj, M.D., Page 10
15. *Your Body's Many Cries for Water,* by Dr. F.Batmanghelidj, M.D., Page 18
16. *Your Body's Many Cries for Water,* by Dr. F. Batmanghelidj, M.D., Page 56
17. www.nytimes.com/2009/12/17/us/17water.html?pagewanted=1&_r=2
18. www.usatoday.com/news/nation/2008-03-10-drugs-tap-water_N.htm
19. articles.mercola.com/sites/articles/archive/2010/12/18/distilled-water-interview.aspx
20. *Postmaster* magazine Boulder CO, 10/1/98

CHAPTER 8

SLEEP TO BURN FAT

I told you this book would be different from other weight loss books. I've already told you in the chapter on water how you can get energy from a substance with zero calories – water. Now, while most diet books go on and on about exercise, I will explain how getting the right amount of quality *sleep* is highly important to getting and staying slim.

The body can maintain optimum weight only if it is receives proper care and attention. Because I knew how important getting enough sleep is, I realized that it would affect weight gain. So I figured that if I went looking for some scientific papers to back up this theory, I would find them. And sure enough, I found this one:

ONE HOUR'S LESS SLEEP CAN MAKE A CHILD TWICE AS FAT!

Children can stay slim by having a full night's sleep. Scientists at Pittsburgh University discovered that just *one hour's less sleep* could mean a child would be *twice as fat*. Researchers monitored the sleep patterns of 335 children aged 7 to 17, reports The Sun. Dr. Xianchen Liu, who led the study said it was due to "biological changes as a result of sleep deprivation". Larger children slept for an average of 22 minutes less than normal weight kids. They also had shorter REM sleep. They also discovered that *sleep loss changes hormone levels.*

Now, if that works for children, it will work for adults as well, although possibly to a lesser extent. But since there's no money in telling people to sleep more, it's unlikely that:

a) Anyone will pay the hundreds of thousands of dollars for a study.

b) You will be told about it.

Here's more data that backs up my claim that lack of sleep contributes to fat gain: University of Chicago researcher Esra Tasali notes that waistlines in modern societies started to expand when people started to sleep less. Today, the average "sleep deficit" is about two hours per night compared with 40 years ago[2]. That is a huge amount! Two hours less sleep each night! In *Mastering Leptin*, Byron Richards says that:

SLEEP IS THE MOST IMPORTANT TIME FOR BURNING FAT

Sleep is the most important time for burning fat[3]. In addition, lack of sleep:

1. Increases levels of cortisol, the stress hormone that makes you fat, especially in the belly.

2. Causes high levels of cortisol, which makes you crave carbohydrates and fats[4].

Anything that affects the efficiency of your body, will eventually affect your ability to reduce weight. So, we need to understand a bit more about something most of us take for granted because it seems so simple. In fact, it turns out that sleep is anything but simple.

Dr. Dement wrote a brilliant and very important book on sleep called *The Promise of Sleep: A Pioneer in Sleep Medicine explores the Vital Connection between Health, Happiness and Sleep*[5]". Most of the information in this book is unknown by most people, including the vast majority of doctors. And yet it is vital to health and wellbeing, so much so that lack of this knowledge not infrequently leads to death.

I highly recommend that you read this book. This aspect of our lives is vital to understand.

I have found from muscle testing and questioning clients in my kinesiology practice the very same thing that Dr. Dement found from his 50+ years of studies on sleep: That a major and common cause of many health and emotional problems is not getting enough sleep, as well as not getting enough uninterrupted sleep. Maybe sleep seems to be so simple, and that is why it is overlooked as a cause of so many apparently complicated problems, like obesity.

You may have already heard that in five years of training your average doctor gets only 0 -12 hours training on nutrition. (So how on earth can they think they are experts on weight loss? I have had clients tell me that their doctor told them "It doesn't matter what you eat!" How can that kind of thinking give good advice for fat reduction?). Therefore it may come as no surprise to you to learn that the average doctor also receives only 0 - 2 hours of instruction on sleep problems during those five years.

This is a good system if you control a multinational drug company that makes trillions of dollars from people with health problems. People will then think they need lots of drugs and operations to get better, rather than something as simple as an improvement in their sleep.

Dr. Dement has done a great job of breaking free of his training as a doctor by researching sleep. However, it is a great pity that he is still affected by his training enough that he seems to think that drugs are often the best, if not the only, solution.

Most people think that when we are asleep, the brain is resting and doing virtually nothing. It was Dr. Dement who discovered the shocking truth, that the brain is as active during sleep as it is during the day!

Most of us think we go gradually to sleep. But Dr. Dement found that this is not the case. The brain produces different brain waves when you are awake and when you are asleep. There is no in-between area. You are either awake, or you are asleep.

During the first period of deep sleep, hormones such as growth hormone and prolactin are released. Growth hormone helps build new cells but it is also important in rebuilding old, damaged cells, and is therefore important in staying young, and reducing fat.

SLEEP DEBT

Perhaps the most amazing of Dr. Dement's findings is that we carry around a sleep debt. Most people need 7-9 hours of sleep a night, *not counting* the time it takes to fall asleep. However, if you miss any sleep, then you 'owe' your body that much sleep. **The body keeps an exact account of how much it is owed!** This debt is added up for at least two weeks and probably a whole lot longer. We don't know if sleep debt carries over for more than two weeks, because so far no studies have looked at this. Could we possibly still owe our body sleep from times of little sleep that happened 20 or more years ago? It is possible. No wonder so many people are so tired! And when we are tired, we are more likely to eat something that will give us a chemical 'lift', like sugar, coffee or fried foods.

The time it takes you to go to sleep is in direct proportion to your sleep debt. If you fall asleep faster than 15-20 minutes, you are sleep deprived. This is assuming your brain is not being interfered with by things such as caffeine during the day or looking at a bright light (such as a computer screen) the hour before bed.

If you fall asleep within 5 minutes you are severely sleep deprived. 10 minutes is borderline.

Accumulated lost sleep must be paid back. And it seems that it might have to be paid back hour for hour. Unfortunately, short naps don't seem to make much difference. The body wants full sleep cycles of at least around one and a half hours.

So, if someone who needs 8 hours of sleep gets only 6 hours of sleep a night, after five days they owe their body *ten hours* of sleep! So sleeping in on the weekend does not pay off the sleep debt. What is needed is a change in lifestyle. Turn off the television and computer and get to bed earlier every night.

Some times when people have had very little sleep over a number of days, and they finally get an extra long sleep, when they wake up they feel terrible. These people sometime then say something like "I slept too much". That is not true. The truth is that they have just started to pay off an enormous sleep debt. You cannot pay off a large sleep debt in one, or even two, nights' of sleep. What they need is more sleep on an ongoing basis, especially getting to bed earlier, rather than just sleeping in. Hopefully the following information will motivate you to get more sleep:

DANGER AND DEATH FROM SLEEP DEPRIVATION

1. Newspapers blamed much of the Exxon Valdez disaster, America's 2nd Worst Oil Spill (after BP in the Gulf of Mexico), on the captain who had ingested some alcohol. But the captain was not on the bridge when the accident happened, and was not to blame. The final report told what really happened. The captain worked out a plan to keep the ship safe, and handed over command to the third mate and left the bridge. The third mate had slept only 6 hours in the previous 48 and was *severely sleep deprived*. He ordered the ship to starboard (to the right), but did not notice that the autopilot was still on, and the ship did not turn.

Twice the lookouts warned the third mate about the position of lights marking the reef, but he didn't change or check his orders. His brain did not interpret the danger in what they said. When he finally realized the autopilot was on and turned it off, and tried to turn the ship around, it was too late. Lack of sleep was the cause of the disaster.

2. The explosion of the space shuttle *Challenger* was also found, in the final report, to have been due to mistakes caused by severe sleep deprivation of the NASA manager.

3. A Stanford professor was in a bike and swimming race that lasted a number of days. He got very little sleep at night during that time, but then he got nine hours of sleep a night, for two nights. Most people would assume that he therefore had no sleep debt. However, an extra two hours of sleep is not enough to pay off as large a number of hours of missing sleep as he must have had. He woke up feeling alert and drove home. But coming down a mountain his massive sleep debt started to kick in. He started to yawn and his

eyelids felt heavy. He did not think of pulling over and taking a nap.

He saw a sign that there was a restaurant several miles ahead, and he thought he would get some coffee there. Right after that he fell asleep for a moment, and woke with a start to find that he had drifted onto the oncoming lane. He jerked the wheel to the right, but the road went to the left and he went over a 30 foot cliff. The car went upside down. His right arm was injured and completely paralyzed, but amazingly he survived.

4. A woman named Helen was worried sick about her husband who had just been called unexpectedly away to active military duty in the Middle East. At the same time her brother-in-law went to hospital in critical condition for a heart problem. Helen's sister left Helen with her three children, so Helen then had four children to look after. Not surprisingly, Helen lay awake on her own for three nights without sleep, worrying about her husband. Helen became utterly exhausted. She knew she had to get to sleep, and asked her doctor for a sleeping pill. The doctor refused.

Dr. Dement explains how in emergency situations like this, it is wise to have a sleeping pill, and there are in fact some now available that don't seem to hurt people as much. Although I hate drugs with a vengeance and think they should always be a last resort after trying kinesiology and other natural methods, I can see that in an emergency, a few nights with a sleeping pill really was what was needed.

After another sleepless night, Helen was so utterly exhausted that she could hardly look after herself, let alone the four children. She called her mother who lived 200 miles away and arranged to bring the children to her and stay with her mother. Helen started to feel some relief knowing that help was at hand. But now there was less stress to keep her awake. The sleep debt that had been mounting over the past four nights began to assert itself.

In mid afternoon (when we are at our lowest due to circadian rhythms) Helen was driving through a small town and did the unthinkable. She drove through a red light. Helen still does not remember approaching the town or seeing the light, but she does remember the nightmare of the squeal of brakes as a pickup truck smashed into the side of the car.

Miraculously, no one was killed, but all sustained injuries of varying severity. The car was totally destroyed.

Lack of sleep doesn't just make people fall asleep at the wheel. It can also do what happened to Helen. It can stop brains from working properly. Your brain needs to be working correctly if you are to reduce fat. Dr. Dement also goes on to explain how many serious accidents in hospitals are also related to sleep deprivation. Anytime that some one has trouble sleeping for a full night, for more than a night or two, they and those around them are in *great danger*.

Tests show that people are terrible judges of how likely they are to fall asleep. So if you become drowsy at any time during the day, resolve to be cautious in hazardous situations. Have a nap before you drive. If your eyelids are heavy and you are driving, stop and take a nap. Even a few minutes can make a big difference. If your sleep debt is large enough, no amount of will power or caffeine will be enough to keep you awake.

When a car crash is attributed to alcohol, the real culprit, or a major part of the problem, is usually sleep debt. Alcohol plus sleep debt greatly increases the effects of alcohol. Australian researchers found that after 17 hours awake, at 1.00 am, a sleep-deprived group had the same test scores as drinking volunteers who had blood-alcohol levels of 0.05 percent. After 24 hours awake, the sleep-deprived group had the same coordination deficits as those with blood-alcohol levels of 0.1 percent! Remember: *Drowsiness is red alert!*

LACK OF MOTIVATION MAY BE LACK OF SLEEP

You need motivation to reduce fat. Dr. Dement found that one of the first things to go when sleep is shortchanged is motivation. Now, how are you going to maintain new habits for a beautiful, thin, strong body, if you aren't motivated? You won't. You have got to get more sleep.

Anyone who is feeling a little poorly due to lack of sleep will be less motivated, and hence, less able to do what they need to do to have a thin body. So add two or more hours of sleep a night until you catch up on your debt and see your motivation improve. Keep doing so until it takes you at least 20 minutes to fall asleep, without caffeine in the day, or looking at a computer in the hour before you go to bed.

Another benefit of more sleep is that it can improve your creativity, by improving your motivation. After decades of study, Rothenberg found that the one trait that all highly creative people have in common is motivation. It is a myth that creativity arrives like a bolt of lightning out of the blue. Rothenberg demonstrated that almost all creative acts come after long, sustained struggle that requires motivation and perseverance.

CAN YOU SLEEP LESS?

While there are people who try to teach how to do with less sleep, Dr. Dement found that sleeping less is seldom a good idea, and virtually impossible in the long run. People who are lacking sleep don't think as well and make mistakes. Little mistakes can turn into serious or even fatal mistakes. All the studies done show that no one can train themselves to deal with less sleep, in order to get more work done. Every individual needs a specific amount of sleep, and this amount *cannot be altered*. It's analogous to your body temperature – it *has* to be at 98.6°F. for you to be healthy. The few people who really can do with only a few hours of sleep without detracting from their performance did not learn how to do that, they were born that way.

Muscle testing from someone who has been trained correctly can give you a good indication of how many hours of sleep your body wants each day right now, and when your sleep debt is paid off.

THE BIOLOGICAL CLOCK

If we have sleep debt, why aren't we sleepy all day long? This is because there is another mechanism which works against the one whose purpose it is to put us to sleep when we need it. That is the biological clock, which is also called a circadian rhythm.

There are two main times when your body clock will make you extra alert: In the morning when you wake up, and in the very late afternoon or early evening, around 6 pm, with the peak at possibly 9 pm. It is at its lowest around mid day, the time when many societies traditionally took (or still take) a siesta.

Now, some people may ask, what is the point of having increased energy between 6 and 9 pm? I believe that at that time we are meant to be in bed! Note that all daytime animals, which easily maintain ideal body shapes, go to bed at sunset and get up at sunrise, and that for millennia, when people were not over-weight, that is what people did. I believe that this extra energy is meant to be used, not for surfing the internet or going out to dinner, but for healing, and for burning fat.

AN HOUR'S SLEEP BEFORE MIDNIGHT IS WORTH TWO HOURS AFTER MIDNIGHT

This is a common saying in the healing world. I have found this to be true for myself. This extra energy before midnight explains this belief. I believe that getting to sleep, not just going to bed, several hours before midnight is important for fat reduction. This is probably not what most people want to hear. But I suggest that you try this. Get to bed by 9 pm. And if you wake up 'too early', get up and start your day.

INSOMNIA

More than a third of Americans suffer from insomnia, with 42 million prescriptions for sleeping medications filled in 2007[6] (and medications make you fat, as you will see in the chapter on drugs). Now, since nearly everyone has caffeine, and caffeine, even in small amounts, causes insomnia, why don't doctors prescribe zero caffeine rather than drugs? Maybe because they are themselves addicted to caffeine, and can't face the truth of how bad it is, apart from the fact that they won't benefit financially from that advice. I will show you other ways that caffeine makes people fat in the chapter on caffeine.

However, once you give up caffeine, there can still be other causes for insomnia. Dr. Dement found independently what most kinesiologists already know from muscle testing – what looks like just one particular symptom like "insomnia" can in fact be a number of different kinds of problems, and have many different causes. Giving one symptom – "insomnia" - one label, gives us the wrong impression that we are dealing with just one symptom and one cause.

Dr. Dement also says that insomnia is not a disease – it's a symptom. It's a pity that he didn't take the next step in realizing that *all* diseases are symptoms of the body trying to heal itself. (For example, a fever is the body trying to kill bacteria. Giving a person a drug to bring down the fever can allow the bacteria to breed even more).

Dr. Dement says the cause of many cases of persistent insomnia can be problems with the biological clock. If the person has problems falling asleep, then they may be being affected by their biological clock becoming more alert in the evening. He says that one remedy for this is sitting in front of a lot of bright lights in the morning (your computer screen does this).

I would suggest some other possible remedies that he may not have mentioned. One is to make sure you do not look at a computer for at least one or even two hours before you go to sleep. Darkness helps your body to produce melatonin and to get you to sleep. Several studies have shown that a melatonin deficiency is associated with weight gain[7]. The darker your room, the better. Even a tiny, tiny, tiny night light or a crack of moonlight through the curtains can help keep you awake, or not sleep properly. And if you have a smoke detector with one of those small battery status indicators, try putting a shield of black cardboard or black art foam between the indicator and yourself (make sure you do not block the smoke sensor). These bright LED indicators are especially troublesome in hotels, so be sure to take your sleeping goggles with you when you travel.

In fact, it's quite possible that the increase in computer usage is a contributing cause to the increase in obesity, because a study on the effects of lighting on mice found that mice under a bright light at night gained a massive 50% more weight than those in darkness[8]!

Dr. Dement says that the biggest challenge to treating insomnia is persuading doctors and even the people who have insomnia that it is a *serious* problem. He says that when they do treat insomnia with pills, it is usually an antidepressant and not the new generation of sleeping pills that were developed specifically for insomnia.

I myself would never take drugs, but that is because I have always been able to heal any problems with kinesiology and other natural methods. However, while I normally never recommend drugs because there are spiritual as well as health ramifications, perhaps it would be beneficial for some people to follow Dr. Dement's advice and take Ambien should they find themselves in the position where they haven't been able to sleep for several nights, since a few nights without sleep can cause accidents which kill the person and others. Dr. Dement says that Ambien is a short-acting hypnotic that does not induce tolerance and has little or no potential to become addictive. Also, it is metabolized in the body overnight.

I personally would not take any kind of hypnotic drug because any kind of hypnosis shuts down the conscious mind and / or can open us to being affected by negative energies. But when it is an emergency, this may be the only alternative for some people.

TIPS ON GETTING TO SLEEP

If you are like some people, you may find it hard to get to sleep within the twenty minutes that it is meant to take. Here are some tips:

1. Stop taking caffeine completely. When I was at university, I used to wonder why I couldn't get to sleep till 2 am. Only now do I realize that 6-8 coffees a day will do it! Even just one cup with caffeine in the day can keep you awake at night, and/or stop you from having deep sleep, which is when you burn fat.

2. I learned this from a seminar I went to. It has worked for me many times. It's the old 'counting sheep' but with some important changes:

Imagine on the right hand side of your mind there is a field full of 100 sheep. Look at each sheep and imagine you see the word 'SLEEP' shorn into their sides in big letters. Then sheep #100 walks slowly to the middle of your field of view. Again, see the word SLEEP on her side. She jumps over a low jump. Again, see the word SLEEP on her side. Then she walks over to the left side of your mind - see the word SLEEP - and see the sheep curl up and go to sleep.

Then repeat for sheep #99 and so on.

If you do this fully and slowly, chances are you won't even get to #80.

3. Turn the brightness on your computer screen down as much as you can. Plus do not look at your computer screen for two hours, not just one, before you go to sleep. That bright, white light will trick your brain into thinking it's the middle of the day. TV does not seem to be as bad as a computer screen, possibly because there's not as much white color.

4. Read a *non-fiction* book before going to bed. Not a book that gets you really 'into' it, so you don't want to put it down. Reading a book with big words or concepts that you don't fully understand will put you to sleep very fast, as your brain ties up parts of itself ('attention units') and tries to figure out what the words mean. I will be surprised if you can read more than one or two pages of any of Buckminster Fuller's books without falling asleep – that has sure worked for me in the past!

5. Get a kinesiology balance and see if your cloacals are in balance. The cloacals are an energy system that cannot be seen, related to the Central nervous system, and are greatly involved with sleep. Having your cloacals in balance can make a big difference to sleep, which can help you to reduce fat. Further information is available in the chapter on Kinesiology.

DEPRESSION

Dr. Dement says that much insomnia is caused by psychological problems, such as depression. It is a shame that he does not mention that one researcher found that a major cause of depression is caffeine[9]

Caffeine stops your body from having proper deep sleep, which is necessary for fat loss, as well as wellbeing. I will talk more about caffeine in its own chapter.

REST IS DIFFERENT FROM SLEEP

A lot of people confuse rest with sleep. They are very different from each other. Certainly, if you are not getting enough sleep, extra rest is better than nothing. But your body wants *both* rest and sleep. Make sure you get enough sleep. But, also, several times a day, take some time out to lie down or at least sit down and do and think nothing. Give your brain a rest, as well as your body. A 20 minute lie down in the middle of the day to rest your spine is an excellent thing to do.

GOOD SLEEP IMPROVES OUR MOOD

Study after study shows that good sleep gives us good, positive feelings and moods. These are necessary if we are to be happy with eating healthy food, giving up toxic food and doing the gentle exercise that I will discuss in later chapters.

In addition, study after study shows that our bodies can never adapt to short sleep. Sleep debt makes us feel and act lousy. However, we often don't realize that it is lack of sleep causing the bad feelings, because clock-dependent alerting masks this effect at certain times of the day. During the hours when your body is experiencing clock-dependent alerting, you will feel okay and maybe even good. But when the clock-dependent alerting drops off, the effects of sleep debt will be felt even more.

If you have children who are grumpy or unhappy at any time in the day, or overweight, see what giving them 10-12 hours of sleep every night (in addition to the time it takes them to get to sleep), does for them.

Do the same for yourself. Lowering sleep debt can make people thinner, as well as smarter and motivated. *Plenty of good sleep is vital for fat loss.*

GET A LATEX PILLOW

Here is a tip that is relatively cheap that can help you to improve your sleep right now. Get a latex pillow. Your head is buried in your pillow for one third of your life. You don't want to be inhaling any molecules of artificial substances, and as few molecules of anything at all. I have seen how a latex pillow can stop a person make "snuffling" sounds overnight.

REFERENCES

1. *Source*: 2008, an article on the Ananova website, which is now web.orange.co.uk/p/news/uk_world?menu

2. Breitbart.com. 7/1/05.

3. *Mastering Leptin*, Byron Richards CCN, page 257

4. From an article quoting www.shuteye.com and the American Council on Exercise, National Sleep Foundation

5. *The Promise of Sleep: A Pioneer in Sleep Medicine explores the Vital Connection between health, Happiness and Sleep*, by Dr. Dement, M.D., Ph.D., 1999

6. chriskresser.com/10-ways-stress-makes-you-fat-and-diabetic

7. www.naturalnews.com/032285_melatonin_weight_gain.html

8. www.dailymail.co.uk/femail/article-2046500/Lose-weight-going-diet-forget-calorie-counting.html

9. *Caffeine Blues*, by Stephen Cherniske, M.S., Page 110

CHAPTER 9

CLEANSING REACTIONS FROM DETOXIFYING

If you do any of the things suggested in this book, then it is very likely that your body will start detoxifying. This is great, because it's something your body needs to do in order for it to burn fat.

However, most people are not trained in the knowledge of natural health, and don't always know that sometimes things have to get worse before they get better. Therefore, when they give up toxins and eat more nutritious food, and they experience the effects of detoxification, they give up before they experience the benefits. It's a lot like giving up drugs – it gets worse before it gets better. In fact, since caffeine *is* a drug, and a number of substances in the food we eat act like drugs on the brain, it's no wonder that giving these substances up is very like drug withdrawal.

Right now, there are lots of toxins stored away in various parts of your body, especially the fat cells. Once you start ingesting less toxins, and doing more positive things for the body, your body can start to get rid of these toxins. Fresh-squeezed juicing will almost certainly do this for at least the first few days.

Unfortunately, while the toxins may appear to not be affecting you while they are 'safely' stored in a fat cell, you may experience some uncomfortable symptoms while the toxins make their journey from the cells out through the lymphatic system and eventually out of the body. The main ways the body gets rid of toxins are:

- Poo it out.
- Pee it out.
- Sweat it out.
- Put it in mucus to cough or sneeze out.
- Put it in skin cells to slough off.
- Vomit it out.

When the body does this, you can experience symptoms such as:

1. Tiredness. Your body is using the extra energy you have given it to get rid of toxins and save its life. It has less energy to spare for you to do what you may want to do. Get to bed earlier. Sleep in if possible. Plus have rests during the day.

2. Headaches. If this happens, having an extra glass or two of water can sometimes help. They should not last more than a day or two.

3. Weird pains that can appear and disappear in the oddest places, often from old injuries.

4. Rashes & skin eruptions. The body is working to get rid of toxins via the skin. For example, there is an area around my right ring finger which had rashes and flaking skin a number of times when I did different kinds of detoxing, including fresh-squeezed juicing. When I asked my body what caused this, I immediately got a picture of a pewter ring that I got when in Greece when I was 12 years old. I then learned that pewter contains lead, which is very poisonous. The rashes were my body's way of getting rid of the lead.

5. Diarrhea. It should not last long.

6. Strong emotions, possibly combined with memories of some

past painful event.

However, I will add a proviso. If you react to something *instantly*, especially with nausea or hives, then that is very likely an allergic response to something that is toxic to you in the substance you just ate, rather than a sign of detoxifying. Do not eat it at all, and see your health practitioner immediately.

The fact that a *healthy* food can cause *negative* symptoms for a short period of time does not seem to be as widely known as it should be. For example, I read a book by a doctor about foods that cause allergies. He assumes that any food that makes you feel bad when you eat it, automatically means that particular food is not good for you. This is not necessarily so.

Here's an example. My naturopathic teacher told us a story of a client he had, who was a farmer, and used to stir the vats of pesticide that he sprayed on his crops with his bare arms. Substances are absorbed through our skin, so you can imagine how toxic he was! The farmer said that he could never eat fresh oranges. If he did, he broke into a rash. That is to say, he considered the oranges as more dangerous than the pesticides. While some people are allergic to oranges (especially bottled orange juice), it is quite likely that in his case, the extra nutrients and alkalinity from the oranges gave the body what it needed to expel some of the pesticides from his body, in the form of rashes.

Pain is an interesting thing. Some people tend to think that doctors know all about pain and what to do about it. However, pain is an *energy*. It cannot be seen with any of our current medical instruments. I wish I was paid for every client who has told me that they had a pain, and that they paid for many, many medical tests, and the doctors "could not find anything wrong."

I believe that pain is the body's way of telling us that something is wrong, and that pain is often associated with toxins. For example, one day I got the most excruciating, appalling, pounding pain in my gall bladder area. It attacked me in waves. I understood for the first time why people might rush off to hospital to get their gall bladder cut out when this happened. Fortunately, I knew about natural health by then. I thought over what I had eaten to find out what could have caused this. The *second* that I remembered that I had eaten something I had not eaten before - some big, super thick, deep-fried potato wedges from a fast food store - and I thought that was probably the cause, and I apologized to my body for eating them, the pain went away, and did not return. My body had got my attention and got my promise to not eat them again.

People involved with natural health call all of these unpleasant side-effects a "healing crisis". The idea is that things have to get worse before they get better. Think of it as being like a spring-clean of your house. There will be mess everywhere, and things certainly look messy before it gets to the stage where things are cleaner than they were before. However, a healing crisis should not last more than a few days, and maybe only hours. If it's longer than this, something else may be involved. You may be eating something that you are allergic to, or you may need to see a doctor. If it is really too uncomfortable, then it may be a good idea to lessen whatever changes you were doing that caused the detoxification.

Remember, when you spring clean a house, or spring-clean your body, things will get worse for a short while, before they get better.

CHAPTER 10

PARASITES MAKE YOU
FAT AND HUNGRY

"Alert! Parasites are making up to 32% of women fat and tired!" headlined an article by *First* magazine[1]. Here are parts of that article:

"The scientific community has made a breakthrough that could free millions of women from stubborn pounds. But chances are, you've never heard of it. That's because few doctors are even aware that the problem exists in North America, nor do they appreciate the tremendous impact it's having on our health and our weight."

This is a gross, very tough subject to talk about. It makes most people feel squeamish, and I am one of them. But, please, be brave and read on, because this is a very important subject, not just for your weight but also for your health[2].

Parasites are anything that live in our bodies, that do not help our bodies. These can be different worms, fungi, bacteria or viruses, in different areas of the body. Most are microscopic. Parasites take from us, and give nothing in return.

I knew from my own knowledge and observations that parasites cause weight gain. So it was nice to see my beliefs backed up in the article in *First* magazine. For example, it said:

'As many as 73% of infected people struggle with symptoms, yet they have no idea that a microscopic intruder is to blame. And since most doctors get little or no training in parasitology, they frequently overlook even the classic signs, notes Ann Gittleman Ph.D."

The article goes on to describe the main ways that parasites affect weight and health:

1. They *block the absorption of nutrients*, by inflaming the digestive tract.

2. They trigger *yeast overgrowth*, by hindering good bacteria.

3. They *acidify body systems.* This damages organs and nerves. (Once again, anytime your body is not at peak efficiency, weight gain is likely). To make it worse, the body moves the acid into the fat cells. (This backs up what I said earlier: your body uses the fat cells as a place to dump toxins. The more toxins you have, the more fat cells you need for garbage dumps).

4. They slow down your organs. They do this by excreting waste products which your liver and kidneys have to deal with. (Therefore, the liver has less energy available for dealing with toxins, and is more likely to dump them in fat cells).

I will add one more very important way that parasites are making people fat. They produce *ammonia*. Ammonia inside your body alone can make you fat. In addition, high levels of ammonia in the brain can also cause insomnia[3]. If you wake up in the night and can't get back to sleep for hours, it's possible that this is caused by parasites. Getting a full night's sleep is essential for fat loss.

The *First* magazine article describes a 2-week cleanse that 'makes weight loss effortless', designed by Ann Gittleman Ph.D. (www.UniLey-Health.com). Here are some examples of success stories:

- Catherine, 225 pounds, lost 85 pounds to go to 140 pounds.
- Georgia, 197 pounds, lost 65 pounds to go to 132 pounds.
- Shelly, 185 pounds, lost 57 pounds to go to 128 pounds.

I know from personal experience how parasites make a huge difference to weight loss because of what happened to me around 1995. I used to be hungry a *lot* of the time. I probably ate more than most people. I could never miss meals. After 6 pm, I would be ravenously hungry. If I did not eat dinner around this time, I would get quite emotional. Then that year, a new book came out – *The Cure for All Diseases*, by Dr. Hulda Clark. While the title is not totally correct, as the information in it is not the only thing one needs to do for health, this is still a very important book that I highly recommend. It has much information about parasites and pollutants that I cannot include in this book.

Dr. Clark claims that we *all* have a lot of parasites inside us. And that all diseases, including cancer, are caused by a parasite, plus a pollutant. The pollutants that help the parasites to live in us are solvents (like cleaning fluids & alcohols) and heavy metals (I will talk more about heavy metals in another chapter).

Dr. Clark also claims that it is relatively easy and inexpensive to kill the parasites and remove the pollutants. Her books have many case histories which are evidence to the truth of her findings.

Hulda Clark attended the University of Minnesota, studying biophysics and cell physiology, and received her Doctorate degree in physiology in 1958. In 1979 she left government funded research and began private consulting on a full time basis.

I reasoned that since I had grown up surrounded by animals – many cats and dogs, plus horses, chickens, guinea pigs and other animals - that it was quite possible that I had a lot of parasites inside me. The fact that just thinking about parasites made me want to be physically sick, was also an indication that there was something inside me that should not be there. (I believe that if you are feeling queasy right now, that's a big clue that *you* have parasites). So I went on her herbal parasite program, which consists of a herb called wormwood (it's called that because it kills worms), black walnut extra strength tincture and ground cloves. It costs around $40. (A tincture is a plant concentrate in water and alcohol. An extract is a plant concentrate in water and alcohol that is 3 to 8 times stronger than a tincture. We personally use an extract, rather than a tincture, for our parasite program.)

Amazingly, within days, my hunger *decreased by about 2/3*!!! For the first time in my life I was able to go to 9 pm without eating and not get upset! (Not that I am recommending that. To keep slim, one should have an early dinner). This made total sense. Parasites eat your good nutrition, which makes our bodies crave food, to replace what was taken. They cause us to have malnutrition, even if we are very overweight.

And in addition, they release ammonia and other substances into our bodies as one of their waste products. That is, they pee ammonia into your body. This puts incredible chemical stress on our bodies, which damages our bodies and makes us want to ingest food to dilute the ammonia.

More and more people are coming to realize that Dr. Hulda Clark was correct in thinking that virtually all of us have many different kinds of parasites inside us, even if we have never been around animals. Parasites are throughout our bodies, not just in the intestines. This should not be any surprise to us, because every farmer knows that his animals get worms, and he regularly gives them substances to kill off the worms. So why don't humans? The eggs are in the air around us, and on objects like furniture. If you have ever had pets or other animals around you, then the chances of having higher numbers of parasites, or more species, increases dramatically. If you've kissed an animal, you absolutely have parasites.

In 1979 a British study reported on 600 former prisoners from World War II. These men had been stationed in the Far East. Thirty years after the war, 15% were still infected with a parasite called *Strongyloides* that they had contracted during the war. This means you could have eaten contaminated meat 30 years ago, and still be hosting the tapeworms or other types of parasites that were in that meat. If you've travelled to third world countries, the chance that you have parasites is very high.

Despite their almost invisibility, small parasites can be extremely dangerous. Microscopic parasites can destroy calcium lining in your bones, eat the myelin lining off your nerve cells (causing breakdown of the brain-nerve connection) and even inhabit the liver, colon and other areas causing major discomforts and problems.

When we think of parasites, we tend to think that they make people thinner, because of all those pictures of starving Africans. But that happens only when people have virtually no food at all. In the developed nations, parasites are making people fatter. This is because the parasites are eating a person's good nutrition, and leaving the junk behind. That is causing massive malnutrition, which causes people to eat more, because the body must have the many different vitamins, minerals, essential fatty acids, protein and other substances to perform the thousands of different chemical reactions it needs to function properly.

In an earlier book, *The Cure for All Cancers*, Dr. Clark found that in 100% of over 100 cases of cancer there was both an intestinal parasite and propyl alcohol in the liver. If people killed the intestinal parasite by a simple herbal program (`parasite cleansing') and removed the cause of the propyl alcohol, the cancer went away.

To quote from her books;

"For many years we have all believed that cancer is different from other diseases. We believed that cancer behaves like a fire, in that you can't stop it once it has started. Therefore, you have to cut it out or radiate it to death or chemically destroy every cancerous cell in the body since it can never become normal again. Nothing could be more wrong! And we have believed that cancers of different types such as leukemia or breast cancer have different causes. Wrong again!

In this book you will see that *all cancers are alike*. They are all caused by a parasite. A single parasite! It is the *human intestinal fluke*. And if you kill this intestinal parasite, the cancer stops immediately. The tissue becomes normal again. In order to get cancer, you must have this parasite.

How can the human intestinal fluke cause cancer? This intestinal parasite typically lives in the intestine where it might do little harm, causing only colitis ... or irritable bowel syndrome, or perhaps nothing at all. But if it invades a different organ, like the uterus or kidneys or liver, it does a great deal of harm. If it establishes itself in the liver, it causes cancer!

It only establishes itself in the liver in some people. These people have propyl alcohol in their bodies. All cancer patients have both propyl alcohol and the intestinal fluke in their livers. The solvent propyl alcohol is responsible for letting the fluke establish itself in the liver. In order to get cancer, you must have both the parasite and propyl alcohol in your body".

AFTER DESCRIBING THE FLUKE AND HOW IT GETS INTO THE LIVER, HULDA CLARK WRITES;

"Clearly you must do three things:

• Kill the parasite and all its stages.
• Stop letting propyl alcohol into your body.
• Flush out the metal and common toxins from your body so you can get well.

We have been taught to believe that every parasite is so unique that a different drug is required to kill each one. The better drugs, such as Praziquantel™ and Levamisole™ or even Flagyl™ and Piperazine™, can each kill several worm varieties. But this is just not practical when dozens of different parasites are present. It would be best to kill them all together even though only the intestinal fluke is causing cancer...

It is not unusual for someone to have a dozen (or more) parasites out of the 120 parasites I have samples of. ..You can assume that you, too have a dozen different parasites....

We are heavily parasitized beings! Our bodies are large enough to provide food and shelter for lots of these free loaders. If they were settled on the outside, where we could see them, like lice or ticks, we would rid ourselves in a flash... But what about *in* our flesh? V. ⌣ cannot see inside ourselves, so we mistakenly assume that nothing is there...

- I have seen that: Eczema is due to roundworms.
- Seizures are caused by a single roundworm, *Ascaris*, getting into the brain.
- Schizophrenia and depression are caused by parasites in the brain. Asthma is caused by *Ascaris* in the lungs.
- Diabetes is caused by the pancreatic fluke of cattle, *Eurytrema*, in the pancreas.
- Migraines are caused by the threadworm, *Strongyloides*.
- Acne rosacea is caused by a *Leishmaina*.
- Much human heart disease is caused by dog heartworm, *Diro-filaria*, in the heart. And the list goes on.

Getting rid of all these parasites would be absolutely impossible using clinical medicines that can kill only one or two parasites each. Such medicines also tend to make you quite ill....Imagine taking ten such drugs to kill a dozen of your parasites! Good news, perhaps, for the drug makers but not for you.

Just three herbs can rid you of over 100 types of parasites! And without so much as a headache! Without nausea! The herbs are:

- Black Walnut Hulls (from the black walnut tree).
- Wormwood (from the *Artemesia* shrub).
- Common Cloves (from the clove tree).

These three herbs must be used together. Black walnut hull and wormwood kill adults and developmental stages of at least 100 parasites. Fresh ground cloves kill the eggs.

Only if you use them together will you rid yourself of parasites. If you kill only the adults, the tiny stages and eggs will soon grow into new adults. If you kill only the eggs, the million stages already loose in your body will soon grow into adults and make more eggs. They must be used together as a single treatment." (Note: Hulda Clark says that extra herbs are required for tapeworm).

In the case of cancer, how does the fluke get from the intestines (where it is relatively harmless) into the liver? Dr. Clark believes that people with cancer also have propyl alcohol in their liver. Propyl alcohol is the antiseptic commonly used in cosmetics. Also, it is a pollutant in cold cereals and other products, especially those with flavorings. The eggs of the intestinal parasite hatch into small living forms called miracidia. In healthy people, the miracidia are killed by the liver. But somehow, when propyl alcohol is present, the liver loses its ability to kill the hatchlings. So they stay in the body, grow up and reproduce themselves.

She goes on to describe how the three herbs should be taken, and how they work for successful parasite cleansing. It's called the "Hulda Clark herbal parasite program". She also has a program for parasite cleansing for pets, to keep them healthy and to prevent you from getting re-infected, because parasites are everywhere.

THE HULDA CLARK HERBAL PARASITE CLEANSE

CAUTION: NOT TO BE USED BY PREGNANT WOMEN OR YOUNG CHILDREN

Here is the Hulda Clark herbal parasite program for **adults**, from *The Cure for All Diseases*[4]. You may start to feel a lot better and less hungry after just six days on this program, when the adult parasites will be killed. The whole family should do this program at the same time, to prevent reinfection, provided children are old enough. Reduce quantities by weight for children. It is best if this is done in combination with use of the Hulda Clark zapper (see information below), followed by taking probiotics to replace any good bacteria that get killed by the zapper. If you can't obtain the herbs in capsules, you can buy empty vegicaps and a manual capsule machine to help you to fill them. This information is provided to illustrate ease of use. If you wish to utilize this program, please read Dr. Clark's book yourself. If you have any questions about this program, please see Dr. Clark's book and your doctor.

QUANTITY FOR AN ADULT	BLACK WALNUT HULL TINCTURE EXTRA STRENGTH	WORMWOOD CAPSULES - 300 mg	GROUND CLOVES CAPSULE Size 0 or 00
DAY	# of Drops, 1 time a day, before a meal	Capsules, 1 time a day, before a meal	Capsules, 3 times a day, at meal times
1	1	1	1,1,1
2	2	1	2,2,2
3	3	2	3,3,3
4	4	2	3,3,3
5	5	3	3,3,3
6	2 teaspoons	3	3,3,3
7	Now once a week	4	3,3,3
8	None	4	3,3,3
9	None	5	3,3,3
10	None	5	3,3,3
11	None	6	3
12	None	6	Now once a week
13	2 teaspoons	7	
14	None	7	
15	None	7	
16	None	7	
17	None	Now once a week	

QUANTITY FOR AN ADULT	BLACK WAL-NUT HULL TINCTURE EXTRA STRENGTH	WORMWOOD CAPSULES - 300 mg	GROUND CLOVES CAPSULE Size 0 or 00
DAY	# of Drops, 1 time a day, before a meal	Capsules, 1 time a day, before a meal	Capsules, 3 times a day, at meal times
18	None	None	3
Maintenance - Choose any day of the week to take all ingredients on the one day			

Notes:

Black Walnut should be "Black Walnut Green Hull Tincture Extra Strength." We personally use "Black Walnut Green Hull Extract", which is stronger.

Capsules should be vegicaps (plants), not gelatin (from animals).

Cloves must be fresh ground in a spice grinder, not from the supermarket.

PARASITE PROGRAM FOR PETS

Pets have more parasites than us, and we get a lot of parasites from pets, or people with pets. Please, do not ever kiss your pets! Generally, cats are worse than dogs. Pets are part of the family and should be kept as clean and healthy as yourself. Here is the recipe for a 10 pound pet. Double for a 20 lb pet, etc:

1. **Parsley Water.** Cook a big bunch of fresh parsley in a quart of water for 3 minutes. Throw away the parsley. After cooling, you may freeze most of it in several 1 cup containers. This is a month's supply. Put 1 tsp. parsley water on pet's food.

Pets are so full of parasites, you must be even more careful to not deparasitize them too quickly. The parsley water is to keep the kidneys flowing so well that dead parasite refuse is eliminated promptly.

(*Note: It may be good for you to have some as well*).

2. **Black Walnut Hull tincture** (regular strength only): 1 drop on the food. Don't force them to eat it. Count carefully. Do cats only twice a week. Dogs daily, work up to 1 drop a day per 10 lb dog.

If the pet vomits or has diarrhea, this is extremely infectious and hazardous to you. Do not let a child clean it up. Pour salt and iodine on the mess and leave for 5 minutes before cleaning up, whether inside or outside. Clean your hands with diluted grain alcohol (1 part alcohol: 4 parts water) or vodka. Not isopropyl alcohol. Be careful to keep all alcohol out of sight of children.

Start wormwood a week later.

3. **Wormwood**. Open a 200-300 mg. wormwood capsule and put the smallest pinch possible on their dry food. Do this for a week before starting the cloves.

4. **Ground cloves**. Must be fresh ground, not from supermarket. Use a spice grinder. Put the smallest pinch possible on their dry food. Keep all of this up as a routine so that you need not fear your pets. Also, notice how peppy and happy they become. Go slowly so the pet can learn to eat all of it. To repeat:

Quantities are based on a 10 LB. cat or dog. Multiply for a larger pet.	P a r s l e y Water	Black Wal-nut Green Hull Tinc-ture - Regu-lar Strength	Wormwood Capsules - 300 mg.	G r o u n d C l o v e s - Size o or oo
Week	Teaspoons on food	Drops on food, cats twice/week, dogs daily	Open cap-s u l e s - s m a l l e s t pinch on food	Open cap-sules - small-est pinch on food
1	1			
2	1	1		
3	1	1	1	
4	1	1	1	1
5 and on-ward	1	1	1	1

Notes:
Black Walnut should be "Black Walnut Green Hull Tincture, regular strength."
Capsules should be vegicaps (plants), not gelatin (from animals).
Cloves must be fresh ground in a spice grinder, not from the supermarket

THE ZAPPER

In *The Cure for All Diseases*, Dr. Hulda Clark also gives instructions on how to build a device called a 'zapper' which she says can *electrocute parasites*, including bacteria and viruses. I believe that it is a very good idea for everyone to use a zapper every now and again, in addition to taking the three herbs. Hulda Clark zappers can often be purchased on www.ebay.com. Generally, the zapper should be used daily for several weeks. Don't use it forever because it can also kill the good bacteria in your gut. Take some probiotics (available from your health food store) after zapping, to replace any good bacteria that got killed by the zapper. However, please note that the zapper is not a substitute for the herbal parasite cleanse. Each of these methods does something different.

Basically, the zapper is a *low-frequency signal generator*. In a way, this technology is a revival of some of the technology of the great Royal Raymond Rife, who cured virtually all diseases in the early 1900's, until the Medical Mafia shut him down. At the back of *The Cure for All Diseases* Dr. Clark lists the frequencies needed to kill particular parasites.

There were times in the past when we got the flu, and when we zapped we got well within one hour! One time it took two days to get well, even with zapping - but we learned later that many others in town were sick for 5-6 weeks! Zapping has also helped me to get rid of headaches quickly, when water alone was not enough.

There was a time when we sold zappers, but the FTC (Federal Trade Commission) sent out a letter telling us and other suppliers who sold zappers to not sell them. So you know they must be good! Government agencies love to help the drug companies to get rid of any competition. There were all kinds of testimonials to the power of the zapper, and no one was hurt by them. One man on the internet reported how he healed himself of multiple sclerosis (which is meant to be incurable) by zapping and removing his mercury amalgam fillings. He then gave a speech to the multiple sclerosis society[5]! His reward? In his own words:

"The MS Society didn't want me to finish my speech in 1997, despite the fact that they had invited me there to express my views freely. I had made no agreement with them ahead of time to pander to them and they had no inkling of what I was about to say. They had never received such a direct message before ... My speech was a full frontal assault on their culture of immorality. They heckled me and tried to shout me down."

Naturally the MS Society had to heckle him - MS is big business.

The strange question is, why on earth don't doctors tell us that parasites are a major cause of disease, weight gain, tiredness and brain fog? Surely somebody must know this? My naturopathic teacher David Bridgman told us how a butcher told him how when they cut open the organs of animals, the parasites go running all around the place! While many parasites are microscopic, some of them are not! I believe the plain answer is again, money. You have read that Hulda Clark says that everyone who has cancer has a parasite. About one in three Americans will get cancer. The average cancer patient pays over $300,000. Add similar amounts for heart disease, plus money for diabetes and the list goes on and on. Now you know why you weren't told about parasites, because three simple herbs can kill them.

DIATOMACEOUS EARTH - FOOD GRADE

CAUTION: NOT TO BE USED BY PREGNANT WOMEN OR YOUNG CHILDREN

There is another supplement which is wonderful at killing parasites, and that is Diatomaceous Earth - Food Grade. It is sometimes called "Fossil Shell Flour", because Diatomaceous Earth is a remarkable, all-natural product made from fossilized diatoms. Diatoms are microscopic water plants. Diatomaceous Earth is mostly composed of silica, which helps grow strong bones, skin, nails and hair.

Diatomaceous earth has many uses, including as a very effective natural insecticide for the garden, where it kills pests, but not earth worms. It is wonderful for improving the health of animals, so long as it's food grade.

Food grade diatomaceous earth has been used for at least two decades as a natural wormer for livestock. Only now are more people starting to use it on themselves as well. Some people believe diatomaceous earth scratches and dehydrates parasites. Some scientists believe that diatomaceous earth is a de-ionizer or de-energizer of worms or parasites. Some believe that it cuts up the insides of the parasites with its microscopic razor edges. No one really knows why it works so well, but regardless, people report definite control.

To be most effective, food grade diatomaceous earth must be fed long enough to catch all newly hatching eggs or cycling of the worms through the lungs and back to the stomach. A *minimum* of 60 days is suggested by many, *90 days* is advised for lungworms.

Food grade diatomaceous earth works in a purely physical/mechanical manner, not "chemical" and thus has no chemical toxicity. However, it is so effective at killing parasites that I must add this warning:

Warning: Start off with it *very slowly*. No more than 1/8 teaspoon for an adult the first few days. I say this because I read one account of a man on the internet who took several teaspoons initially, and collapsed and had to go to hospital. This was presumably because, like many people, he was loaded with parasites, and when the diatomaceous earth killed a bunch of parasites, his body got overloaded with toxins. You must give the body time to remove the dead bodies of the parasites slowly. Some people recommend taking several months to work up to one or two tablespoons a day, for adults.

When my husband and I started on diatomaceous earth we felt *very* tired the first few days. This is a sign of detoxification. The body uses extra energy to remove the extra toxins that are coming out. The saying is that detoxing is like cleaning house - it looks worse before it looks better. But after that, we noticed a *great* improvement in mental clarity and energy. It was as though a 'brain fog' that we did not even know we had was lifted.

Mix it in water, or water with a little juice. It seems to work best if you have it apart from food, like after you drink water in the morning, but before you have any food. Some people recommend taking it three times a day.

You can buy Food Grade Diatomaceous Earth for as low as $2 a pound on www.ebay.com! It **must** be food grade or it may contain dangerous toxins. I really believe that this is one of the most beneficial of all health supplements for reducing weight and improving health.

You can also give Food Grade Diatomaceous Earth to your pets. Notice how glossy their coats become. Do the same as was recommended for the Hulda Clark herbal parasite cleanse - start with a week of parsley water before you give any. Then give the very smallest amount possible and increase the amount very slowly over the next 6 weeks.

WARNINGS:

1. Diatomaceous Earth must be **FOOD GRADE**.

2. Not be used by pregnant women or young children.

3. To help you remove the dead parasites, drink some parsley water before and during your cleanse. Cook a big bunch of fresh parsley in a quart of water for 3 minutes. Throw away the parsley. After cooling, you may freeze most of it in several 1 cup containers. Drink at least 1 tsp. for every 10 lb of body weight.

4. Diatomaceous Earth Food Grade **MUST** be taken initially in **VERY SMALL DOSES.** If you don't do this, too many parasites can die at once and the body can get overloaded trying to get rid of all the bodies. Start with **1/8 tsp.** or less for an adult, and increase very slowly every few days. Some people recommend taking several months to work up to taking one to two tablespoons a day for adults, and one teaspoon for children.

5. Diatomaceous Earth can be constipating. Make sure you drink 6-8 glasses of water a day, including 1-2 before breakfast. Increase the amount you take very slowly, and spread it out throughout the day.

6. Do not inhale. Dust may cause eye and respiratory irritation. Keep out of reach of children.

7. Detoxification of parasites often causes feelings such as tiredness and headache for a while. If this happens, drink plenty of water and get more sleep. You can also reduce the amount you are taking and work back up to it later.

8. Clean up your pets as well. Start off with a week of parsley water to flush out the kidneys. Then, so that you don't kill too many parasites at once and stress the body out, start with the very lowest amount possible, and increase gradually over a six week period.

You're not fat. You have parasites. Parasites make the body toxic by eating your good nutrition, peeing ammonia in your body and by damaging it directly. This stops the body from working at full efficiency. It also makes you feel bad. So many people have had parasites for so long, that they think that feeling bad is 'normal'. Feeling bad encourages a person to crave junk food and drink. Kill your parasites with herbs, diatomaceous earth food grade and other natural remedies, and do the same for your pets, and you may be shocked to discover how happy and energetic and unhungry you become.

REFERENCES
1. *First* magazine 10/30/2006
2. *First* magazine, USA. 10/30/06
3. *The Cure for All Diseases*, by Dr. Hulda Clark, 1995, page 243
4. *The Cure for All Diseases*, by Dr. Hulda Clark, 1995, page 341
5. zap.intergate.ca/speech.html

CHAPTER 11

DRUGS ARE FATTENING

We have been told over and again that only calories and lack of exercise make us fat. The truth is, toxins make you fat. There are few things the body finds as toxic as drugs, whether prescription or otherwise, even though they have almost zero calories. This is because drugs force the body to do things it does not want to do. That's how they work. They are not nourishing the body to do a better job.

An article by Roger Dobson published in the UK *The Independent*[1] backs up my claim that drugs are fattening:

"Huge weight gains reported by patients on prescription drugs

Thousands of people who take prescription medicines for everyday conditions are gaining large amounts of weight (up to 22 pounds) as an unexpected side effect...

All of the patients they studied, on medication for conditions as diverse as diabetes, epilepsy, depression, high blood pressure and schizophrenia, showed evidence of weight increase....

A team from Glasgow University and Glasgow Royal Infirmary reviewed and analyzed data on drug use by more than 25,000 people to quantify the effects of prescription drugs.....

Olanzapine and clozapine, drugs used for psychiatric conditions, resulted in the most weight gain - up to 22 pounds in 52 weeks. Insulin for type 2 diabetes was found to increase weight by up to 13.2 pounds, while some drugs for depression added up to 8 pounds, and some for high blood pressure led to gains of up to 3 pounds. A heart drug added 5 pounds, while some treatments for epilepsy added more than 12 pounds, and some bipolar drugs led to weight gains of around 8 pounds.

The researchers say that many other drugs which are being pre-scribed and have not been investigated may also have an effect on weight."

In 2008 a huge 48% of Americans used at least one prescription drug. A massive 11% used five or more prescription drugs[2]. This is hardly sur-prising when you realize that most doctors have only two main prod-ucts to sell their customers: drugs and operations. If you go to a drug dealer or butcher, you will not be offered the chance to buy spinach.

Since drugs are fattening, and we want you to get thin, it will be important to teach you some things about drugs that the Medical Ma-fia[3] do not want you to know.

While people like to say things like "medicine makes you well", the truth is that medicine is just drugs, and drugs are not active. They don't do anything by themselves. They are passive chemicals. It is the body which is active. If the drugs did the work, then a drug for diar-rhea would have little effect on a healthy person, more effect on a sick person, and cause the most amount of diarrhea in a corpse. The op-posite is what happens. A healthy body gets diarrhea because the body knows that the drug is bad for it, and wants the drug out of the body as quickly as possible.

The disadvantage with drugs is that they don't address the cause of the problem. Drugs are chemicals which control, rather than help the body. This is why drugs *always* have side-effects. It is just that the doctor decides which side-effects he/she thinks are needed. However, there will always be side-effects that are not wanted, like weight gain, that go along with the side effect that is 'desirable'. This is because you are messing with the body's infinitely complicated balance of nutrients and chemical reactions, by adding toxic chemicals to it.

And you are doing nothing to correct the *cause* of the original problem.

For example, if a doctor decides that the blood pressure is too high, he may give a drug that forces the body to lower the blood pressure. However, the blood pressure may be raised because the blood vessels are lined with bad fat and other foreign substances, and the heart actually *has* to raise the blood pressure, to work harder to get blood to the various parts of the body. The body is making the best of a bad situation.

Another example: If a person has a headache, a doctor will usually give a person a drug to mask the pain. However, he seldom asks questions to find out what may be causing the pain. I have found out from experience that in many cases, possibly as high as 50%, that when someone has a headache, if they drink 1-2 pints of good water, their headache is gone within 20-30 minutes. The pain was caused by dehydration, and toxins which the body couldn't flush out of the system. You may be surprised when you discover how few people drink the recommended (even by doctors) 6-8 glasses of water a day. Many drink none or almost none at all! The fact that these people are alive is a tribute to the body's fantastic ability to make the best of a bad situation.

I wish I was paid for every client who came to me and said that they had a health problem, and had spent a lot of money getting tests done for the problem, and the doctors found nothing wrong with them. Pain does not register on a machine. But *you* know it's real. Pain is the body telling you that something is wrong, and needs fixing. But instead of addressing the cause, many times the medical system works to mask the problem. That way, the problem still exists, so they can continue to profit from it.

The medical system is saying that it knows more about your body than your body does. Well, the amazing thing is that your body managed to grow from a microscopic cell into a full-grown body, with everything in the right place (two legs, two arms, two eyes, one heart, one set of lungs etc. - all working perfectly - and all bodies looking much the same as each other) without any advice from a doctor.

If you think that taking herbs instead of drugs is okay, please think again. As Dr. Keith Scott-Mumby so accurately says in *DietWise*, herbal remedies act the same as drugs do. They are just less toxic. The only time when this does not apply is when you are eating herbs that don't have strong medicinal actions, and instead support the body with good nutrition, such as parsley and basil. If you have been taking a strong acting spice or herb for a long time, consider that perhaps your body has become allergic to it, and this is causing side effects, including extra fat.

The 'symptoms' we perceive as 'disease' are actually the very processes the body uses to restore balance, and thus health, to an out of balance system. What are the symptoms of 'disease' (dis - ease)? Amazingly they are few in number:

THE ONLY SYMPTOMS OF DISEASE

1	Pain
2	Hardening (sclerosis)
3	Discharge
4	Necrosis (tissue breakdown)
5	Swelling
6	Inflamation (redness)
7	Increased temperature
8	Nerve Signaling Problems

We are led to believe that there are many different diseases requiring many different treatments. The truth of the matter is that there are many different parts of the body, with many and varied functions, and if any of the above 'symptoms' occur in those parts the condition seems different only because that part or system has a different function.

For example, Bronchitis is an inflammation in the bronchial tubes. The symptoms are coughing, pain, discharge and temperature increase - but no bowel spasms, diarrhea or intestinal bloating. Colitis is an inflammation of the colon. The symptoms are abdominal cramps, loose stools, discharge of mucus and some bloating - but no coughing, chest pain or breathing difficulties. Why? The bowels can't cough and the lungs don't pass stools.

This is why many different and apparently unrelated conditions in the body improve or disappear when we restore the structural, chemical and emotional contexts to balance.

WHAT HAPPENS IN ANY 'DIS-EASE' - AND WHY ALL DISEASES ARE SIMILAR

The body has two responses to the introduction of a threat to its structural, chemical and emotional health. The first is resistance, which is active and in many cases dramatic actions, such as rashes, swelling, fainting or vomiting.

As resistance is expensive of energy, and the body does not have a limitless supply of energy, resistance cannot be maintained indefinitely. If the attack continues, the body's enthusiasm for resistance sadly gives way to the apathy of toleration or adaptation. The spirit of the fight is lost and acceptance of unsuitable things lays the foundation for chronic illness and inevitable death. The body degenerates in the following order. Virtually all body problems can be located in the following eight steps:

1. Enervation

Lack of energy, locally or generally, due to going out of balance by exceeding the biological laws by having too much or too little oxygen, pure water, wholesome / unwholesome food and drinks, exercise, rest, sleep, sunshine, emotional poise or electrical disturbances.

2. Toxemia

The lack of energy has reduced elimination of waste and thus toxins begin to build up. The person is tired and feels sluggish.

3. Irritation

Waste has reached irritant proportions. The body may initiate a resistance at this stage if there is some energy to do it with. Otherwise passive acceptance, stiffness, pains and deposits remind one that all is not well.

4. Inflamation

Irritation and toxemia have reached threatening levels, so energy must be mustered from within to activate the inflammation process, which means more blood (redness), more white cells (pus and discharge) and more lubrication and neutralization (mucus).

That is, the immune response is in full swing, and the body is actively resisting and processing. Depending on where the inflammation occurs, it is usually labeled as an "itis", for example appendicitis, colitis, tonsillitis.

Unfortunately, at this point the process may be suppressed with drugs (more toxemia), or the energy reserves may fail and the body changes out of desperation to an adaptation/toleration mode.

5. Ulceration or Necrosis

There is even more tissue breakdown in whatever area of the body it begins. There is not enough energy or materials to repair with.

6. Induration (Hardening)

This is a hardening, thickening or toughening of tissue (e.g. arthritis). It is the body's desperate attempt to stop the extreme breakdown of cells. This is adaptation/toleration at its peak.

7. Fungation

The induration of tissue has reduced the oxygen to the tissues by reducing blood circulation. The resultant build up of waste causes this new stage.

Organisms such as yeasts, fungi, bacteria and protozoa find the environment most favorable for feeding and production. They in turn create more toxins to the already overburdened system.

8. Cancer

The cells find themselves cut off from the oxygen they love, so in order to survive they must alter their function by becoming an-aerobic, which leads to them becoming independent and cancerous.

The immune system is too tired to deal with the situation, and the final take over of the body is beginning. And yet, this is still an intelligent process, designed to maintain life in a situation that is way from ideal.

THE SOLUTION

If you are taking drugs, or medicinal herbs, the solution it is to solve the cause of the problem. The drugs have not healed the problem, or the problem would be healed, with no side effects, and you would be able to stop taking the drugs after a while. They have masked the symptoms. So it's time to look for new solutions, so that you can heal the problem and stop taking the drugs, with the help of your doctor, which are contributing to fat gain.

Our bodies replace and replenish themselves, atom by atom. For example, you have new taste cells every two weeks (which means you can re-train them to enjoy healthy food), new lungs every six weeks, new blood every four months, a new liver every 150 days and new bones every ten years. It has only *just* been discovered that the heart replaces itself at least three or four times in a lifetime[4]. (Maybe one day they will also find out that the same applies to brain cells). Therefore, we have the ability to reverse the above changes. One of the first steps that need to be taken is to restore the energy in Step 1.

I have found through personal experience and the experience of thousands of others, that this can be done by improving diet through the methods described in this book, through kinesiology, and generally by studying and applying the laws of natural health. If we fail at that, all else fails. I will explain in the chapter on kinesiology what kinesiology is and how it can help to heal.

REFERENCES
1. *The Independent.* 24 June 2007. news.independent.co.uk/health/article2701322.ece
2. www.cdc.gov/nchs/data/databriefs/db42.pdf
3. *Medical Mafia*, by Guylaine Lanctot, 1995
4. www.dailymail.co.uk/health/article-1219995/Believe-lungs-weeks-old--taste-buds-just-days-So-old-rest-body.html

CHAPTER 12

KINESIOLOGY AND MUSCLE TESTING YOUR SECRET WEAPON FOR FAT LOSS

Kinesiology is a brand new technology which helps the brain to 'rewire' the body energetically. It is amazingly efficient at balancing the body, so that it can return to excellent health, energy and emotional strength. Therefore, it is a powerful tool to help you to get thin, provided it is done correctly. It stands apart from any other type of health technology largely due to its revolutionary use of muscle testing.

I have used kinesiology to help many people heal pain, health and emotional problems that they had for years, even decades, within just 2-3 sessions. Not uncommonly, weight loss was a lovely 'side-effect'. If you are taking drugs, which we have seen are fattening, then kinesiology is something I suggest you look into, because getting off the drugs (with your doctor's help) is something that will help with your fat loss. In addition, accurate muscle testing can help to identify the particular foods that your body is allergic to, and giving up those foods can greatly accelerate fat loss.

I will give one example of how kinesiology can create miracles: In the very good book *A Revolutionary Way of Thinking*, Dr. Charles Krebs tells how when he was a fit 35 year old, he had a diving accident, and was told that he would be a quadriplegic for life. But using kinesiology, he now leads a perfectly normal life!

There are two different definitions of "kinesiology". The term "kinesiology" which I use is that which is connected with Specialized Kinesiology and Academic Kinesiology (which includes Applied Kinesiology). It always includes manual muscle testing. It is not to be confused with another definition of "kinesiology", which is that which is taught in some colleges and does not include muscle testing.

When you muscle test a person properly for different foods, the person you test will not be able to hold up their arm when they hold a piece of a food that is toxic for them, beside their cheek, no matter how strong they are. This works also by just saying the name of the food being tested. This is because the brain stops sending electrical signals to the muscle you are testing. No longer is a food "bad" or "fattening". It is now *weakening*. No one wants to be weak. Somehow, this process makes a person just automatically start to steer away from unhealthy and fattening foods, and want to eat more nutritious foods, just like God intended.

As a person gets more and more specific communication back from their body through kinesiology sessions, they often begin to take more and more responsibility for their own health. Plus they have more knowledge of how to do that. When a big, tough guy sees that a puny girl can easily push his arm down when he says "alcohol" or "sugar", he often begins to think seriously about giving them up. Many people don't feel like giving up harmful habits because someone else has told them that they should, but when their own body starts telling them in no uncertain terms that those habits are weakening it, then that is another matter.

However, kinesiology goes beyond muscle testing. It also includes corrections which balance the body energetically so that different systems can work more efficiently. The brain allows you to become aware of energetic imbalances and blockages. It then rectifies these. It is not uncommon for people to notice an immediate absence of pain in the troubled area during a session. Within a few days many other symptoms often go away as well. Even better, the symptoms often stay away, provided the person no longer does the thing that caused the problem in the first place. This can be a great help for fat loss.

When we are tired, hurting or feeling negative emotions, it can be more tempting to eat something that is toxic. Kinesiology can help a person to improve all of these symptoms. Even better, it helps to balance the body's energies so that the body can work more efficiently. For example, if there is a blockage in the large intestine energies, the person might become constipated. This causes a back log of toxins, and makes it much harder for the body to burn fat. I have not seen a client who was constipated who I have not been able to help using kinesiology, combined with improvements in diet.

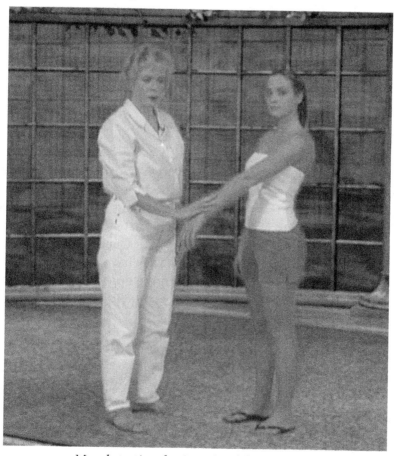

*Muscle testing the Anterior deltoid muscle
from "Perfect Health with Kinesiology and Muscle Testing"*

If you are the kind of person who has "tried everything" including all kinds of doctors and natural healers for a particular problem, including fat loss, then you are typical of the kind of clients who I have seen, and been able to help with kinesiology.

Kinesiology is a truly 'wholistic' system, because it looks at the *whole* person (not just at selected parts). When you step on a cat's tail, it's the other end that screams. That is, the whole body affects the whole body.

In addition, kinesiology looks at *all* types of stresses which can cause disease. They include emotional, nutritional, structural and electrical stress.

The basis of kinesiology is that the body is like an electrical piece of equipment, which is controlled by an incredibly complex computer, namely the brain. The brain is continually in communication with each of the approximately 639 muscles in the body, and it knows exactly what it needs and in what priority.

FOURTEEN MUSCLE BALANCE

There are many kinesiology balances which can help you to reduce fat. For example, there is a balance called the Fourteen muscle balance. This balance is based on Chinese medicine. Each of the fourteen muscles that are muscle tested, relate to a particular organ or system in the body. For example, if a person has their Quadriceps muscles out of balance, not only may they find that they have difficulty climbing stairs, because this is a major muscle in the upper leg, but the small intestine will also be out of balance, because it is energetically connected to the small intestine.

THE BODY CLOCK

The Fourteen muscle balance is based on the body clock. We have all talked about how our "body clock" gets messed up when we travel long distances by air. What not so many people know is that ancient Chinese mapped this clock. It includes the energy flows in the main meridian systems during a 24 hour time period.

Central Nervous System	Governing (Spinal Cord)
Heart	Gall Bladder
Small Intestine	Liver
Bladder	Lung
Kidney	Large Intestine
Circulation Sex	Stomach
Triple Warmer (hormones)	Spleen

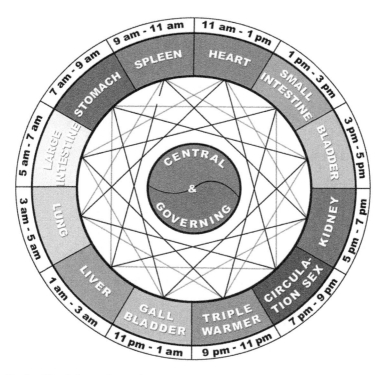

The Body Clock based on the Meridian System from Chinese medicine from "Perfect Health with Kinesiology and Muscle Testing"

MERIDIANS – PATHWAYS OF ENERGY

Energy flows continuously around the body in an unbroken flow like a river, on invisible pathways called meridians. These meridians form the meridian system. The meridian system is the basis for acupuncture.

ANTERIOR TORSO MERIDIANS

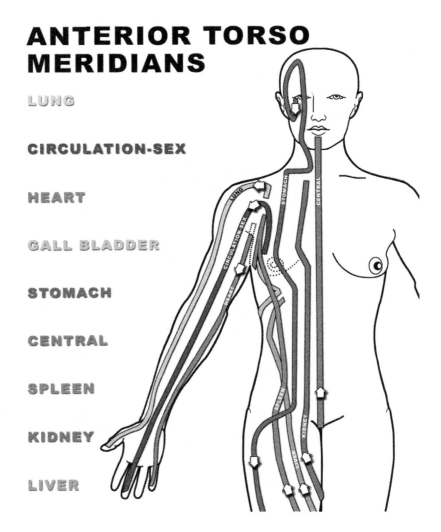

The Anterior Torso Meridians, from
"Perfect Health with Kinesiology and Muscle Testing"

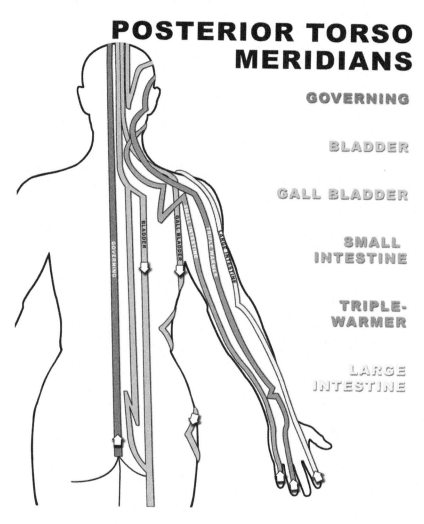

The Posterior Torso Meridians, from
"Perfect Health with Kinesiology and Muscle Testing"

HEAD MERIDIAN RELATIONSHIPS

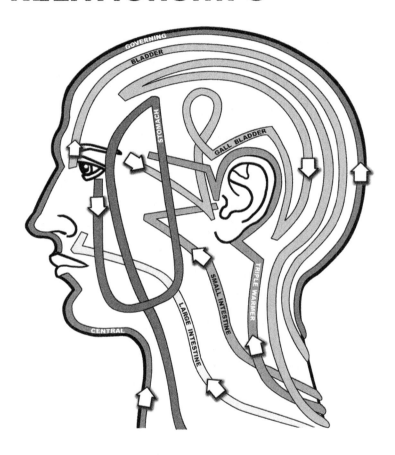

*The Head Meridian Relationships, from
"Perfect Health with Kinesiology and Muscle Testing"*

Each meridian is associated with a particular organ or system of the body. Each item on the body clock is associated with a particular meridian in the body. For example, the central nervous system, in the middle of the wheel, is associated with the supraspinatus muscle.

At particular times of the day, more energy flows to one meridian, and hence to one organ, than at any other time of the day. If you look at the wheel you will see that at 1 to 3 pm, the small intestine meridian receives more energy than any other meridian. Then at 3 to 5 pm, the bladder meridian receives more energy than any other meridian. Then at 5 to 7 pm, the kidney meridian receives more energy than any other meridian. And so on around the clock until you come again back to the small intestine meridian.

Look again at the body clock. Notice how different lines go to different organs? When an organ receives maximum energy, the organ that is opposite that organ on the wheel receives minimum energy. For example, 11 am to 1 pm, most energy goes to the heart. At the same time, the least amount of energy goes to the one opposite the heart, which is the gall bladder.

Note that at 1 to 3 pm most energy goes to the small intestine. Also, at this time the least amount of energy goes to the liver, because the liver is directly opposite the small intestine on the clock. This is why people get more drunk from alcohol at lunchtime, than at any other time of the day. At this time of day, the liver has less energy available, and the liver is the organ that has to detoxify the alcohol. Another interesting correlation is the time when most heart attacks tend to occur, which is in the middle of the night, when the heart energy is at its lowest.

In the middle of the circle are central and governing. Central is short for the central nervous system and governing is the nervous system related to the spinal cord.

THE CLOACALS

If you are one of those people for whom "nothing works" for your health problems, and you are also extra low in energy, then it's quite possible that an energy system called the "cloacals" is out of balance. This is the most powerful kinesiology correction of all, and one that can cause miracles. The cloacals is an energy system that is related to the autonomic nervous system, which controls many actions of the human body. This control happens without the person having to think about it, such as heart rate and digestion. The cloacals is part of Applied Kinesiology. It is unknown by the medical system, and even by most kinesiologists.

If anyone has ever had a time when they were healthy, and then *almost overnight* started having all kinds of awful symptoms, including weight gain, it is quite likely that one of two things happened:

1. They picked up a parasite. Particularly suspect this if the person travelled to a foreign country. Please see the chapter on parasites for more information.

2. Their cloacals went out of balance as a result of extreme stress. The stress could have been:

- Emotional, such as divorce or death of a loved one.
- Physical, such as a car crash or difficult birth.
- Chemical, from something extremely toxic to the body, such as a vaccination.
- Electrical, such as an electric blanket or eating microwaved food.

Unlike most energy systems in the body, the cloacals do not seem to be good at getting back to balance by itself with a good night's sleep. I have had clients whom muscle testing indicated that they had their cloacals out of balance since they were born, often because of a difficult birth.

The cloacals are part of what kinesiologists call the centering system. The test to see if the centering system is in balance is simple. As always, the tester must do the six pretests first to make sure that all muscle tests are valid. (There are many people who think that they know how to muscle test, but since they don't do the pretests, their results are invalid). The tester then warns the person of what they are about to do. The tester then gives the person a light slap on an upper arm, and then muscle tests the other arm. If the arm tests weak, that means that the simple slap was more stress than their body could handle and the centering system is out of balance. Once the appropriate Kinesiology correction is applied to the body, and the test is repeated, the arm will stay strong when the body is given another light slap.

Anyone who has "incurable" health problems and very low energy, as well as fat that refuses to budge, quite possibly has their cloacals out of balance. Rebalancing the cloacal system can help to heal and to reduce fat, because the cloacal system controls and regulates most, if not all, of the major fluctuating qualities and quantities in the body. The cloacals seem to work by acting as a reference point for the autonomic nervous system, which has the main job of maintaining stability within your body. Therefore, with the cloacals out of balance, a person will be continually out of balance. Their body is like a 'leaf in the wind', affected greatly by even the smallest stresses, and not able to completely heal itself fully, even with good food and sleep.

In addition, the person may be operating on a shocking 30 – 70 % of normal body energy levels. In this case, there is little energy available for any needed healing or fat reduction, and a person can feel so lousy that foods like ice cream become a lot more attractive.

For example, if the cloacals are not working properly, a few of the things that may not be as efficient as possible are the following:

- Body fat.
- Hormone levels.
- Metabolism.
- Blood sugar levels.
- Body energy levels.
- Emotional stability.
- Allergic responses.
- Bladder.
- Bowels.
- Reproductive organs.
- Pregnancy.
- Sexuality.
- Blood pressure.
- Body temperature.

- Speed of healing.
- Immune efficiency.
- Brain chemistry.
- Learning abilities.
- Co-ordination.

The good news is that a good kinesiologist can put the cloacal system back into balance. People sometimes notice an immediate improvement in their symptoms. In cases where people feel worse for a few days after having their cloacals back in balance, it is a symptom of the body using the extra energy available to it to heal some major problems, which previously the body did not have the energy to do.

You can learn this yourself, because I teach the cloacals correction in my DVD training system, *Perfect Health with Kinesiology & Muscle Testing*. I also teach that to get a *permanent* healing you may need to do more than just put the cloacals back in balance. If the cloacals do not stay in balance during the weeks after rebalancing them, as they should, then the kinesiologist needs to use muscle testing to locate the cause of why the cloacals would not stay in balance.

I have found that the cause can be many different causes, all of them extremely stressful to the body. Some causes have been major emotional shock like death of a loved one, or divorce of parents, a car crash, having something terrible happen in childhood, being born by "western" birthing methods, having a baby – or even what would appear to be not too stressful, but obviously is from how it puts the cloacals out of balance - being vaccinated, using an electric blanket or eating microwaved food.

Once you get the cloacals to be in balance, and to remain in balance, you may get a surprise at the list of symptoms which is improved if not fully healed. I used to cry much too very easily before I found kinesiology, and it was all because my cloacals were out of balance. Now I cry only for beautiful things. It's also likely that this is one of the reasons why I used to eat huge amounts of food, and now do not eat nearly as much, at the same time that I no longer experience constant hunger.

The cloacals correction is explained in the *Basic Applied Kinesiology*

Workshop Manual by Gordon Stokes and Mary Marks, which is unfortunately currently not available. A very strange thing is that, while the cloacals is the most important Applied Kinesiology correction of all, it is not described in the *Applied Kinesiology Synopsis* by Walther. However, I teach this correction in my DVD training system *Perfect Health with Kinesiology & Muscle Testing*.

Unfortunately, you cannot do kinesiology on yourself, because a broken computer cannot fix itself. Your brain is the computer. You need to have someone else work on you. Because it can be difficult finding a good kinesiologist to work on you, my husband and I spent four years creating *Perfect Health with Kinesiology and Muscle Testing*, which is designed for ordinary people to learn, not just professional natural health practitioners, so that they could improve their health. More information is available at www.PerfectHealthSystem.com and www.PerfectHealthDVD.com.

As a wife and mother, I do not know how other people manage to raise a healthy, happy, thin family without the tools that kinesiology provides, and that I teach in my DVDs. If you want to reduce your fat, and 'nothing works', then I highly recommend that you learn kinesiology with someone close to you, so that you can work on each other, or find a good kinesiologist to work on you. Kinesiology really can be your "Secret Weapon" for fat loss.

CHAPTER 13

LEPTIN - THE FAT HORMONE

A hormone is a chemical made by one part of the body, that affects other parts of the body. Generally, only very small amounts are needed to cause the desired effect. Hormones function like chemical messengers. Leptin is the *most important hormone* in the body[1]! And yet, science has begun to understand leptin only recently. Understanding leptin is essential for reducing fat. I'll do my best to give you a very brief summary of leptin. In addition, I strongly urge you to read the excellent book *Mastering Leptin* by Byron Richards, from which most of the following information comes. Another good book for understanding leptin is *The Rosedale Diet* by Dr. Ron Rosedale. There is a great deal to know about the complex relationships between leptin and the body, and what you eat and do.

Leptin is the hormone secreted by fat cells. That means that you definitely don't want to liposuction it away. Since science has only just started to learn this most important fact about the human body, I wonder how many other facts about the human body and diet we don't yet know?

Leptin regulates other hormones, including thyroid, adrenal, pancreatic and sex hormones[2]. Leptin is involved with insulin, cardiovascular health, the immune system, bones and many other things.

Leptin was not discovered until 1994[3] and few people, including doctors, so far know about it, although this situation is changing. Fat cells are not just for storage of fat and toxins. They are a major controller of health for the human body[4]. No wonder I shuddered when I once saw on television some people getting liposuction.

Leptin communicates with the brain. When the brain senses that leptin levels are going up and down at a normal rate, then it believes that there is no need to store fat[5]. Leptin also tells the body when to burn fat, and when to feel hungry[6]. But if you are thinking that all you need is a shot of leptin, think again! It was found that people who are overweight have too much leptin. This is because the delicate balance of leptin has been thrown out of balance[7]. (There's that word again - 'balance'. Remember how we "balance" energies in kinesiology?)

When the balance of leptin is thrown out of balance, we say the person has **leptin resistance**[8]. Leptin is meant to have a rhythm of highs and lows each day, but with overweight people, this rhythm has been lost. When there is leptin resistance, the body keeps the metabolism low, and stores extra energy as fat. It's kind of like keeping the body hibernating. A lot of people these days believe they have thyroid problems, but the ultimate cause of this is leptin resistance[9].

High levels of carbohydrate raise leptin levels quickly. And high levels of carbohydrate lead to leptin resistance. However, what many people do not know is that *too much protein* is just as bad, because the extra protein is converted into carbohydrate[10].

Stress should release energy from the fat cells. But if the stress is constant, from a fat cell's point of view, it is like being yelled at too often. The fat cells become 'numb' to the signals. Leptin resistance is the result[11]. Leptin resistance can happen from any kind of stress, including chemical stress from caffeine or alcohol. That means, those morning cups of coffee and nightly sips of wine with your dinner, could be making you fat.

A secret to living a lot longer is to eat less food. Too much food is toxic, because it overloads the body. In studies, dozens of species of animals, including worms, rodents and monkeys, have had their caloric intake reduced by one third, at the same time that they were given extra nutrients. Those animals lived 30-80% longer. That is the equivalent of a human living 160-220 years old[12].

But you can eat less only if you are not hungry. Leptin is the hormone that tells you when you are hungry. Here are some of the rules for burning fat by getting your leptin working properly[13]:

1. Eat three meals a day.

2. Reduce the amount of carbohydrate you eat, especially cooked potato and grains. Particularly never eat any wheat. More on this later.

3. **Don't snack,** even on healthy foods. This is one of the most important rules. This disrupts the whole system of hormones and leads to leptin and insulin resistance, and makes you fat. If you must have a snack, it should only be raw seeds or nuts (e.g. pumpkin seeds, almonds, brazil nuts).

Studies on mice showed that after 100 days, mice that snacked throughout the day got fat, but mice that were only able to eat for 8 hours and then fasted for 16 hours weighed a massive 28% less[14]. Constant eating leads to fat. So eat only three times a day.

4. Dinner should be at least three hours before you go to bed, the earlier the better. And then do no snacking on anything until breakfast. *When* you eat, can be more important than what you eat.

5. If you absolutely must have something toxic and fattening, make sure it is eaten only at lunchtime. Dinner should be smaller than lunch. Lunch is the time your body will find it easiest to deal with toxins and extra food, rather than turn it into fat.

6. Get some exercise. It's not about burning calories. Regular unstressful exercise is very important for keeping leptin working properly. The longer you exercise, the better your leptin will be. Please see my chapters on walking and a simple resistance exercise you can do in your bedroom.

7. Increase the amount of good fats and oils you eat, especially Omega 3's, in the form of raw seeds and nuts. Please see the chapter on fats and oils for more information.

8. Get as much sunlight as you can, without burning, in addition to taking a Vitamin D supplement. Vitamin D deficiency causes leptin resistance[15]. Who would have thought that not having sun could make you fat? This is a good example of how everything affects everything else. I will talk more about Vitamin D in its own chapter.

9. Do not ingest substances which stress your body, such as alcohol and caffeine. For more information, see chapter 25 on coffee and caffeine.

You're not fat, you have leptin resistance. Real fat loss comes with long term changes to what you do, not from short diets. As you read this book and make changes to how you look after your body, it is important to keep your new habits for at least three months, before you decide whether or not you want to continue with them. This is partly because when we decrease body fat, the first fat to go is usually internal, around the organs, rather than the fat we see.

REFERENCES

1. *Mastering Leptin,* by Byron Richards CCN, 2002, 3rd edition 2009, pg. 4
2. *Mastering Leptin,* by Byron Richards CCN, 2002, 3rd edition 2009, pg.4
3. *Mastering Leptin,* by Byron Richards CCN, 2002, 3rd edition 2009, pg. 23
4. *Mastering Leptin,* by Byron Richards CCN, 2002, 3rd edition 2009, pg.23
5. *Mastering Leptin,* by Byron Richards CCN, 2002, 3rd edition 2009, pg. 24
6. *Mastering Leptin,* by Byron Richards CCN, 2002, 3rd edition 2009, pg.28
7. *Mastering Leptin,* by Byron Richards CCN, 2002, 3rd edition 2009, pg. 30
8. *Mastering Leptin,* by Byron Richards CCN, 2002, 3rd edition 2009, pg. 30
9. *Mastering Leptin,* by Byron Richards CCN, 2002, 3rd edition 2009, pg. 34
10. *The Rosedale Diet,* by Dr. Ron Rosedale M.D., page 13
11. *Mastering Leptin,* by Byron Richards CCN, 2002, 3rd edition 2009, pg.41
12. *The Rosedale Diet,* by Dr. Ron Rosedale M.D., page 43

13. *Mastering Leptin*, by Byron Richards CCN, 2002, 3rd edition 2009, pg. 114
14. *Cell Metabolism*, May 2012
15. *Mastering Leptin*, by Byron Richards CCN, 2002, 3rd edition 2009, pg. 183

CHAPTER 14

TOXIC FOOD #1
ASPARTAME IS EXTRA FATTENING

It may come as a shock for you to learn that one of the most fattening things you can ingest is *diet* drinks, foods and powders. Since I already knew that it's toxins that cause weight gain, I was not surprised to see that a recent study showed that saccharin and aspartame cause more weight gain than sugar[1]!

Aspartame is the worst, but I believe that all other artificial sweeteners will be found to do similar damage to the body. Aspartame is so bad that they have to keep giving it new names to trick you into drinking it. Product names include NutraSweet, Equal, Spoonful, Canderel, Benevia and AminoSweet. Never ingest anything that has a registered trademark ® symbol after its name, which lets you know it's not part of nature.

To make matters worse, Aspartame is very addictive. There have been cases of people getting more upset at not being able to get a diet coke in the morning, than not being able to have coffee! Aspartame is addictive because it is an "excitotoxin". That is, it 'excites' your brain cells. It is also a carcinogenic drug that interacts with virtually all drugs[2]. The fact that it is addictive may make it tougher for you to give it up, but you must be strong and do that if you want to get thin, and to live a long and healthy life. Just knowing that it is addictive can give you the extra strength to go without it long enough for the cravings to leave, which could be three weeks to two months.

Dr. Sandra Cabot[3] has over 30 years clinical experience. She says about aspartame:

> "After having been consulted by thousands of overweight people suffering with problems concerning the liver and/or metabolism I can assure you that aspartame will not help you in any way, indeed it will help you to gain unwanted weight. This has been my experience, and there are logical reasons to explain the fattening and bloating effects of aspartame.
>
> When you ingest the toxic chemical aspartame it is absorbed from the intestines and passes immediately to the liver....The liver then breaks down ... aspartame to its toxic components - phenylalanine, aspartic acid and methanol (wood alcohol). This process requires a lot of energy from the liver which means there will be less energy remaining in the liver cells. This means the liver cells will have less energy for fat burning and metabolism, which will result in fat storing.
>
> Excess fat may build up inside the liver cells causing "fatty liver", and when this starts to occur it is extremely difficult to lose weight. In my vast experience any time that you overload the liver you will increase the tendency to gain weight easily."

Note that Dr. Cabot indirectly backs up my claim that it is mainly toxins that cause weight gain, rather than simply calories, because the main job of the liver is to break down all toxins, and when it can't do this, it stores them in fat cells.

Please note that a similar thing could be said of all artificial sweeteners. Anytime you 'trick' the brain into thinking something is sweet when it is not, there will be problems. I believe it's even possible that this includes stevia. After all, it sure tastes like aspartame.

Would you believe that the FDA (Food and Drug Administration) lists 92 symptoms from aspartame[4]? And that these include weight gain and *death*?

Nutrasweet was not approved until 1981, in dry foods. For over eight years the FDA refused to approve it because of the seizures and brain tumors it produced in lab animals. The FDA continued to refuse to approve it until President Reagan took office and fired the FDA Commissioner who wouldn't approve it. Dr. Arthur Hull Hayes was appointed as commissioner. Even then, there was so much opposition to approval that a Board of Inquiry was set up. The Board said: "Do not approve aspartame". Dr. Hayes then overruled his own Board of Inquiry.

Shortly after Commissioner Arthur Hull Hayes Jr. approved the use of aspartame in carbonated beverages, he left for a position with Searle's Public Relations firm. Searle is part of Monsanto, which created aspartame.

If you react to aspartame, you are one of the 'fortunate' ones, because you might have worked out that it was bad for you, and thus avoided it. Unfortunately, for most people, it appears that aspartame causes slow, cumulative damage. It may take one year, five years, ten years, or forty years, but it seems to cause some reversible and some irreversible changes in health over long-term use.

10% of aspartame produces methanol, which is also called wood alcohol and is a deadly poison. Methanol was the poison that has caused some alcoholics to end up blind or dead. Methanol breaks down into formic acid and formaldehyde in the body. Formaldehyde is a deadly neurotoxin. That means that it is a poison that affects the nerves. Anything that affects your nerves is going to make you fat, because it affects the delicate balance of the body, as well as the liver. Even the Australian Cancer Council has said that there are no safe levels of formaldehyde. That indirectly means there is no safe level of aspartame.

The most well known problems from methanol poisoning are vision problems. Formaldehyde is a known carcinogen, causes retinal damage, interferes with DNA replication, and causes birth defects. Due to the lack of a couple of key enzymes, humans are many times more sensitive to the toxic effects of methanol than animals. Therefore, tests of aspartame or methanol on animals do not reflect the full danger for humans.

The absorption of methanol into the body is sped up considerably when aspartame is heated to above 86°F (30°C). In 1993 the FDA did an evil act by approving aspartame as an ingredient in numerous food items that would always be heated above this temperature, such as Jello.

Even more evil, in 1996, without public notice, the FDA removed all restrictions from aspartame, allowing it to be used in everything.

The truth about aspartame's toxicity is far different from what the NutraSweet Company would have you believe. In February of 1994, the U.S. Department of Health and Human Services released the listing of adverse reactions reported to the FDA (DHHS 1994). Aspartame accounted for more than 75% of all adverse reactions reported to the FDA's Adverse Reaction Monitoring System (ARMS). By the FDA's own admission, fewer then 1% of those who have problems with something they consume ever report it to the FDA. This balloons the almost 10,000 complaints they once had to around a million.

However, the FDA has a record keeping problem and they tend to discourage or misdirect complaints, at least on aspartame. The fact remains, though, that most victims don't have a clue that aspartame may be the cause of their many problems! Many reactions to aspartame are very serious including seizures and death.

Those reactions include the following. A number of these relate to weight gain directly, although I imagine that you would not want any of the other symptoms either. Please always remember that the whole body affects the whole body. Any problem in another part of the body can affect your ability to reduce fat.

FDA LISTS 92 SYMPTOMS FROM ASPARTAME

- Abdominal Pain.
- Anxiety attacks.
- Arthritis.
- Asthma.
- Asthmatic Reactions.
- Bloating, Edema (Fluid Retention).
- Blood Sugar Control Problems (Hypoglycemia or Hyperglycemia).
- Brain Cancer.

- Breathing difficulties.
- Burning eyes or throat.
- Burning urination.
- Can't think straight (It's hard to shop and eat right if you can't think right).
- Chest Pains.
- Chronic cough.
- Chronic fatigue (You will eat more when you are tired).
- Confusion.
- **Death.**
- Depression (You will eat more when you are depressed).
- Diarrhea.
- Dizziness.
- Excessive thirst or hunger (Especially for carbohydrate, the most fattening kind of food).
- Fatigue.
- Feel unreal.
- Flushing of face.
- Hair loss or thinning of Hair.
- Headaches / Migraines.
- Hearing Loss.
- Heart palpitations.
- Hives (Urticaria).
- Hypertension (High blood pressure).
- Impotency and sexual problems.
- Inability to concentrate (So you are more likely to eat the wrong things).
- Infection susceptibility.
- Insomnia (You burn most fat when you sleep).
- Irritability.
- Itching.
- Joint pains.
- Laryngitis.
- "Like thinking in a fog".
- Marked personality changes.
- Memory loss.

- Menstrual problems.
- Migraines & severe headaches.
- Muscle spasms.
- Nausea or vomiting.
- Numbness or tingling of extremities.
- Other allergic-like reactions.
- Panic attacks.
- Phobias.
- Rapid heart beat.
- Rashes.
- Seizures and convulsions.
- Slurring of speech.
- Swallowing pain.
- Tachycardia.
- Tremors.
- Tinnitus.
- Vertigo.
- Vision loss.
- Weight gain.

Aspartame is chemically addictive, so do not be surprised if you have resistance to giving it up. But give it up you must. Please realize that it may take at least sixty days without any aspartame before you see a significant improvement.

Check all labels very carefully, including vitamins and pharmaceuticals. Look for the word "aspartame" on the label and avoid it. Also, it is a good idea to avoid "acesulfame-k" or "sunette."

Avoid getting nutrition information from junk food industry Public Relations organizations, such as the International Food Information Council (IFIC), or organizations that accept large sums of money from the junk and chemical food industry, such as the American Dietetic Association. It's not information, it's propaganda, to make money.

SEE WHAT ANTS DO TO ASPARTAME

It turns out that ants are smarter than us in some aspects. I had heard of a woman who made up ant poison from aspartame. So when we were in Florida in a house that was being invaded by ants, I decided to make up some ant poison of my own. I decided the best way to get them to eat it was by mixing it with raw honey. I mixed roughly 3 or 4 parts raw honey to 1 part aspartame (Nutrasweet from the supermarket) and put it out in a toy baby saucer for them.

Sure enough, pretty soon, the saucer was full of dead ants. If it can kill ants, it can kill you.

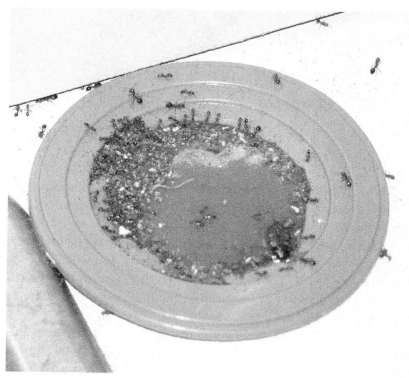

Later on, I put a small amount straight onto the floor. But this time, I got quite a shock when, later on, I glanced at the mixture. The ants had done something very strange to it...

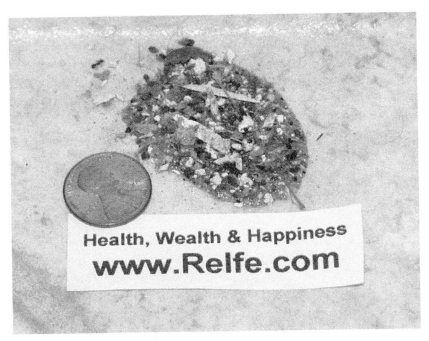

Health, Wealth & Happiness
www.Relfe.com

You see in the above picture that the ants covered up the aspartame mixture! Presumably this was done as a warning to other ants - "Stay away from this! It kills you!"

I was amazed that they had managed to find so many bit and pieces of stuff to cover it up with. The floor looked clean. You will notice that there are very few bodies in the second picture. I guess they got the message. After I saw this, I noticed in the first image that there are also some bits of debris there as well.

The moral of the story: In some respects, ants are smarter than people. People continue to suck down diet drinks. And if you stop and tell them that it's bad for them, or fattening, they look at you as though you are crazy. Anthony Robbins has said that the most powerful form of "proof" is "social proof". That is, if enough people do something, it must be good. Unfortunately, with regard to aspartame, this is not the truth. And because of its addictive nature, not enough people are willing to look into this. In fact, aspartame should be totally illegal.

I have also used a raw honey & aspartame mixture for killing cockroaches. There are some big ones in Florida! We once were in a house where they kept coming in from outside. Normal poison baits didn't make much difference, and we didn't want to spray because we didn't want to harm ourselves. I didn't find out how effective it was in actually killing roaches, although we did get a few bodies after we put it out, but it sure did slow them down. Normal cockroaches are way too fast for me to catch them with a wet paper towel (although my husband manages it), but once they have had a few days of raw honey & aspartame, they are *so slow* that I just have to bend down, catch them in the wet paper towel and drop them in the toilet. The aspartame made them sick enough to be caught easily. We don't want you to slow down like they did!

To help you give up aspartame, I thought I would include the following story:

SUCCESS STORY OF PEOPLE WHO GAVE UP ASPARTAME[5]

"Dear Betty, in October of 2001, my sister became very ill. She had joint pain, stomach spasms, headaches, blurred vision, slurred speech, memory loss etc. She started going to the doctors.

Because of her stomach spasms, they diagnosed her with Krohn's Disease. She had no symptoms of it, but they felt they had to label her with something. She could barely walk, and great depression set in, her menstrual cycle was way off and she often felt dizzy.

She is a single mother. It took everything she had in her to keep her job. Barely able to get out of bed in early March 2002, she felt she was dying, and decided to put her home, life insurance, and custody of her younger children in her older daughter's name. She wanted one last hooray, so she planned a trip down to Florida, knowing she'd be going in a wheelchair.

She was due to arrive in Orlando on March 22, 2002. March 15, 2002 she was scheduled for a biopsy at the hospital in which her daughter took her too. At this time the doctors had her on a cocktail of 24 different prescription medications...

So, on Tuesday March 19, 2002, I called my sister to see how things went at the biopsy. She told me they ruled out Krohn's Disease, and said they told her she had multiple sclerosis (MS). Then it clicked. My friend had sent me an email on the nutrasweet thing, and I asked my sister if she drank diet soda. She told me she did drink diet pepsi and while I was on the phone with her, she was getting ready to crack one open.

I told her to stop drinking the diet soda and any other stuff with aspartame in it.

She called me the next day...32 hours later...she was crying. I thought, *"Oh no,* what happened?" But she was crying with joy... she was *walking* again, and her stomach stopped having spasms. She said she felt much, much better and has not had one diet soda in 32 hours. I thought WOW...this is unreal. She took the email to her doctor that day. He was amazed at her recovery, gave her a big hug, and informed her that he was going to contact all his MS patients to find out about their diets. I live in Florida, so when my sister got here on March 22, 2002, we went dancing and she didn't need a wheel chair...

Thank you so much for saving my sister's life. God Bless all of you....
Marcy Nolan"

"Hi Dr. Hull, I just want to let you know what has gone on with me since I no longer use any aspartame. I have been off all of it for 7 weeks now and I am starting to feel so must better. No leg problems, No bad headaches, No more dizziness, No more feeling bad. I am so glad. I have been on this stuff for years and I did not know it was from aspartame. Thank you for all your help".[6]

Dr. Hull, been off aspartame now since 7/10/09. ... Was reading about all the problems it causes and it sounded like me. I've had problems with my knees for about a year. The doctor kept saying I had a little arthritis and I was aggravating it so he'd give me a shot. I had itching without rash, irritability, depression, headaches, and weight gain, etc. Two days after no aspartame I was walking without a limp & pain in knee, no headaches, no acid reflux pills every day and my list goes on. I don't feel like I got one foot in the grave now. I really feel good. All the money I've spent on going to the doctors for help. If the President would get this poison off the market maybe people wouldn't be going to the doctor so much".[7]

"I gave up aspartame 6 months ago. It has been a difficult journey but I am glad I braved the hard times. When I gave up my favorite diet cola the cravings diminished and I lost 8 pounds in 3 weeks. My appetite for nourishing foods has increased and I truly feel better. I can be a foodie *and* manage my weight better without my favorite diet cola. Score![8]"

"I made a decision to give up soda. It has not been easy. I love diet soda! But I am doing it! ... About 7 years ago I gave it up and combined with diet and exercise, I lost over 40 lbs in 4 months! :")[9]

In addition to poisoning your body and overloading your liver so that it cannot burn fat, when sweet taste stimulates the tongue, the brain programs the liver to prepare for the acceptance of new energy in the form of sugar. However, if sweet taste is not followed by real nutrients, an urge to eat will be the outcome. The liver produces the signals and the urge to eat. The more a sweet taste is ingested without real food with calories, the more there is an urge to eat.[10] This is one reason why I suggest you avoid stevia as well.

Tardoff and Friedman have shown that this urge to eat more food after artificial sweeteners can last up to one and a half hours after the sweet drink!" [11]

Please do not consume any artificial sweeteners. Make sure you take a magnifying glass with you when you go shopping. Read every label. Aspartame is hidden in more products than just drinks.

WARNING! SPLENDA IS NOT SO SPLENDID

Don't go thinking you can replace aspartame with, say, Splenda. All artificial sweeteners will cause similar problems to aspartame. It may have a "splendid" sounding name, but Splenda is also a potential poison. Splenda contains the drug sucralose, another toxin you must avoid totally. In fact, the chemists who invented sucralose were originally researching insecticides when they discovered by accident that it tasted sweet. More ant poison! One chemist likened Splenda to a drug that "explodes internally"[12], because it causes that much damage.

SUCRALOSE IS IN DRINKING WATER!

Here's a weird piece of information: A scientific paper published in 2001 reported that Sucralose "has been shown to be a widespread contaminant of waste water, surface water and ground water." That is, it's in your drinking water[13]! This is yet another reason why you must get a reverse osmosis water filter.

Please see the list of sweeteners that you should and should not have at the end of the chapter on sugar.

REFERENCES
1. *Appetite* January 1, 2012, Volume 60, Pages 203-207
2. *Aspartame Disease: an Ignored Epidemic*, www.sunsentpress.com by H. J. Roberts, M.D. , 1000 page medical text on this plague. *Excitotoxins: The Taste That Kills* by neurosurgeon Russell Blaylock, M.D., www.russellblaylockmd.com
3. Mission Possible Australia, www.liverdoctor.com

4. Mark Gold mgold@tiac.net, researcher for twenty years on such subjects. Information originally appeared on www.dorway.com

5. Dr. Betty Martini, D.Hum, Founder, Mission Possible International, 9270 River Club Parkway, Duluth, Georgia, 770 242 - 2599. www.mpwhi.com

6. canidoit.org/aspartame-personal-testimonials

7. canidoit.org/aspartame-personal-testimonials

8. marystuart.hubpages.com/hub/Diet-Colas-and-Weight-Gain

9. www.healthybranscoms.com/2012/03/giving-up-soda-for-good-bring-on-water.html

10. *Your Body's Many Cries for Water.* by Dr. F.Batmanghelidj, M.D., pg. 108.

11. *Your Body's Many Cries for Water.* by Dr. F.Batmanghelidj, M.D., pg. 108.

12. thepeopleschemist.com/splenda-the-artificial-sweetener-that-explodes-internally/

13. Environ Sci Technol. 2011 Oct 15;45(20):8716-22. doi: 10.1021/es202404c. Epub 2011 Sep 26.

CHAPTER 15

TOXIC FOOD #2
EXCITOTOXINS: A MAJOR CAUSE OF OBESITY

Monosodium Glutamate (MSG) and aspartame are part of a group of toxic chemicals called "Excitotoxins". Excitotoxins are chemicals that stimulate brain cells so much that you think that food tastes better than it really does. Unfortunately, they also stimulate the brain so much that the brain cells *die*, within hours.

Food is meant to support your body. How can a body function if what you eat kills brain cells?

CHINESE FOOD MAKES YOU FAT

The excellent book *Excitotoxins*[1] by Brain Surgeon Dr. Russell Blaylock, M.D., goes into great detail about excitotoxins. He talks about how scientists, in order to create test animals, consistently create short, grossly obese mice and rats by giving them MSG, or by giving it to pregnant mice to make their babies obese. If this poison creates obese mice, isn't it obvious that it will create obese humans?

MSG is in a lot of restaurant and fast food meals, as well as processed foods, because it's very addictive. It keeps people eating more, as well as coming back for more. That's profitable.

But it gets worse. A lot worse. Here are some important reasons why you need to get MSG and other excitotoxins totally out of your diet forever:

MSG DESTROYS CELLS IN A CRITICAL AREA OF THE BRAIN - THE HYPOTHALAMUS, AFTER JUST ONE DOSE

Remember that sentence. That is terrifying. The hypothalamus is tiny – no larger than the fingernail of your little finger. Yet it controls most of the most important systems in the body, including consciousness itself. Some that relate directly to fat gain and fat loss are:

- Appetite.
- Growth.
- Hormones.
- Metabolism.
- Sleep cycles.

How terrible that this vital part of the brain should be *seriously* damaged because some corporations want to make more money.

HOW NERVES SEND MESSAGES

A signal is sent along a nerve by electrical means. But when one nerve ends and another begins, there is a small gap between the two nerves, that the electric signal cannot cross. To keep the signal travelling from one nerve to the next, chemicals are sent across the gap. These chemicals are called neurotransmitters (because nerves are neurons). Some neurotransmitters are the amino acids glutamate, aspartate and cysteine. When everything is in balance, everything is fine. But when we eat or drink unnaturally high concentrations of these amino acids, the nerves fire off too much, so they die.

Glutamate is the most common neurotransmitter. It stimulates the brain, much the same way that cocaine does[2].

In 1968 Dr. Olney of Washington University in St. Louis fed doses of MSG similar to those found in human diets to various species of animals[3], and found that doing this destroyed nerve cells in the hypo-thalamus, and made the animals short and obese. What do you think was the reaction to his results? Instead of being acclaimed as a hero for saving lives and health, he was viciously attacked by groups who claimed to have results proving otherwise. As usual, every one of the attacks came from groups who directly or indirectly profited from sell-ing the product involved.

Here's two good examples of how so-called 'scientific' experiments will falsify the truth. Two studies that tried to prove that MSG is really safe did the following[4]:

- The scientists fed so much MSG to the baby animals tested that the babies vomited it up. Naturally they did not absorb most of it.

- Other scientists gave an additional drug to the animals, that blocked MSG brain damage, at the same time they were test-ing to see if MSG could cause brain damage.

This story gets much, much worse. We are not mice. Humans are much more sensitive to MSG and other excitotoxins than any other species. It is the high concentrations of glutamate that do the damage, because that is what excites the nerves. After eating MSG, humans had a massive[5]:

- 5 times more glutamate than mice!
- 20 times more glutamate than monkeys!

Unfortunately, no one tells pregnant or breastfeeding women about these problems. Pregnant monkeys and rats who had MSG had babies with brain damage. Note that brain damage can be in great or small amounts. One cause of children being fat or having mental, educational or health problems is from mothers having MSG and other excitotox-ins such as aspartame when pregnant or breastfeeding – for example, eating out or having diet foods. And later on when the children eat processed foods directly.

If you did this, please don't feel bad about it. You were a victim of corporate manipulation. The important thing is to realize that there is a war going on right now about health, and you are a casualty of it. Please make sure that the buck stops here, right now. Look to the future and do the best you can to educate others so that this does not happen again to future generations.

If you think this happened to you or your children, don't despair, the body has an amazing ability to heal itself. The brain has over 100 billion nerve cells. Nerves are continually being replaced, hundreds of times in a lifetime[6]. Plus, unlike a computer, the brain can change its nerve pathways and circuits when it needs to bypass damaged areas. The process of molding the brain continues throughout life. While most brain growth occurs in the first 6 or 7 years, with 80% of the weight growing in the first 4 years, restructuring occurs right up to old age.

CHANGE YOUR MIND. CHANGE YOUR BEHAVIOR

But in order to heal, each person must have *zero* excitotoxins for the rest of their life, huge decreases in other toxins and massive increases in nutrition from sources such as fresh, daily juicing and raw plants. In addition, pray for a miracle, while you take action to lead a better life.

People who don't prepare their own meals from whole ingredients are not just getting fat. They are getting closer and closer to death. In addition, they are getting less and less intelligent, whether they know it or not, because they are killing their brain cells.

The scary thing is that if we keep doing the same things we are doing now, there will come a time when people are so stupid that they are unable to learn the things that they need to do to get their brains working properly. And their children will have even worse problems. You think you've seen big people? You haven't seen anything yet. Unless poisons like excitotoxins are prevented from being added to the food supply, a lot of people are going to get enormous – and there will be more and more of them.

The effect of excitotoxins is cumulative. A person may not notice signs of brain damage until they are old, and then probably no one will realize that the dementia and senility that sets in then was the end result of lots of doses of excitotoxins.

The amount of MSG has doubled every decade since the 1940s. No wonder people are fat and sick. MSG and other excitotoxins are found in most:

- Diet foods!
- Soups.
- Canned foods.
- Chips.
- Fast foods.
- Restaurant meals, especially Cajun & Chinese meals.
- Frozen foods.
- Ready-made dinners.

MSG is not the only taste enhancing food additive that kills nerves. There is a whole class of chemicals that do much the same. Here are more things that MSG and other excitotoxins, such as aspartame, do:

- They are toxic to the retina of the eye. Young animals given MSG had virtually all of the nerve cells in the inner layer of the retina destroyed.

- Exposure to excitotoxins early in life could cause brain defects, that result in learning and behavior problems. (Note: If you can't control what your children eat, please research the immense benefits of homeschooling).

Go to your kitchen and check the cupboards and the fridge. You will see that MSG is in most processed food. Just a few examples are Campbell's soups, Hostess Doritos, Lay's flavored potato chips, Top Ramen, Betty Crocker Hamburger Helper, Heinz canned gravy, Swanson frozen prepared meals and Kraft salad dressings, especially the 'healthy low fat' ones.

The items that don't have MSG often have instead what is called Hydrolyzed Vegetable Protein. While that may sound healthy, Dr. Blaylock says that Hydrolyzed Vegetable Protein is also very dangerous.

WHAT IS HYDROLYZED VEGETABLE PROTEIN?

Sounds healthy, doesn't it? In fact, it's made from vegetables that are unfit for sale, that are selected because they have high glutamate concentrations. They are boiled in acid, then have caustic soda added to make a brown sludge that collects on the top. This is scraped off and dried. It is high in the three excitotoxins:

* Glutamate.
* Aspartate.
* Cystoic acid, which converts to cysteine.

Plus, it has several substances that cause cancer. It is shocking to see just how many of the foods we feed our children everyday are filled with this stuff. They hide excitotoxins under many different names in order to fool those who catch on.

But it doesn't stop there. Ask at the restaurants and fast food outlets what menu items have MSG. If they say they don't use MSG, ask for the ingredient list. If they will provide it, you will likely see MSG and Hydrolyzed Vegetable Protein are everywhere. It's probably the most important of the 'secret herbs and spices' in Kentucky Fried Chicken (KFC). That is why it's 'finger-licken good'. It's is also a major contaminant of Cajun & Chinese dishes.

So why are excitotoxins in so many of the foods we eat? They are not preservatives or a vitamin. They are added to food for the addictive effect it has on the human body. It makes you eat more. 'Betcha can't eat just one', takes on a whole new meaning where MSG is concerned! Plus it makes an inferior, poor tasting food able to be sold.

And we wonder why the nation is overweight at the same time that school results are going down. The MSG manufacturers themselves admit that it addicts people to their products. It makes people choose their product over others, and makes people eat more of it than they would if MSG wasn't added. That makes MSG a drug, not a food.

But MSG is not just fattening because it makes you eat more. It's also fattening because it's super toxic.

There are at least 70 different kinds of excitotoxins found in food.

Aspartame (nutrasweet) is also an excitotoxin. MSG, aspartame other excitotoxins are often in diet foods and drinks, which makes them extra fattening as well as bad for you.

Excitotoxins kill brain cells, and the effect is cumulative. While they are obviously going to hurt small children, they are also a major cause of mental diseases in the elderly. Just like with caffeine, excitotoxins cause strokes. A stroke occurs when a blood clot blocks an artery (a blood vessel that carries blood from the heart to the body) or a blood vessel (a tube through which the blood moves through the body) breaks, interrupting blood flow to an area of the brain. When either of these things happen, brain cells begin to die and brain damage occurs[7].

But it's not just the big, horrendous strokes you should be concerned about. Dr. Blaylock explains[8]:

"While major strokes do occur frequently, much more often we see minor strokes. These may be so small that the person is not even aware that they have occurred. Usually they develop deep in the ... brain and involve tiny blood vessels rather than major arteries to the brain. We call these *silent strokes*. What makes them important is that they produce "holes" in the blood-brain barrier. These holes can act as leaks in the blood-brain barrier that allow ... *toxic substances to enter the brain.*"

Silent strokes are likely a major cause of senility and diseases such as Parkinson's and Alzheimer's.

Please, get all excitotoxins out of your life forever. Many ingredients hide MSG in them, because consumers are waking up to the fact of how fattening and dangerous MSG is. Many of these substances are 12-40% MSG.

DO NOT EVER EAT THE FOLLOWING EXCITOTOXINS

- Aspartame.
- Autolyzed Yeast.
- Calcium Caseinate.
- Hydrolyzed Oat Flour.

- Hydrolyzed Plant Protein.
- Hydrolyzed Protein.
- Hydrolyzed Vegetable Protein.
- Kombu (this was the original 'taste enhancer', which caused the creating of MSG, because it has extra high levels of glutamate).
- Monosodium Glutamate (MSG).
- Plant Protein Extract.
- Sodium Caseinate.
- Textured Protein.
- Vegetable Protein.
- Yeast Extract.

The following frequently contain MSG, and should also be avoided:

- "Spices" (the manufacturer should say *which* spices).
- Bouillon.
- Broth.
- Flavoring.
- L-cysteine (in some breads).
- Malt extract.
- Malt flavoring.
- Natural flavorings (you will see a lot of this in health food stores).
- Seasoning.
- Soy milk.
- Miso.
- Soy sauce.
- Soy Protein Concentrate / Isolate.
- Stock.
- Whey Protein Concentrate.

This is a long list. As you can see, once again, it really means that you need to spend time making your own food from scratch. While there will be an initial learning curve that you have to get over, just keep going. Eventually you will do it easily, and as you see the results you will be so thankful that you put in the effort to do so.

REFERENCES

1. *Excitotoxins*, by Dr. Russell Blaylock, 1997
2. *Excitotoxins*, by Dr. Russell Blaylock, 1997, page 31
3. *Excitotoxins*, by Dr. Russell Blaylock, 1997, page 36
4. *Excitotoxins*, by Dr. Russell Blaylock, 1997, pages 56,57
5. *Excitotoxins*, by Dr. Russell Blaylock, 1997, page 216
6. *Excitotoxins*, by Dr. Russell Blaylock, 1997, page 63
7. www.stroke.org/site/PageServer?pagename=stroke
8. *Excitotoxins*, by Dr. Russell Blaylock, 1997, page 108

CHAPTER 16

TOXIC FOOD #3
WHEAT: THE FAT FOOD

Dr. William Davis, author of *Wheat Belly*, has seen time and again that many people, who give up wheat totally, lose 10 pounds in just 14 days[1]! He has seen thousands of people lose 50 – 100 pounds in a year, just by giving up this one food[2]!

"Many people who follow a wheat-free diet lose weight even while consuming the same number of calories", says Savill and Hamilton, authors of *Lose Wheat, Lose Weight*[3].

Even if you are addicted to wheat, as most people are, if you want to get thin, the one food that you absolutely must give up, is wheat. In fact, it's so toxic that even if you are thin, you should give it up anyway, because it could easily be affecting your brain. While all grains are fattening because they are acid-causing (whereas vegetables, fruits, nuts and seeds are alkalizing), and are high in carbohydrates, wheat is super fattening because today's modern wheat is nothing like God intended. It has been changed so much genetically that it is no longer the original wheat which our ancestors ate.

This applies whether the wheat is white or whole wheat. Yes, whole wheat is better than white flour for most people, but both are super fattening because the plant they come from is so toxic.

Much of the information in this article comes from the very good book *Wheat Belly* by Dr. William Davis M.D. This is an excellent book to learn about how fattening and toxic wheat is, and I urge you to read it (although the author obviously has things to learn about other toxins, since he recommends that people eat other toxic & fattening substances, for example, Splenda, chocolate and microwaved food).

The original wheat was the emmer variety, called einkorn. It had only 14 chromosomes. Today's wheat has a whopping 28 chromosomes. It's a totally different plant. This change started only in 1943 (when almost everyone was naturally thin) by the Rockefeller Foundation[4], the same family who enriched themselves by creating a monopoly of American medicine and drugs in the 1920s, with funding of the Flexner report. The Flexner report falsely claimed that natural health therapies were quackery, and also centralized the power of independent doctors. When vast changes were made to wheat with the publicized goal of increasing yields and qualities suitable for factory processing, not one test on animals or humans was made to see if this was a good or safe idea. We now know that it was definitely not safe.

To give you an idea of how crazy modern wheat is, after einkorn was crossed with goatgrass (*Aegilops speltoides*) to produce modern wheat, depending on the type of wheat produced, a whopping 5-14 % of the proteins in the new offspring are not found in either parent. How is that possible?

Dr. Davis, who knows that he is sensitive to wheat, did an experiment on himself:

1) He baked some bread made only from einkorn flour – the original wheat. He ate 4 oz. and noted symptoms. His blood sugar rose by 26 mg/dl. He felt no symptoms, including no sleepiness or nausea.

2) He baked some bread made from whole wheat flour. He ate 4 oz. and noted symptoms. His blood sugar rose by a massive 83 mg/dl (that's three times the difference!). He then became extremely nauseated for 36 hours, got stomach cramps, restless sleep and clouded thinking, so much so that he could not understand research papers he was reading.

Millions of other people are also sensitive to wheat. They just don't know that wheat is a major cause of their list of weight, health and mental problems. And even those who don't have symptoms showing yet, don't know that their lives could be so much better without this genetic atrocity in their diet.

One of the main reasons why wheat is so very fattening, as well as super toxic, is that it has a high glycemic index. The glycemic index is a number which tells you how much a food increases the level of blood sugar in your blood. The higher the blood sugar levels in your blood, the more fat your body will make. Plus the more hungry and tired you will be later on.

In addition, when blood sugar goes up quickly, your pancreas has to produce a lot more insulin. If you do this too many times, the pancreas gets worn out, which then causes diabetes. Diabetes is serious. More limb amputations are performed for diabetes than any other non-traumatic disease[5].

One slice of whole wheat bread has a higher glycemic index than table sugar! The glycemic index of whole wheat bread is 72. Sugar is 59[6]. The shocking truth is that two slices of whole wheat bread raises blood sugar more than most sodas or candy bars[7]!

And that is partly why Dr. Davis has had diabetics become non-diabetics by removing carbohydrates, especially wheat, from their lives[8]. How strange then that the American Dietetic Association recommends that you do the opposite – that you should eat lots of 'healthy' whole grains. Or do they perhaps know what they are doing? Could this fact from their own website *possibly* have anything to do with it? – The cost of diabetes in the U.S. in 2007 exceeds $174 billion each year[9]. Somebody gets that money. This means that they are either stupid, or greedy and evil. Take your pick. If they are doing this on purpose, and I believe they are, then it makes organized crime look like kindergarten.

As Dr. Davis says in his book *Wheat Belly*, which I urge you to read, especially if you are diabetic or could have heart disease:

"*Ignoring* ADA diet advice and cutting carbohydrate intake leads to improved blood sugar control...dramatic weight loss, and improvement in all the metabolic messiness of diabetes such as high blood pressure and triglycerides[10]".

Other ways in which wheat is a major cause of obesity are:

1. Wheat causes a two hour roller coaster of satiety and hunger, that causes constant snacking, and 'ups and downs' in energy. (The substance in wheat that does this is called amylopectin A[11]).

2. Wheat stimulates appetite in yet another way, because it has substances which mimic morphine.

3. Do you find it hard to give up wheat? You are not alone. There's a reason for that. Chemicals in wheat act like opiates and get into the brain[12]. These chemicals are called exorphins. These opiate-like chemicals keep you addicted[13]! No other grain does this. (Although, as we see in the chapter on dairy, cheese also has opiate-like chemicals).

Give up wheat totally. Hang on for a few days to get through the drug withdrawal symptoms, and see if you don't start to feel happier and calmer, and think and sleep better. In fact, wheat can even cause hallucinations, delusions, social detachment and even suicide attempts[14]! (So it makes sense that giving up wheat is also an essential part of healing autism, Attention Deficit and Hyperactivity-ADHD). Even if you don't experience these effects – the exorphins are still there and doing something to your brain, including mild euphoria followed by the drug-addicts 'crash'.

4. Fat deposited from eating wheat is especially likely to be in the belly[15].

5. 80% of the protein in wheat is gluten, which is why it makes baked goods so fluffy. It's like glue (which, not surprisingly, is something your body does not like). Gluten damages the lining of the intestinal walls, causing digestive problems which can lead to all manner of symptoms, including fat gain. People who experience major

problems from this are said to have celiac disease, but gluten is probably toxic in some way to most, if not all, people. Bad as this is, gluten is only one of the many problems with wheat.

Columbia University found that when people with celiac disease eliminated wheat, the frequency of obesity was cut in half within a year[16]. Nothing else was changed except for cutting out wheat and gluten.

ALLERGY = TOXIN = FAT

There's more. Dr. Keith Scott-Mumby, author of *Diet Wise*, estimates that 80% of us are allergic to wheat and / or dairy. Anything that you are allergic to, is toxic to you, and can easily make you fat. Some reasons why wheat is so extra allergy-causing are:

1. Modern wheat is capable of producing an astonishing 23,000 different proteins[17]! You could be allergic to *any one* of them. Anything that causes an allergic reaction can make you fat.

2. We eat way too much of it. The more you eat something, the more likely you will become allergic to it.

3. A lot of us were given wheat before we even had teeth. That is, before our digestive system was strong enough to handle it.

Also, consider this: Your body really would prefer things that are easy to digest, like fruit, nuts and seeds. Can you eat raw, whole wheat grains like you can an apple or spinach leaf? No. Since we can't do this, it's likely that our bodies are not designed to digest it.

How's this for a winner? People who cut out wheat reduce their total daily calorie intake by 350 to 400 calories, without even trying[18]! This backs up the main premise of this book: To get thin, you must focus on toxins instead of counting calories. This statistic gives you an idea of how removing a toxic food ends up causing you to naturally cut down on overall food intake.

Wheat is a good example of how big organizations secretly work for the pharmaceutical companies. You can see just how evil wheat is, because it has been so majorly changed from its parents. And yet, the American Heart Association, the American Dietetic Association and the American Diabetes Association all keep saying, over and over, that people should eat "more healthy whole grains[19]." What a great marketing scam!

This is so evil when one considers that a fat belly is not just a problem of looking good. A fat belly means that the *organs* have a lot of fat. This is called "visceral fat". A fat belly means that the liver, kidneys, pancreas, intestines and heart are all fat[20]! This is very bad for your future life projection and quality of life, for many reasons. For starters, this means that they don't work as well as they should. And another, they find it harder to produce the substances which normally protect you against heart attacks[21] and other health hazards.

Plus, as I discuss in the chapter on "other toxins", when you have a fat belly, you make more estrogen – which makes you fatter, whether you are female or male. This is also how men develop male breasts.

In *Diet Wise*, Prof. Keith Scott-Mumby M.D. gives some wonderful case histories of people who give up particular foods, often wheat and dairy, and get amazing improvements in health & mental symptoms. For example:

> "Arthur in his 60s was so weak he lay in bed over 20 hours a day. After one month of giving up wheat totally, as well as a couple of other foods, he was able to travel. Eventually he became fitter than men ten years younger than him."

If you need any more incentive to give up wheat for life, consider this amazing fact: Wheat can cause death! Worse than peanuts! Many people who may not appear to have celiac disease, still test positive for antibodies against gluten. And the number of these people is rising over time. One study found that for these people (and you could be one of them), eating wheat causes a 29% increased chance of death from acute allergic reactions. Eating pumpkin or apples does not do that. Another study found that people with celiac disease had 30% more chance of developing cancer[22].

Learning what you must not eat can take a bit of doing for some people. I shared with a lady some ways to get thinner, including to give up wheat. She told me that she had done that, when her husband, who was within ear shot, laughed out loud, and turned her in – "What about the macaroni and cheese? And the wraps?" She had not realized that these contained wheat because they contained "white flour". White flour is wheat, with the nutrition removed. Strangely enough, some people are less allergic to white flour than whole wheat flour, probably because some of the proteins which cause allergies have been removed, but because it has almost no nutrition in it, we should not eat it either.

That means, you must not eat anything that lists any of the following words under "ingredients":

- Enriched flour.
- Wheat.
- White flour.
- Wheat flour.
- Whole wheat.

Unfortunately, if you look at what most people have in their shopping trolleys, you will see that they buy many different products that are simply different ways of repackaging wheat, including:

- Bagels.
- Bread.
- Breakfast cereals.
- Buns.
- Cookies.
- Cous cous.
- Crackers.
- Croutons.
- Hot dog buns.
- Muffins.
- Pasta of all shapes.
- Pita bread.

- Pizza.
- Pretzels.
- Rolls.
- Spaghetti.
- Stuffing.
- Wraps.

Please stop buying these things, whether or not they are whole grain, and instead buy the foods listed in the shopping list chapter.

Here are some great testimonials from Amazon.com for the book, *Lose the Wheat, Lose the Weight*, by Dr. William Davis:

- "I started my journey with high blood pressure, 260 pounds, in my mid forties... I started walking 4 miles per day in an effort to increase calorie burn, but weight was not coming off. I was a wheat junkie - bagel on way to work - glycemic crash mid-morning, sub or sandwich for lunch - glycemic crash mid-afternoon, followed by wheat pasta and garlic bread for dinner - vicious cycle. I was tired all the time. I ...feel I had developed gluten sensitivity over the years and as the author claims, the wheat we eat today is genetically far removed from historical grain stocks. So, I figured, what the heck did I have to lose but some weight. The first week was a little rough, adjusting to new products from the local health food store. I quickly started feeling more energy and by day 5 it was like a wheat hangover was gone - no more lethargy, no more post nasal drip making it hard to sleep at night. Fast forward 3 months and I have shed 35 pounds, and feel like I am 30 again."

- "I've now been wheat free for three weeks ... and I've lost 7 pounds. That may not sound like much of an accomplishment, until you consider: - I am 6'4", and have been stuck at around 210 pounds for over two years. I have not been able to lower my weight by dieting or exercise. - 210 is only 20 pounds over my goal weight of 190. And everybody knows how difficult it is to lose those last 10 to 20 pounds---especially at my age (61). - I have not exercised for the past three weeks.

Update: It's now been nearly three months since I went wheat-free, and I've lost 16 pounds, which is about 1.2 pounds per week. So you might think, "Hey, that's no big deal--you could have lost that much weight without really trying." But you'd be wrong. Way wrong. As I stated before, I was stuck at 210 for over two years. Dieting and exercising did nothing to reduce my weight. I had hit a plateau and was going nowhere. Now, in just three months, I'm down another 16 pounds, to 194! I'm within four pounds of my goal weight!... My body fat is now at 14%!"

Here are even more great testimonials to the massive benefits of giving up wheat from *Wheat Belly*, also by Dr. William Davis:

- At age 61, Celeste weighed 182 pounds. After 3 months of no wheat, she reduced by 21 pounds. After 14 months wheat-free, she reduced by a total of 55 pounds to achieve a weight of 127 pounds, which she had not weighed since her 40s. Plus she reduced her waist by 12 inches and was back in U.S. size 6 dresses[23]!

- Geno, 5'10" and 322 lb, reduced his weight by 64 pounds and 14" off his waist in 6 months with no wheat. He went on to reduce a total of 104 pounds in a year[24].

- Wendy, at 36 years old, had ulcerative colitis so badly that she was preparing to have her colon replaced with a bag. (This is a bad thing to do, as you will read in my chapter "Keep your organs"). Even though she had been tested as "not a celiac" she gave up wheat at the suggestion of Dr. Davis. After 3 months, her colitis went away, and she lost 38 pounds[25]!

WHEAT CAUSES HEART ATTACKS & STROKES

Wheat causes high levels of LDL (low-density lipoprotein) particles, which is a major cause of *heart disease*. The drug industry has found it profitable to name a high LDL problem as a high cholesterol problem. That's because in the old days they could not measure LDL directly, so they measured cholesterol instead, because it was vaguely related. However, today there is no excuse for testing cholesterol, and instead going straight to the real problem – LDL. If you are told your cholesterol is high, get your LDL levels measured[26].

High LDL causes plaque in the blood vessels, and therefore causes heart attack and stroke. What triggers the production of LDLs the most? Carbohydrates, particularly wheat.

In fact, it has recently been discovered that fats *do not* increase LDL levels, because when LDL levels go up from diet, the body stops making its own LDLs. But carbohydrates which have *no* fats stimulate insulin, which in turn triggers fatty acid synthesis in the liver, which greatly raises triglycerides. High triglyceride levels cause high LDL levels[27].

So, if you, like many people, have high triglycerides, it's not giving up good fat that is going to help you. Quite the reverse. It's cutting down on carbohydrates, especially wheat, but also grains, potato and sugar. Dr. Davis has found that low-fat diets, where people swap fats for carbs, *raise* triglyceride levels from 150 mg/dl up to *thousands* of mg/dl[28]! That is, some "heart-healthy" foods like whole wheat bread cause heart disease!

Therefore, to save your heart, you must give up wheat. This is the one thing that is missing from the otherwise good documentary *Forks over Knives* where Dr. Colin Campbell found from the China Study that to get thin and healthy, people need to have a "Whole, foods, plant-based diet". The words "whole-foods, plant based diet" appears to include whole grains. However, Denise Minger found that Dr. Campbell's conclusions were incomplete. Minger found that the data showed that wheat was even more of a problem for obesity and cancer than animal protein[29], [30].

Don't expect the medical industry which makes over $273 billion a year in the USA on heart disease[31], and more for cancer, or the government that is run by lobbyists for the drug companies, and doesn't want to have to pay social security for decades, to be in a hurry to tell you this.

Wheat can be hidden in all kinds of things, including drugs and vitamins. A man came to Dr. Keith Scott-Mumby who was over weight and had several heart attacks. He knew he was allergic to wheat, but he did not know that some of the vodkas that he drank were no longer made of potato, but from wheat. He gave up the vodkas that were made from wheat and lost fifty pounds! It is amazing that even alcohols made from different raw material, have different effects.

If you have children who are acting up, this could easily be due to wheat. Wheat has exorphins that act like opiates. That is, wheat affects the brain in a similar way to drugs. It affects our brain, thoughts, emotions and body in a multitude of ways. It can even cause brain damage. We will never know how many old people with dementia would still be thinking clearly if they had never eaten wheat[32]. Try going totally wheat-free for at least three weeks and note the results. Write the results down so you remember them. Wheat is so toxic that it is something that no one should have in their house.

A NOTE ABOUT WHEATGRASS JUICE

Like most people who are into natural health, at one time I thought wheatgrass juice was great. However, I became suspicious of wheatgrass when, like so many others, I and my husband experienced instant nausea when we drank some, even when it appeared to have no mold on it. As I said in the chapter on healing crises, if you get an instant reaction to something, that is not from cleansing. Cleansing is when the body takes nutrients and uses them later on to remove toxins from the bodies. *Instant* nausea is quite different. That is the body telling you in no uncertain terms that what you are eating is very bad for you.

Now, some people say that wheatgrass juice nausea is from mold on the wheat and that the mold is safe. What rubbish! Any mold that causes instant nausea is obviously toxic. However, it's possible that there is more to people's reactions against wheatgrass juice than just mold, especially when there are so many stories from the old days of the healing abilities of wheatgrass. To understand the truth, consider the history of wheatgrass juice:

Wheatgrass juice became popular with the publication of Ann Wigmore's book *The Wheatgrass Book* in 1985[33]. Wigmore learned about it from her grandmother who used grasses to heal wounded soldiers in

Europe during the First World War (1914-1918). Ann later did her own experiments with grasses and found that wheatgrass was the best of all the grasses, and gave miraculous results in healing.

Remember that wheat *used* to be healthy, but once the Rockefeller-led organizations changed it in 1943, gradually it became more and more altered and more and more toxic. Therefore, I believe that the reason for some people's reaction against wheatgrass juice is an allergic reaction against the 23,000 different proteins that can be in modern wheat, any one of which you could be allergic to, especially in concentrated doses. The main benefit of drinking wheatgrass juice is that it contains raw chlorophyll, so instead of wheatgrass, just juice different plants that are leafy and green (kale, parsley, spinach, bok choy etc.)

GOVERNMENT SUBSIDIES MAKE YOU FAT

A major reason why there is so much wheat in food, is because farmers receive billions of dollars from the government to grow it[34]. That is, the government takes your tax dollars, and uses it to grow toxic wheat, genetically modified corn and soy, as well as meat and dairy from animals that are fed these plants. This fattens and kills people, and fills up the hospitals with people with heart attacks and diabetes. I hope this fact makes you angry enough to make some major changes to your life.

Wheat is so addictive, that just having one cookie could see you back on the wagon, with the pounds coming back on again. Do your best to never have one bite. You might think like some people – "There's nothing left to eat!" But before you do that, please go to the chapter called "shopping list" and get shopping. The key to making this plan work for you so that you get thin for life is to already have all the good food you need in your house. If you have to look up a recipe, and then shop for that recipe, then it becomes way too complicated, and you won't do enough of it to replace all the wheat and other toxic food you have been used to.

Once you have bought plenty of food from the shopping list, here is all you have to do before any meal: Just look at what food you have, go to a search engine on the internet, put in "recipe, vegan" or "recipe, raw" and list some of the items you want to use, and see what comes up. You can also go to my recipe chapter. It will help you to give up wheat if, as soon as possible, you make some delicious, easy-to-make grain free walnut Bread, which is in that chapter.

Eventually you will learn to prepare food without recipes - you just throw it all together! The key is in having the right ingredients available with you in the first place.

You're not fat. You're eating food that is addicting. You may be surprised to find that, after getting over the first few days of drug-withdrawal symptoms, life without wheat becomes easier, rather than tougher.

REFERENCES

1. *Wheat Belly*, William Davis M.D., 2011, page 69
2. *Wheat Belly*, William Davis M.D., 2011, page 70
3. *Lose Wheat, Lose Weight*, Antoinette Savill & Dawn Hamilton Ph.D., 2001
4. *Wheat Belly*, William Davis M.D., 2011, page 23
5. *Wheat Belly*, William Davis M.D., 2011, page 101
6. *Wheat Belly*, William Davis M.D., 2011, pages 8-9
7. *Wheat Belly*, William Davis M.D., 2011, page 33
8. *Wheat Belly*, William Davis M.D., 2011, page 9
9. www.diabetes.org/advocate/resources/cost-of-diabetes.html
10. *Wheat Belly*, William Davis M.D., 2011, page 106
11. *Wheat Belly*, William Davis M.D., 2011, page 35
12. *Wheat Belly*, William Davis M.D., 2011, page 49
13. *Wheat Belly*, William Davis M.D., 2011, page 43
14. *Wheat Belly*, William Davis M.D., 2011, pages 46- 47
15. *Wheat Belly*, William Davis M.D., 2011, page 36
16. *Wheat Belly*, William Davis M.D., 2011, page 67
17. Exploring the Plant Transcriptome through Phylogenetic Profiling. *Plant Physiology* Vol. 137, 2005; pg. 3. Also www.greenmedinfo.com/blog/wheat-contains-not-one-23k-potentially-harmful-proteins
18. *Wheat Belly*, William Davis M.D., 2011, page 68
19. *Wheat Belly*, William Davis M.D., 2011, page 59
20. *Wheat Belly*, William Davis M.D., 2011, page 60
21. *Wheat Belly*, William Davis M.D., 2011, page 61
22. *Wheat Belly*, William Davis M.D., 2011, pages 88-90

23. *Wheat Belly*, William Davis M.D., 2011, page 57

24. *Wheat Belly*, William Davis M.D., 2011, page 71

25. *Wheat Belly*, William Davis M.D., 2011, pages 86-87

26. *Wheat Belly*, William Davis M.D., 2011, pages 147-148

27. *Wheat Belly*, William Davis M.D., 2011, pages 150-153

28. *Wheat Belly*, William Davis M.D., 2011, page 155-156

29. *Wheat Belly*, William Davis M.D., 2011, page 160-164

30. www.rawfoodsos.com/the-china-study/

31. www.webmd.com/healthy-aging/features/heart-disease-medical-costs

32. *Wheat Belly*, William Davis M.D., 2011, page 166-175

33. *The Wheatgrass Book*, 1985, Ann Wigmore

34. articles.mercola.com/sites/articles/archive/2011/08/03/the-9-foods-the-us-government-is-paying-you-to-eat.aspx

CHAPTER 17

TOXIC FOOD #4
GRAINS

In the chapter on wheat, we looked at how, of all the grains, wheat is the one grain that you absolutely must give up totally for life, if you want to get and stay thin and healthy, because modern wheat has been altered genetically so much from its natural state that it produces a host of really bad symptoms. Just giving up wheat alone can reduce a person's weight by dozens of pounds.

Now, what about other grains? Well, that depends. Some people are able to reduce while having some grains in moderation. But if you have done everything else in this book, and are still not at the size you want to be, or have diabetes, then you may need to give up all grains, if only for a while. Try it for three weeks and see what happens. Even if you have only a remaining 10-20 pounds to lose, this could be the very answer you have been looking for.

It's probably not forever. You should be able to have some grains in moderation when you get to your desired body size, and are in maintenance mode. The exception will be if you have really done way too much sugar and carbohydrates in your life, so it is going to take your body longer to heal.

GRAINS ARE ACIDIC

Remember, anything that is acidic is toxic, and therefore fattening. While some people like to recommend a "whole foods plant based diet", that is not specific enough because that description includes grains, which are acid-causing. Basically the only foods that are alkalizing are vegetables, fruits, nuts, seeds and soaked legumes.

GRAINS HAVE A HIGH GLYCEMIC INDEX

Grains have a high glycemic index, which means that they send your blood sugar levels high. The higher your blood sugar levels go, the more fat your body stores. For example, just one bowl of oatmeal can send your blood sugar from a normal 90 mg/dl to 200-400 mg/dl[1].

High blood sugar causes a host of problems, including hunger, tiredness and fat gain. This is how this happens: When you eat something that raises your blood sugar levels rapidly, you get a 'high' which you can get addicted to. This makes you want to eat more later. Because your blood sugar levels are extra high, your pancreas then produces more insulin than is normal to bring the levels back down. Insulin tells your body to store fat.

The extra insulin disposes of all the extra sugar. But, because there is too much insulin hanging around, the rebound means that blood sugar does not just come back to the normal levels – it now bounces down to too low a level of blood sugar. This is when you get tired and hungry, and are likely to reach for more high-glycemic foods. Insulin is meant to go up and down by only a small amount.

The glycemic index does not tell us the whole picture, because it treats the body as a simple metal engine, rather than a super complicated organic living body, with thousands of different chemical reactions, which hate toxins, and need hundreds of different nutrients that have to be moved around in infinitely complicated ways. However, the glycemic index is still something to keep in mind.

The following numbers are very approximate glycemic indexes for some high glycemic foods, depending on how the food is prepared[2,3,4], Keep in mind that the more you eat, the higher your blood sugar goes.

So, the amount you eat is as important as the glycemic Index.

- Rice, Jasmine (109)[5]. No wonder it's so delicious! Avoid this. Get brown or basmati rice instead. Better yet, get brown basmati.

- Dates (103). However, dates are super high in nutrition. A few dates are much better for sweetening than toxic sugar.

- Potato (82 - 111). Instead have sweet potato (70) or pumpkin (54).

- Rice, White (89). Avoid this. Get brown or basmati rice instead. Better yet, get brown basmati.

- Watermelon (72).

- Wheat (72). Remember that wheat is so toxic that you should avoid it totally.

- Millet (67).

- Rice, Basmati (67).

- Banana (62).

- Sugar (59).

- Rice, brown (50). Soak on the counter, not in the refrigerator, for 24 hours first to alkalize it. You can store it in the fridge for a day or two until ready for use.

If you keep your blood sugar low, you will keep your insulin levels low, and then you will have more glucagon. Glucagon is a hormone which, like insulin, is made by the pancreas. Glucagon tells your body to *burn* fat. Glucagon and insulin work together to keep your body at the ideal weight – if you eat the right foods[6].

HIGH BLOOD SUGAR AGES YOU

Scientists are now studying a fairly new discovery, "Advanced Glycation End Products", or AGEs for short. AGEs, just like their name, age people. AGEs cause major diseases such as diabetes, kidney disease, atherosclerosis, dementia, cancer and eye problems such as cataracts. The higher your blood sugar level, the more AGEs you have in your body[7].

Although scientists have only recently begun to study AGEs, they have already made the grandiose statement that, once they form, AGE's are irreversible[7]. That is typical of the scientific establishment, that still continues to ignore, for example, dozens of natural ways to heal cancer (see www.CancerTutor.org), which don't cost enough to be of interest to the big corporations that rule our countries. What this sentence really means is "we have not yet studied anyone who eats enough raw plant food and juices and avoids enough toxic food to see if we can reverse these", or "We should have a drug to treat this shortly."

After all, doctors only spend about zero to twelve hours or so learning about diet in 5 years of study at university. I even had a client once who said that her doctor told her it did not matter what you eat! How insane! Your body is obviously made from what you eat.

But I digress: You don't want to make AGEs, so you don't want to send your blood sugar skyrocketing by eating a high concentration of grains. The trick with grains is to have them in moderation with other plant foods, if at all.

The study of AGEs is relatively new. However, it is interesting to me that already there appears to be a correlation between the amount of AGE's produced, and how toxic a food is. For example, some of the biggest producers of AGEs are wheat, fructose and cured meats, all of which are extra toxic.

WHOLE GRAINS ARE MORE SLIMMING

The only grains you should eat should be whole grain. Processing removes and alters all the valuable parts that nature included for a reason, because they are needed, even if science has not yet caught up with what God has designed.

SOAK ALL GRAINS AND FLOURS 12-24 HOURS BEFORE USE

There is no contest. Whole grains are much healthier than processed grains, where nutrients are removed, and sometimes chemicals are added. Bugs prefer whole grains for a reason – they know it's more healthy.

However, many people, even natural health people, do not know that whole grains & flours contain phytic acid, which is harmful to health because it combines with minerals in the intestinal tract so that you cannot absorb them. That is, phytic acid blocks the absorption of essential, slimming minerals such as iron, calcium, magnesium and zinc.

Therefore, do what our ancestors did[8]: Whole grains and flours should be soaked for 12-24 hours in good water, to break down phytic acid and other toxins, before use. If you don't do this, or buy processed food that does not do this, essential minerals which you need for fat loss will not be absorbed. The water should be a little warm. If you soak them and aren't ready to use them right away, store them in the fridge for a day or so until you have time to use them.

In addition to breaking down the phytic acid, soaking predigests the grains so that you can more easily absorb nutrients from them. If you do this with oatmeal, you may be surprised at how noticeably much more filling and sustaining oatmeal becomes. Dilute the oatmeal with as many nuts & seeds (e.g. almonds / ground flax seeds) and low-glycemic fruit (e.g. blueberries) as possible, to keep the glycemic index down.

One should also soak legumes (lentils and beans) before using them, because this 'sprouts' the legumes, which breaks down the complex carbohydrates in them and makes them more digestible.

WHICH GRAINS TO EAT?

Do not eat:

- Wheat, ever, because it's super toxic.
- Corn (unless it's organic, because it's genetically modified).
- Jasmine or white rice (Glycemic Index is too high).

Avoid or go very easy on:

- Rye, barley, spelt, triticale, kamut, bulgar. (Eat as little as possible, because they have gluten which damages the lining of the intestines.

- Oats. (They have a high glycemic index. Also some people say that oats have gluten. Dilute the effect by adding lots of nuts, seeds, fruit).

Eat in moderation, if you can reduce weight while doing so:

- Millet (very nutritious).

- Amaranth (very nutritious with a delicious, nutty flavor).

- Quinoa.

- Basmati Rice (Brown is best. Check it's not from a country affected by radiation from Japan or a country that has high levels of lead in its rice such as China, Taiwan, Italy, India and Thailand[9]).

- Buckwheat (technically not a grain, because it's not a grass).

- Teff.

To get thin, have zero wheat and few or zero grains. Instead, buy more vegetables, fruits, nuts and seeds, as listed in the shopping list chapter.

Giving up grains totally can be tough, because while it's not as bad as wheat, they still have a reasonably high glycemic index and therefore cause a rush of sugar in the blood, which is addictive. Stock up on extra fruits, vegetables, nuts and seeds and have as many of these as you wish at meal times. If you need a snack in between meals, make it seeds, nuts or spirulina/chlorella tablets. If you feel giving up grains is tough, as I did, it's not hunger that you feel when you give up grains. It's withdrawal symptoms, similar to drug withdrawal. Don't give up. After a few days, you should feel good.

REFERENCES
1. *Wheat Belly*, William Davis M.D., 2011, page 135
2. *Wheat Belly*, William Davis M.D., 2011, page 34
3. www.mendosa.com/gilists.htm
4. www.health.harvard.edu/newsweek/Glycemic_index_and_glycemic_load_for_100_foods.htm
5. drclay.com/2012/02/jasmine-rice-glycemic-index/
6. en.wikipedia.org/wiki/Glucagon
7. *Wheat Belly*, William Davis M.D., 2011, page 134
8. www.thenourishinggourmet.com/2010/09/reducing-phytic-acid-in-grains-and-legumes.html
9. *Time Magazine Health & Family Website* - healthland.time.com/2013/04/11/high-levels-of-lead-found-in-imported-rice/

CHAPTER 18

TOXIC FOOD #5

GMO FOOD MAKES YOU FAT
(AND CAUSES CANCER)

Possibly the very worst food you can eat, and what people are beginning to realize is a major cause of obesity, are GMOs. And yet, most people still don't know what they are. I have been horrified to meet many people, who regularly shop at health food stores, who have never heard of GMOs.

GMO stands for "Genetically Modified Organism". Another word for it is GE food which means "Genetically Engineered" food. And some people call them "Frankenfoods", named after the Frankenstein monster. The first GMOs were eaten in 1994[1]. This is relatively recent. I believe that GMOs are a major cause behind the reason why it seems that people have grown visibly much larger in just the last few years.

It *looks* the same — the bread, pizza, sodas, corn on the cob. So much of what we eat every day looks just like it did 20 years ago. But something profoundly different has happened without our knowledge or consent. And it's not even labelled. The company Monsanto, which is behind GMOs, has been working vigorously to see to that. You will remember Monsanto as the chemical company responsible for atrocities such as DDT, Agent Orange & PCBs[2].

Proof that GMO food is radically different from normal food was provided in 2012 after the completion of the first long term study of the effect of GMOs. Corn is meant to be healthy for rats, but in the study, rats given even small quantities of GMO corn developed massive cancer tumors as early as four months for males, and seven months for females[3].

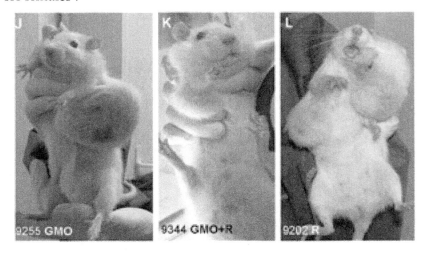

GMO rat tumors from Food and Chemical Toxicology
www.journals.elsevier.com/food-and-chemical-toxicology/

Yet more proof that GMO food is completely different from non-GMO food is provided by a nutritional analysis. For example, normal corn has 437 times more calcium than GMO corn, and 56 times more magnesium[4]. Lack of minerals makes you fat. But that's only the beginning of what's wrong with GMOs.

WHAT IS GMO FOOD?

Genetic engineering is totally different from normal breeding, because it involves taking genes from a completely different species and inserting them into the DNA of a plant or animal. In fact, it doesn't just interbreed similar species. Plants and animals are being bred with virtually any other living thing, particularly *bacteria*.

In the case of GMO food plants, many are made to either drink poison, or produce poisons. The main poison is glyphosate, the active ingredient in Roundup herbicide.

POISON DRINKERS:

The poison drinkers are called herbicide tolerant. They're inserted with genes from bacteria. Do you want to *eat bacteria*? This allows them to survive otherwise deadly doses of toxic herbicide. The plants live, but you get to eat a lot more poison than you would have otherwise.

POISON PRODUCERS:

The poison producers are called Bt crops. Genes from bacteria are inserted into the plant, to make the plant produce poison in every cell.

Remember, you are not fat, you are *toxic*. And GMO poisons are very toxic. So far, much more money has gone into studies which have tried, and failed, to show that GMOs are not harmful, than the reverse. But at least one study has found that animals fed GM corn put on weight, when animals fed normal corn do not[5]. The study was only short term. A long term study would be bound to show even worse results.

GMOS CAUSE ORGAN DAMAGE

Remember, food is meant to nurture organs. And yet, studies on rats have shown that GMOs cause organ damage[6] How are you meant to get thin if your body is not working properly? Answer is - you won't. This includes damage to:

- Liver (Essential for weight loss).
- Kidneys.

- Heart.
- Adrenals.
- Spleen.
- Blood cells.

FOOD THAT CONTAINS GMO POISON

The number of plants that we eat that are genetically modified is growing all the time. As of the time of writing, in the USA, GMO foods are[7]:

- Soy (89%) (soy oil is in just about everything).
- Corn (61% or higher) (GMO sweet corn was started in 2012).
- Canola (75%) (Canola is a fancy name for Rapeseed oil).
- Hawaiian papaya (more than 50%).
- Alfalfa (A major feed source for dairy cows. Started in 2012. Unlike previous GMO crops, alfalfa pollen spreads everywhere, even into organic crops. So possibly even organic dairy is not safe).
- Cotton (83%) (cottonseed oil is toxic in any case. Always avoid it).
- Zucchini and yellow squash (small amounts).
- Sugar. (GMO sugar started in 2008. 95% of sugar beets are GMO. If you must use sugar, make sure it's organic, because GMO sugar cane is expected by 2015[8],[9]).
- Some vitamins.
- Milk and dairy products can contain dangerous genetically modified Bovine Growth Hormone (rBGH).
- Other countries have other GMOs and these could be in American products. For example, Australia imports GMO potatoes and GMO rice, from other countries.

This is why you *must* get a magnifying glass and read every ingredient before purchase. If any of the above words are mentioned, avoid it to so that you can have your natural body back again.

Europe is a little better than the USA, but the trouble is that they import GMOs. Dairy cows in Denmark have been found to have glyphosate, the GMO poison that is in Roundup, in their urine and in their blood[10], at levels that suggest serious cell toxicity. So you know it will be in their milk. To get up-to-date information on what food is GMO in your country, visit www.gmo-free-regions.org. You should also research regularly on the internet to keep up-to-date with the latest foods that have become genetically modified.

OTHER FOODS CONTAIN SECOND-HAND GMO POISON

Even if you think "well, I don't eat any corn, soy or canola" you are probably still eating GMO poison. That is because GMO corn, soy, cottonseed and alfalfa are fed to chickens and animals. Therefore, unless it's USDA organic or wild, you are eating GMOs if you eat:

• Eggs.
• Dairy (milk, cream, cheese, butter, yogurt, ice cream). Plus non-organic milk can contain dangerous genetically modified Bovine Growth Hormone (rBGH).
• Meat, including poultry.
• Farm raised fish or seafood. Even wild caught salmon is not safe, because some of it has been found to be farm raised.

Organic food is meant to be free of GMOs. But we are starting to find out that even this is not a guarantee. It's way too easy to sneak it in. There have been so far at least two instances where GMOs were found in so-called 'organic' food. In each case, this discovery was not made by organizations that should protect you, like the FDA. They were made by independent bodies. Baby food[11] is one, which is really scary. With these kinds of toxins being given to babies, it's no wonder we have obese children now. The only food a baby should have is breast milk and, when ready for solids, homemade baby food (cook it, strain it, freeze in ice cube trays) and reverse osmosis water.

Kashi 'organic' cereal is another. The Cornucopia Institute found that Kashi has high levels of GMOs in it's 'organic' cereal[12]. You may be less surprised at this once you realize that Kashi is not owned by green-thumbed nature-lovers, but by Kellogg's Mega-corporation.

In addition, pollen from GMO alfalfa, which was introduced only in 2012, goes everywhere, so even organic dairy is no longer safe.

GMOs STERILIZE YOUR GRAND-CHILDREN

When Genetically Modified Organisms were first created, some people knew they were very bad. But no one really knew just how bad they are. We know that now. Basically, not only are they contributing to the obesity epidemic, because they are so highly toxic, in the longer term they will **wipe out the human race if not eradicated completely**. Because animals fed GMOs have grandchildren who cannot have children[13]. *No* other food does that! This is proof that we are dealing with something completely different, and evil. Here is some evidence of this:

GMO GENOCIDE

Concerning the experiment carried out jointly by the National Association for Gene Security and the Institute of Ecological and Evolutional Problems, Dr. Alexei Surov had this to say;

"We selected several groups of hamsters, kept them in pairs in cells and gave them ordinary food as always," says Alexei Surov.

"We did not add anything for one group, but the other was fed with soya that contained no GM components, while the third group was fed with some content of Genetically Modified Organisms and the fourth one with increased amount of GMO. We monitored their behavior and how they gained weight and when they gave birth to their cubs.

Originally, everything went smoothly. However, we noticed quite a serious effect when we selected new pairs from their cubs and continued to feed them as before. These pairs' growth rates were slower and they reached their sexual maturity more slowly. When we got some of their cubs we formed the new pairs of the third generation. *We failed to get cubs from these pairs*, which were fed with GM foodstuffs. It was proved that these pairs lost their ability to give birth to their cubs," Dr. Alexei Surov said.

GMO FED GRANDCHILDREN GROW HAIR IN THEIR MOUTHS

Another surprise was discovered by scientists in hamsters of the third generation. *Hair* grew in the mouth of the animals that took part in the experiment! What kind of damage must have been done to these poor animals?

Because I knew that it is toxins that is the main cause of obesity, and that GMOs are super toxic, I did not have to look too hard to find scientific evidence that GMOs contribute to obesity. The following are notes from an interview of Dr. Don Huber, by Dr. Mercola. Dr. Huber is an expert in the areas of science that relate to the toxicity of GMO food. He taught as a staff Professor at Purdue University for 35 years, and over 55 years he has researched how to improve agriculture.

MONSANTO'S ROUNDUP READY CROPS (GMOS) ARE DE-STROYING GUT FLORA, WHICH IS LEADING TO OBESITY[14]

A major modification done to genetically engineered food crops is the introduction of herbicide resistance. Monsanto is the leader in this field, with their patented Roundup Ready corn, cotton, soybean and sugar beets, which can survive otherwise lethal doses of glyphosate—the active ingredient in Roundup.

The working premise is that by making the plants resistant to the herbicide, farmers can increase yields by cutting down on weed growth. This premise has been found to be severely flawed, however, as farmers around the world are now fighting glyphosate-resistant super-weeds at an alarming rate. Dr. Huber explains:

> "You have to realize what an herbicide, or a pesticide, is. They are metal chelators. In other words, they immobilize specific nutrients. It's a compound that can grab onto another element and change its availability to a plant or animal. We have herbicides and pesticides that are quite specific for just one particular essential nutrient like copper, zinc, iron, or manganese.

Glyphosate is unique because it can bind with any positively charged ion. If you look at the essential minerals for plants, you see calcium, magnesium, potassium, copper, iron, manganese, zinc, and all of those other critical transition elements... They all have an ion associated with them. That means Glyphosate binds to all these nutrients, not just one of them. This makes it so much more lethal.

You have to realize that this mode of action immobilizes a critical essential nutrient. Those nutrients aren't just required by the weed, but they're required by microorganisms. They're required by us for our own physiologic functions". (Note: No wonder pesticides make us fat! They cause malnutrition by depriving us of essential minerals that the body will crave - constantly urging us on to eat more until we get them!)

"The nutritional efficiency of GE plants is *profoundly compromised.* Nutrients such as iron, manganese and zinc can be reduced by as much as 80-90%!

Many staunch defenders of genetically engineered foods are under the misconception that GE foods are "better" or have improved nutrition when the exact opposite is true. They also don't understand that the glyphosate residue *cannot be washed off* because it's part of the plant itself.

Furthermore, about 20 percent of the glyphosate migrates out of the plant's roots and into the surrounding soil. Once in the soil, the glyphosate affects beneficial soil microorganisms also. With each new Roundup Ready crop approved, the glyphosate residues in the soil increases, and so it becomes ever more toxic.

The quality of food is almost always related to the quality of soil. The most critical component of the soil is microorganisms. They are even more important than soil nutrients, because it's the microorganisms that allow plants to *use* those nutrients. *Glyphosate is extremely toxic to all of those organisms.*

What we see with our continued use of GMOs is that it is totally eliminating many microorganisms from the soil. We no longer have the same balance that we used to have. Consequently, we see an increase of over 40 new plant diseases. And previous diseases which were not a big problem are now a big problem. The beneficial gut bacteria in humans, which are essential for weight loss, are also very sensitive to glyphosate levels.

Glyphosate nullifies genetic resistance." (Note: This is affecting food production, animals, pets, and people). "For example, toxic botulism is now becoming a more common cause of death in dairy cows whereas such deaths used to be *extremely* rare. The reason it didn't occur before was because beneficial organisms served as natural controls to keep the bacteria responsible for this disease in check. Without them, the bacteria is allowed to proliferate in the animal's intestines and produce *lethal* amounts of toxins."

What a mess! Similar things are no doubt happening to people, which is contributing to obesity as well as disease.

GMOS CAN REMAIN INSIDE US[15]

The only published human feeding study revealed what may be the most dangerous and fattening problem with GM foods. The gene inserted into GM soy transfers into the DNA of bacteria living inside our intestines *and continues to function*[16]. This means that long after we stop eating GMOs, we may still have potentially harmful GM proteins produced continuously inside of us. Put more plainly, eating a corn chip produced from GM corn might transform our intestinal bacteria into living pesticide factories, possibly for the *rest of our lives*.

Realizing that we may all have harmful bacteria in us from eating GMOs a long time ago, I set out to see how this could be healed, after we stop eating GMOs. Obviously, I have no way of knowing if the following is true, but I muscle tested various items, and I believe that Monolaurin would be beneficial in this case. It is made from coconut, and has even been reported to heal Lyme disease[17].

If you need someone to do a whole lot more scientific tests showing the whole picture of how dangerous GMOs are to humans, tests which cost hundreds of thousands of dollars, before you will believe that GMOs are a major cause of weight gain, and death, then you may be waiting a long time before you lose that weight and feel better. While many people now know that Monsanto's GMO crops provide a very real threat to both humans and the environment as a whole, the depth of Monsanto's corruption is often a less covered topic. It has been revealed by WikiLeaks that Monsanto not only has key figureheads stationed in powerful government positions inside the United States, but also has many, if not all, U.S. diplomats on their payroll[18]. Why would the government want this? Could it be because it solves their problem of having "borrowed" social security funds, by killing off old people?

In the bombshell report, the leaked cables reveal that **many U.S. diplomats work directly for Monsanto.** Furthermore, Monsanto also has powerful international people pushing their agenda.

Please, look after yourself. Read all labels. Realize that anything that is toxic, let alone as poisonous as GMOs, messes up your body and causes it to not work properly, and to keep more fat as a place to store toxins it can't deal with.

To get slim, and maybe even to stay alive, please do not eat anything that contains these words:

- Soy (some organic Soy Sauce or Tamari may be okay).
- Corn.
- Canola.
- Papaya (USDA organic is okay).
- Cottonseed.
- Zucchini and yellow squash (USDA organic is okay).
- Sugar (USDA organic is okay).
- Vitamins that have not been certified GMO free.

Eat ONLY USDA organic of the following:

- Eggs (make sure they are free-range as well).
- Dairy* (milk, cream, cheese, butter, yogurt, ice cream).

- Meat*, including poultry.

*With the introduction of GM alfalfa in 2012, even these may not be safe, because pollen from GM alfalfa goes anywhere.

Many products that you would not suspect are made from corn, which is likely GMO[19]. So don't eat foods containing these, unless they are organic & certified GMO free:

- Baking powder (baking soda is corn free).
- Caramel.
- Citric acid.
- Dextrin.
- Golden syrup.
- Maltodextrin.
- Vanilla extract.
- Xanthum gum.

If you eat fish or seafood, please make sure it is not farm raised. It must be ONLY wild caught. Unfortunately, some salmon that was labelled "wild caught" was found to be farm raised.

LATEST NEWS (1) – BEWARE GMO SALMON!

Currently at the time of going to print in early 2013, they are about to produce GMO salmon, called AquaAdvantage Salmon, for humans to eat. As with all genetically modified food, there will be no label that distinguishes this salmon from real salmon. The GM salmon has a growth hormone gene from the Chinook salmon, plus a gene from the eel-like ocean pout that *keeps the growth gene switched on*[20]! These Frankenfish grow twice as big and twice as fast as real salmon. The FDA's own testing showed that it caused increased allergies in humans[21], and yet they still approved it. Wait until people start eating fish with growth hormones that stay switched on forever. Think you've seen fat people? You haven't seen anything yet.

LATEST NEWS (2) – GMOS ARE KILLING BEES

While a few crops, such as corn and wheat, are pollinated by the wind, bees help pollinate more than 90 commercially grown field crops, citrus and other fruit crops, vegetables and nut crops[22], the very foods we need to stay thin and healthy. Keep that in mind as you read:

(1) The government destroyed ten years worth of research proving that Monsanto's roundup is killing the bees[23].

(2) Monsanto bought out the largest bee-research company, Beeologics, which was researching the link between GMOs and Colony Collapse Disorder, which is wiping out bees.

(3) There is a "super-bee patent[24]" for a GM bee that is "pesticide-resistant" – presumably one that can pollinate Monsanto GM foods without dying.

LATEST NEWS (3) - GMOS HAVE VIRUS GENES!

A virus gene that was 'missed' when GM food crops were first assessed, has been found in a massive 54 of 86 GM plants approved for food in the US, including corn and soy. Do you want to eat viruses? What do you think *eating viruses* will do to people? What does this virus do? No one knows! We need to work *with* nature, not mess it up.

All GMOs, including GM trees, need to be outlawed worldwide. [25],[26]. Let's follow the example of Hungary, that not only outlawed all GMOs, but destroyed the 1,000 acres of GMOs that they found growing[27].

LATEST NEWS (4) - MONSANTO PROTECTION ACT PASSES, MARCH 2013

Using the deceptive title of "Farmer Assurance Provision", Sec. 735 was inserted into the federal budget. This lets Monsanto grow what ever GMOs they wish, no matter what they do, and the government and the courts cannot do anything to stop them. Only the president himself can cancel this[28].

LATEST NEWS (5) - AUSTRALIA TO GROW GMO WHEAT, WHICH WILL KILL CHILDREN BEFORE FIVE YEARS OLD

Wheat is already toxic enough, without making it worse. The GM technology silences a gene which the liver needs, and could therefore kill children before they are five[29, 30].

LATEST NEWS (6) - GMO FLAX SEEDS FOUND IN 30 COUNTRIES

The GMO Flax seed came from Canada and is currently found mostly in Europe[31]. It was supposedly destroyed in 2001, but obviously that was not the case.

LATEST NEWS (7) – AMERICA PLANTS RICE WITH HUMAN GENES

The USDA has approved a petition by Ventria to plant up to 3,200 acres of GM rice with human genes in Kansas. The rice is being grown to make drugs. When people ingest this on purpose, or if it spreads into rice grown for food, does that make them cannibals?[32]

LATEST NEWS (8) – RICE IN 30 COUNTRIES IS CONTAMINATED WITH GM RICE

New evidence has emerged suggesting that the entire global supply of rice may have already been contaminated by unapproved, genetically modified rice manufactured by Bayer CropScience. A recent entry in the GM Contamination Register explains that between the years of 2006 and 2007, three different varieties of illegal GM rice, none of which were ever approved for cultivation or consumption anywhere in the world, were identified in more than 30 countries worldwide[33].

HOW TO GROW ALL THE FOOD WE NEED, WITHOUT GMOS

Corporations justify growing GMOs by saying that we need to use GMOs to combat world hunger. This is not true. First of all, most problems of hunger are more to do with distribution than lack of food production. Secondly, birth rates decline greatly wherever electricity and modernization is implemented[34]. Generally, the people who have large families are those without electricity, because they need children to help with survival. Recent research shows that while world population will max out at around 9 billion around 2070, thereafter it will start to fall. By 2200 it will be only around 3.5 billion people[35].

Thirdly, there are ways of growing tons of food which are healthy and high in minerals, and therefore more slimming, which are not currently used by most farmers yet. These methods can achieve record yields, for example, one farmer in India grew 22.4 tonnes of rice on 2.4 acres[36]. They can even grow food in the desert[37]! They work by working with, rather than against, nature. For further information please study:

- Permaculture.
- Biodynamics.
- Biointensive farming.
- SRI (System of Rice/Root Intensification)
- Methods described in *Secrets of the Soil* by Peter Tompkins.
- Methods described in *Back from the Brink*, by Peter Andrews.
- Acres USA magazine. www.acresusa.com.

Just imagine how much extra food there would be if everyone planted just one fruit, nut or olive tree.

FOR MORE INFORMATION ON GMO FOOD

I strongly urge you to watch the excellent, horrifying documentary, *The World According to Monsanto.*

REFERENCES

1. www.bionetonline.org/english/content/ff_cont6.htm
2. en.wikipedia.org/wiki/Monsanto
3. www.thegrocer.co.uk/topics/technology-and-supply-chain/monsanto-weedkiller-and-gm-maize-in-shocking-cancer-study/232603.article

4. www.momsacrossamerica.com/stunning_corn_comparison_gmo_versus_non_gmo

5. www.care2.com/causes/fattening-our-kids-on-gmo-foods.html

6. www.naturalnews.com/027931_GMO_crops_organ_damage.html

7. www.responsibletechnology.org/

8. www.sustainablebusiness.com/index.cfm/go/news.display/id/21828

9. www.cocopalmsugar.sch.ph/node/47

10. www.naturalnews.com/042175_glyphosate_dairy_cows_harmful_effects.html

11. www.organicconsumers.org/articles/article_24414.cfm

12. www.naturalnews.com/033838_breakfast_cereals_GMOs.html

13. www.salem-news.com/articles/april232010/gmfood-russia.php

14. healthimpactnews.com/2011/how-gmo-foods-are-destroying-your-gut-flora/

15. www.newswithviews.com/Smith/jeffrey125.htm

16. Netherwood et al, "Assessing the survival of transgenic plant DNA in the human gastrointestinal tract," *Nature Biotechnology* 22 (2004): 2.

17. www.inspirednutrition.com/3/3_Step_Natural_Answer_for_Lyme_Disease.html

18. mikesanubis.wordpress.com/2012/03/10/monsantos-blatant-corruption-gmo-crops-get-approved-faster-with-new-rule/

19. www.vishniac.com/ephraim/corn-bother.html

20. www.hcn.org/blogs/goat/fda-ruling-on-gmo-salmon-worries-alaska-fishermen

21. www.foodconsumer.org/newsite/Politics/Politics/gmo_salmon_0103120622.html

22. blog.targethealth.com/?p=58

23. www.naturalnews.com/035920_beekeeper_Illinois_raid.html#ixzz1vRmIgAPO

24. maryamhenein.tumblr.com/post/16471484566/the-buzz-behind-the-monsanto-beeolgics-acquisition

25. www.independentsciencenews.org/commentaries/regulators-discover-a-hidden-viral-gene-in-commercial-gmo-crops/

26. www.dailymail.co.uk/news/article-2266143/Uncovered-toxic-gene-hiding-GM-crops-Revelation-throws-new-doubt-safety-foods.html?ito=feeds-newsxml

27. www.planetsave.com/2011/07/21/hungary-destroys-all-monsanto-gmo-maize-fields/

28. www.wakingtimes.com/2013/03/24/senate-passes-monsanto-protection-act-granting-monsanto-power-over-us-govt/

29. www.naturalnews.com/037261_GM_wheat_liver_failure_fatalities.html

30. www.naturalnews.com/040759_GM_wheat_Australia_genetic_pollution.html

31. www.naturalnews.com/040924_GM_flax_GMO_contamination_flaxseed.html

32. www.naturalnews.com/021683_GM_rice_crops.html

33. www.naturalnews.com/041054_GM_rice_food_apocalypse_USDA.html#ixzz2Y19QDaAE

34. www.relfe.com/2009/world_population_growth_energy_solar_renewable_solution.html

35. www.slate.com/articles/technology/future_tense/2013/01/world_population_may_actually_start_declining_not_exploding.2.html

36. www.grist.org/food/miracle-grow-indian-farmers-smash-crop-yield-records-without-gmos/

37. *Greening the Desert*, Documentary by Geoff Lawton, 2001, www.youtube.com/watch?feature=player_embedded&v=xzTHjlueqFI#!!

CHAPTER 19

TOXIC FOOD #6
MEAT IS MAKING YOU FAT

Most people start to panic that they won't get enough protein when they learn that they can get thin and healthy by giving up eating meat. But consider this: A 20 year Harvard study of 120,000 people found that the five most fattening foods are:

- Potato chips.
- Potatoes.
- Sugar-sweetened drinks.
- *Red meat.*
- *Processed meat[1].*

Hmmm... that shows you that meat is not so thinning after all – in fact, it's very fattening. Consider this quote from an article that I was surprised to find on the American Heart Association website:

"Plant Foods Have a Complete Amino Acid Composition", by John McDougall, M.D. ...To wrongly suggest that people need to eat animal protein for nutrients will encourage them to add foods that are known to contribute to heart disease, diabetes, *obesity,* and many forms of cancer, to name just a few common problems[2]."

There are twenty-two amino acids needed by humans. They are all essential for health and fat loss. But only eight amino acids are called "essential" amino acids, because currently a lot of scientists believe that our body cannot manufacture these, and that we need to supplement them from the diet[3].

Currently, many people believe that they need to eat meat to get all the supposed "essential amino acids". If you are one of those people, the following information may come as a shock to you. The idea that we need to eat meat to get enough essential amino acids is an urban myth that is not based on science. The chart on the next page proves that this is false.

This chart is created from figures from the World Health Organization and FDA (Food and Drug Administration). The second row of the chart shows the amount of that essential amino acid that we need[4], [5]. The rest of the information is from figures from the USDA (U.S. Department of Agriculture[6]). They show that all plants - even lettuce - have more than enough protein for us! The essential amino acids are listed on the top row.

Protein does not make protein. Protein is made from amino acids. Plants have plenty of amino acids, as you can see from the graph. If you eat protein, your body has to break it down into amino acids, and then build them up again into new protein. It's a lot easier on the body to just build protein directly from amino acids from plants. Our body builds 50,000 different proteins[7], as well as 5,000 enzymes, from just 22 amino acids[8],[9].

If you think that you won't get enough protein if you don't eat meat and dairy, please stop and think about where this belief came from. Did it come from US nutritional guidelines that we have all been taught since school? Did you know that these guidelines are reformulated every five years? If they were not correct in the past, why should they be correct now?

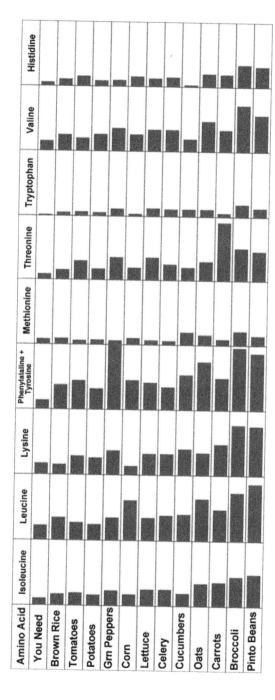

Essential amino acids - Human requirements, and availability in plants

Did you know that US nutritional guidelines are mainly decided by the U.S. Department of Agriculture (USDA)? They decide what food is fed to soldiers and to students, the same children who are now gaining weight every year. The truth is that the USDA is just an organization that works for farmers. Its goal is to make *as much money* as possible for farmers. That's all. Your health and waistline are not taken into consideration.

Dr. Neal Barnard M.D., Medical Researcher & President of Physicians Committee for Responsible Medicine discovered that six of the eleven people on the panel that has the audacity to tell you what you should eat, have direct financial relationships with the food industry. Dr. Barnard had this to say -

"You see government policy in action at school where children are given burgers, cheese and milk. Vegetables and fruit are harder to find. It has nothing to do with the health of the children. It has all to do with the financial health of big agribusiness[10]."

It is shocking for most people to learn that the truth is that human protein needs are actually *very small*. We don't need anywhere near as much protein as we have been lead to believe we do.

How do you know that? You can easily know what your true protein needs are by examining the protein content of human mother's milk. When we are babies we grow faster than at *any other time* in our lives. Therefore, this *should* be when we get the *greatest* concentration of protein. But -

"Breast milk contains a very small amount of protein! Breast milk contains only 2.5-3.5%, depending on the age of the baby[11] Some people estimate this amount at 1-6%".

Realize that even fruit contains roughly the same percentage of protein, on average 1-6%[12]

At the same time that a massive 40% of Americans are not just fat, but obese, degenerative diseases, such as diabetes and heart disease are growing at an alarming rate everywhere. This gives us another clue that it's not just calories that are the problem, it's *what* we are eating. We are told often that obesity causes health problems like heart disease. In fact, the people who spread this 'gospel' have it back-to-front. While obesity does make some degenerative diseases worse, it is not obesity which causes them. Instead, the truth is that the same things that cause degenerative diseases, are the same things that cause obesity.

Degenerative diseases are not ordinary diseases, in that they are not caused by a bug. You can't 'catch' a degenerative disease from anyone. A degenerative disease means that parts of the body have broken down to a great extent and don't work properly. Examples are diabetes, heart disease, Parkinson's disease, Multiple Sclerosis (MS), cancer, inflammatory bowel disease and arthritis. Growing fat is just another indicator of reduced health. When a body is healthy, it maintains an optimum amount of fat and muscle, all the time, just like wild animals do. Your body does not want to look after, and to lug around, all that extra weight.

But we have gone in the wrong direction because we have been brainwashed by agricultural companies who are in collusion with the government, and have taught us for decades that animal protein in the form of meat and dairy is good for us, as well as slimming (so long as it's low fat).

However, major new evidence has surfaced that proves that this is a lie. Some of the information which I am going to give to you comes from the very good documentary *Forks over Knives*, which I strongly urge you to watch.

The documentary centers around the work of two doctors, Dr. Colin Campbell Ph.D., one of the world's leading researchers in the field of diet and disease with Cornell University, and Dr. Caldwell Esselstyn M.D., a top surgeon and head of the Breast Cancer Task Force at the world-renowned Cleveland Clinic. Both of these doctors grew up on a farm. Like most people, both of them originally thought that eating meat and drinking milk was healthy and essential for humans.

But their studies and the results that they obtained eventually changed their minds, even though the animal-protein bias is a tough one to give up. They came to the conclusion that the opposite is true. That to get slim and healthy, all of us must have a whole-foods, plant-based diet, that is also low in packaged oils. (We still need raw, unprocessed oils from eating seeds and nuts).

That means to get thin you should have no, or very limited, meat, fish or dairy, or even eggs (I believe that occasional organic eggs are okay). You will learn in the chapter on dairy why dairy foods are fattening, as well as meat, *even if* they are low-fat, because it is the *protein* which our body considers toxic, and therefore fattening. That's right. Animal protein is a toxin to our bodies.

There is one thing that is missing from *Forks over Knives*. The words "whole-foods, plant based diet" appear to include whole grains. However, Denise Minger found that Dr. Campbell's conclusions were incomplete. Minger found that while the data showed that animal proteins cause obesity and cancer, wheat is an even bigger cause. For more information, please see the chapters on wheat and grains[13].

Forks over Knives concentrates mostly on healing degenerative diseases, such as diabetes and heart disease. But if you watch the DVD you will see how everyone who followed the advice of these two doctors not only healed their health problems, but also lost a lot of excess weight.

ANIMAL PROTEIN DESTROYS ENDOTHELIAL CELLS, WHICH LINE YOUR BLOOD VESSELS

Dr. Esselsytn explains that endothelial cells are the cells that line the veins and arteries. Endothelial cells are only one cell thick. When we are young, if all these cells are spread out, they cover *6-8 tennis courts*. But a diet based on animal protein is toxic to us, because it damages the endothelial cells. This is tragic because the endothelial cells are essential, because they make nitric oxide. Nitric oxide is essential to:

- Keep blood flowing smoothly.
- Dilate blood vessels during activity.
- Inhibit formation of plaque and inflammation.

When you kill endothelial cells from eating animal protein, the arteries harden. This is called plaque buildup or arteriosclerosis.

If you want to lose fat, don't you think it would be a good idea to have healthy blood vessels, where blood flows freely? Obviously, the answer is 'yes'. Unfortunately, older people on a western diet with animal protein tend to have reduced their 6-8 tennis courts' amount of endothelial cells, down to a paltry *one or two tennis courts*.

The good news is that, according to research by Dr. Esselstyn, when people switch to a whole-foods, plant-based diet (that is wheat-free), and low in processed oils, this trend is reversed. The endothelial cells repair themselves! No drugs or surgery will do this.

Here is more evidence that eating animal protein is making us fat. While waistlines have grown, so have the amounts of meat, dairy and processed food consumed by the average American. How does this make sense if animal protein is what we need to get thin?

MEAT

YEAR	LB PER PERSON.
Around 1900	120 LB.
2007	222 LB.

DAIRY

YEAR	LB PER PERSON.
1909	294 LB.
2006	605 LB.

Now, some people will argue that this just means that people are eating more, which means more calories, and that's all there is to it. This is partly true, but why are people eating more? It's partly because they are hungry, because when you eat food that is not what your body wants, it will keep on saying – more food! It can't tell you – "I want chlorophyll, minerals, vitamins, alkaline food and dozens of different micronutrients for my thousands of different chemical pathways!"

It's also because much of the food we eat creates an addiction. Did you ever hear of anyone being addicted to apples or celery?

Only a diet based on vegetables, fruits, nuts, seeds and soaked legumes will do the best job of reducing your hunger. That's because we are naturally plant-eaters. Even though we can be carnivores, we are not meant to be even omnivores. You can tell that by looking at our bodies. If we were wild animals we would eat only plants, like gorillas do.

For example, like other herbivores, we have a long, complex intestine. Carnivores, on the other hand, have a short, straight intestinal tract. That's because they want that rotting meat out of the body as fast as possible. This is not possible in our digestive tracts, which are long and very folded, and therefore obviously designed to digest plant material. That is why many people are constipated (which adds to weight) and have their intestines clogged up with meat that has been there for a long time. Here are more major comparisons, that show that biologically we are meant to eat only plants[14]:

Body Part	Carnivores	Omnivores	Herbivores	Humans
Teeth - Incisors	Short and Pointed	Short and Pointed	Broad, Flattened, Spade Shape	Broad, Flattened, Spade Shape
Teeth - Canines	Long, sharp and curved	Long, sharp and curved	Dull, short or none - Long ones for defense	Short and blunted
Teeth - Molars	Sharp	Sharp blades and/ or flat	Flattened with cusps	Flattened with cusps
Chewing	None. Swallows food whole	Swallows whole or simple crushing	*Extensive chewing necessary	*Extensive chewing necessary
Facial muscles	Reduced	Reduced	Well Developed	Well Developed
Jaw motion	Shearing. Minimal side-to-side motion	Shearing. Minimal side-to-side motion	No shear. Good side-to-side and front-to-back.	No shear. Good side-to-side and front-to-back.

Body Part	Carnivores	Omnivores	Herbivores	Humans
Saliva	No digestive enzymes	No digestive enzymes	Carbo-hydrate digesting enzymes	Carbo-hydrate digesting enzymes
Stomach acidity - with food in stomach	pH equal to, or less than, 1	pH equal to, or less than, 1	pH 4-5	pH 4-5
Length of small intestine	3-6 times body length	4-6 times body length	10-12 times body length	10-12 times body length
Colon	Simple, short, smooth	Simple, short, smooth	Long, complex	Long, with saclike ex-tensions
Kidney	Extremely concentrat-ed urine	Extremely concentrat-ed urine	Moderately concentrat-ed urine	Moderately concentrat-ed urine

(*The extensive chewing that is necessary for digesting plants brings a thought to mind. It's quite possible that we are meant to keep our wisdom teeth, the way that elephants do. Elephants have six sets of molars, so that they can get replacements throughout their life, from the wear and tear of chewing plants. Our teeth do the same as elephants – move down to the front as we wear them away, leaving room for new molars. I believe that wisdom teeth are meant to move down when we have made room for them.)

In fact, our bodies, teeth and digestive systems are very similar to those of chimpanzees and gorillas. Chimpanzees are almost totally vegan, and gorillas are 100% vegan. If you watch a gorilla eating in the wild, they eat tons and tons of green leaves (rather different from the piles of fruit they seem to get fed in zoos).

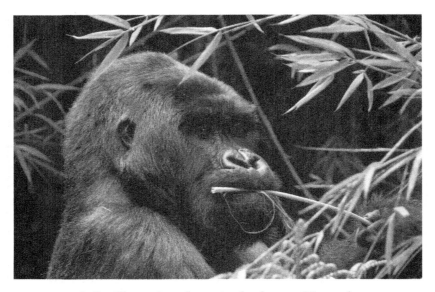

A Gorilla eating plants in the forest of Rwanda

Does a gorilla need a steak to gain more muscle? Apparently not. Gorillas have at least 6 times the strength of a human being[15], and the people at the Jane Goodall Institute in South Africa report that chimpanzees are also this strong.

At Yale, Professor Irving Fisher studied stamina and strength of three groups of men – meat-eating athletes, vegetarian athletes and vegetarian sedentary subjects. You may be shocked to learn that of the three groups compared, the meat eaters showed far less endurance than the vegetarians, even when the vegetarians were leading a sedentary life! Overall, the average score of the vegetarians was over *double* the average score of the meat-eaters, even though half of the vegetarians were sedentary people, and all of the meat-eaters were athletes[16].

Dr. John McDougall studied people on a sugar plantation in Hawaii, and also came to the conclusion that animal protein is the main cause of deadly diseases. He found that weight & health depended a lot on how long people had been in Hawaii and eating a western diet, with meat and dairy. The first generation of Hawaiians from Japan, Philippines, Korea and China were always trim, with no heart disease, cancer or arthritis. They ate only a whole-foods plant-based diet of rice and vegetables (Note: This diet was also wheat-free).

Their children, who had more meat and dairy, in the 80s and 90s, were a little fatter and a little sicker. And the grandchildren who continued to have more meat and dairy were just as fat and sick as anyone in America.

All three of these doctors concluded that most of our crippling conditions could be greatly reduced simply by eating a whole foods, plant-based diet. That is, eating non-refined (preferably), or minimally refined:

- Fruit.
- Vegetables.
- Nuts.
- Seeds.
- Legumes (beans and lentils).

And giving up:

- Animal based foods, such as meat and dairy.
- Processed foods.
- Oil.

The results also show that one should have no wheat, and minimal other grains.

Forks over Knives shows numerous people who switched from a normal western diet with meat, dairy and factory eggs, to a whole-foods, plant based diet, with low processed oil, under the supervision of different doctors. All of the people who needed to lose weight, lost a lot of weight and healed serious health problems. Including:

San'Dera Nation – Had hypertension and diabetes and was seriously overweight. After 20 weeks, she reduced by 45 pounds. After two months her blood pressure was wonderful, and her blood sugar was normal. She had reversed her diabetes! And she had lots of energy which she did not have before. Her message to herself was,

"Win the war. If you lose one battle, do not give in and quit. Get

right back on track, right now."

Joey Aucoin – Went from 220 pounds to 180 pounds in 8 weeks. His big clothes no longer fit him. In addition, he was originally taking 9 pills and giving himself 2 injections each day. He gave up all medications (which caused problems from detoxing for a while). This saved him over $800 in 4 months (more evidence as to why you won't hear the Medical Mafia telling you about why you should give up meat and dairy). After 22 weeks, 26 out of 27 health complaints that he had were healed. Plus he then felt really good, like he had *never* felt in his life before.

Lee Fulkerson – Reduced weight on this plan, even though he was eating more often. He reduced fat from his face, neck and belly, and got more energy. He also gave up coffee, which as you will see in my chapter on caffeine, also helps permanent fat loss.

The documentary also shows an interesting piece with Rip Esselstyn, the son of Dr. Esselstyn. Rip was a plant-based professional triathlete, who went on to become a firefighter. He tells the story of how in Austin, Texas it's considered 'manly' to eat meat. One day the firefighters had a bet to see who had the lowest cholesterol. They were shocked to find that one of their firefighters, James Ray, had a cholesterol level of 344, which meant that James could have dropped dead at any moment. In fact, while firefighters look, and have to be, super fit, to carry all that gear up as many as 20 flights of stair, 52% of firefighters die, not from fires, but from heart disease, in the line of duty.

So all the firefighters, as a show of solidarity, and to save James's life, went on a plant-based diet. Within just three weeks James's cholesterol dropped to just 148 points, nearly half the original reading.

If you think that you need animal protein to build muscle, and that there is not enough protein in a plant-based diet, you really should watch *Forks over Knives,* and watch this hugely muscular man, Rip Esselstyn, climb UP the fireman's pole all the way to the high first floor, with arms only, no legs(!), saying over and over:

"REAL MEN EAT PLANTS. REAL MEN EAT PLANTS. REAL MEN EAT PLANTS"

Pam Popper N.D. explains in *Forks over Knives* how at the Wellness Forum in Columbus, Ohio, they have a lot of young people come to them who have only one thing wrong with their health, and that is excess weight. And once they go on a whole foods, plant based diet without toxins, they achieve a normal weight, at the same time that their energy, complexion and ability to think improves.

MASSIVE STUDY IN CHINA

Massive evidence that meat and dairy cause health problems was shown in the *Atlas of Cancer Mortality in China*, printed in 1981. In this study, 880 million people were studied in every county in China, by a massive 650,000 researchers. While all the people were genetically the same, some areas of China had 400 times the levels of cancer mortality as others did.

Dr. Campbell & Dr. Junshi Chen Ph.D.[17], looked at 367 different variables that could have caused these massive differences. It took years to analyze the data. They studied 94,000 correlations between diet and disease. From this they came to one simple conclusion: That a diet based on animal products caused disease, and that a diet based on whole plant-foods caused health. (Note: The data also shows that people must also give up all wheat[18]). Obesity is part of disease. Being slim is part of health. Here are some quotes from the movie:

Dr. Campbell: "I know of nothing else in medicine that can come *close* to what a plant-based diet can do. I can say this with confidence. Our national authorities are squirreling this concept from the national conversation, in order to *protect the status quo*. I really believe if everyone would do this, we could cut healthcare costs by 70-80%. That's amazing."

Dr. Terry Mason M.D.: "You can eat yourself into poor health and early death, or you can eat yourself into good health and a long healthy life. And that road is on a plant-centered dietary pattern."

In fact, overconsumption of animal protein presents a far greater threat to our health than not getting enough. This is partly because animal protein is acidic, and our bodies need to be alkaline to be thin and healthy. A body that has too much protein is too acidic and too toxic. The truth is, it's practically impossible to not get enough protein, and actual cases of protein deficiency are almost nonexistent in our culture.

When people say "I'm craving protein", often what they are really craving are good fats, because good fats are essential for our brains and nerves.

Also, I do believe that one day science will find that there is something addictive to eating meat. It may seem a crazy thought, but maybe we get addicted to the hormones and energy that are associated with the extreme terror an animal feels when it is killed. Animals know what's coming at the abattoir. For example, when one pig screams when its throat is cut, they ALL start screaming. The noise must be something quite devastating to experience.

MEAT ANIMALS ARE FED FRIGHTENING STUFF

Are you imagining that the cow, pig or chicken you ate was grazing on a lovely, green pasture before it had its throat cut? That only happened a long time ago. Now, animals are raised in cruel factories, and are fed, in addition to genetically modified corn, soy and alfalfa, animal feed that is partly composed of the products from rendering plants, an invisible industry which is worth billions of dollars worldwide.

One estimate states that 40 billion pounds a year of slaughterhouse waste like hooves, eyeballs, brains, bone and animal guts, as well as supermarket waste, and even in some states euthanized dogs and cats, are rendered every year for animal feed[19]. Only half of a cow and one third of a pig gets used for people to eat. The rest gets used for something, including crayons, makeup, shampoo and soap[20]. A lot also goes into animal feed, because it's cheap, and there would be a massive health problem if you put it all in landfills.

Inspectors of animal feed check only for things like protein content.

They seldom if ever check for levels of poisons. Cows, pigs and chickens are no longer vegetarians. They have been forced to be carnivores. Eating a carnivore is a bad idea, because toxins get concentrated the higher up the food chain you go.

Unfortunately, it gets even worse. There are reports, which I find hard to discount, that in order to keep costs down, workers don't always remove the plastic wrapping or styrofoam from the rotten supermarket meat. In it goes, along with the plastic garbage bags that the dead pets came in from the vet and animal shelters. Same with the flea collars on the dead dogs. And since the euthanized cats and dogs were killed with a poison, you can end up eating that as well.

It gets worse the more you research this. For example, the latest report says that chickens are fed over *twenty* drugs including *Prozac*[21]!

No wonder that the breast milk of vegetarian women has only 1-2% of the pesticide contamination that is the national average for breast-feeding women on a flesh-centered diet[22]. This is a shockingly high difference. If you absolutely insist on eating meat at some time, it absolutely *must* be organic. Please watch the excellent documentary *Food Inc.* and you will see the absolute necessity for this. For example, they show that meat is so contaminated now with E.Coli, that they have to treat it with *ammonia*! But note what Dr. Campbell said in *Forks over Knives*, that it's not just about the quality of the food. Animal protein creates problems that plant protein does not.

PROTEIN AND THE AMINO ACID "CONSPIRACY"

- We need a lot less protein than we have been lead to believe.

- Protein does not make protein. Protein is made from amino acids. Plants have plenty of amino acids. If you eat protein, your body has to break it down into amino acids, and then build new protein later on. It's a lot easier to just build protein directly from plant amino acids.

- According to the Max Planck Institute, cooking destroys about half of the protein. You can eat raw plants, but not raw meat.

- Plants have all the protein that you need, in the form of amino acids. Plus a whole lot of other nutrition and a lot less toxins.

Unlike what some people believe, it is not necessary for all eight of the essential amino acids to be present in one food or even within one meal in order to obtain our full protein needs. The body has its own amino acid pool to draw from, to supply amino acids which may be missing from dietary sources. This fact is proven by observing patients after lengthy fasts who exhibited not a protein deficiency, but a restored protein balance.

If you have a lot of variety of plants in your diet, you will have all the amino acids you need, all the time.

"Adding fruits and vegetables to a low-fat diet lessens abdominal obesity, lowers glucose, insulin, blood pressure and weight ....The same low-fat diet without fruit and vegetables (did not). In one study, subjects on a diet of micronutrient-rich ... reduced central obesity 80% more than those on a non-micronutrient diet[23]."

IT'S REALLY MEAT THAT'S INCOMPLETE!

When you think about it, it's ridiculous to single out protein as *the* nutrient we need, because it's just one of the dozens of nutrients your body needs. Why aren't we declaring meat to be an incomplete vitamin? Because it is. For example, beef is completely devoid of Vitamin C, an essential nutrient without which you'd die. And beef doesn't just have a lower level of this essential nutrient, it has *zero*.

No combination of meat will make a complete vitamin, since every single kind of meat has zero Vitamin C. And it's deficient in other vitamins as well. So while plants *aren't* actually deficient in protein, meat is *definitely* deficient in vitamins. But I'm sure you never heard about vitamin deficiency in animal foods. All you've heard about is the supposed deficiency of protein in plants.

I will give more information on the "perfect protein" myth in the chapter on raw food.

NO SEAFOOD

Fish and other seafood is just about as bad as meat, because it is still animal protein, and nowadays fish has its own set of problems including:

- Dr. Mercola reported that mercury is present in nearly all fish[24]. There is no safe level of mercury. This includes both salt and fresh-water fish. Some fish, such as tuna, are carnivores, and therefore have higher concentrations of toxins, including mercury.

- There are numerous reports of radiation contamination in Pacific seafood, from the Fukushima disaster in Japan.

- Seafood from the Gulf of Mexico is contaminated from the BP oil disaster and the poisonous dispersant Corexit, and will be contaminated for decades if not centuries[25].

- Fish fraud is off the scale these days. A new two-year study by the non-profit group Oceana found that one-third of fish in restaurants, supermarkets and sushi was consistently mislabeled wherever they looked[26]. For example, pricey wild-caught Alaskan salmon can be farmed Atlantic salmon from Chile, and therefore it could be fed any amount of GMOs and other toxins. The same study found that 55 of 66 white tuna samples from sushi restaurants turned out to be escolar, an eel-like fish. While it supposedly tastes good, it's obviously toxic, because it contains an oil that can cause diarrhea and gastrointestinal distress for several days.

AGEs AGE YOU

If you need more convincing to give up on eating meat and fish, then please keep up to date on the latest research about AGEs (Advanced Glycation End Products). AGEs age you. They also cause a huge number of health problems including joint problems, stiff arteries, dementia, eye problems, arthritis and serious complications that arise from diabetes, such as blindness.

The foods richest in AGEs are animal products (e.g. meat and cheese) and especially those heated to *high temperatures*. Broiling or frying increases AGE content by over *1,000 times*. Plus the longer you cook, the more AGEs you get. Therefore, it is a great shame that the government promotes meat-eating, by subsidizing it with taxpayers money. You will see how they do this in the *Food Inc.* documentary. 30% of the land base in the USA is under corn (mostly GMO corn), which is super cheap *only* because of money from the government. That is, taxpayers are paying for massive, cruel factory farms where animals are fed corn, not grass, and which keep the price of meat artificially low.

I digress again – back to the production of AGEs from cooking. You can eat raw plants, but you can't eat raw meat. Correction – it is physically possible, but not advisable, because it's a perfect way to get a host of parasites. I was horrified when I saw a travel documentary where the travel expert Rick Steves ate a raw beef dish in a restaurant in France. Just because the French have a reputation for being gourmet does not mean they should not question what they eat.

Please, question everything. Who benefits financially from telling you what you should eat? Is there a better way?

It can be hard for a while to give up eating meat, I know. I used to eat it, but only because my parents taught me to do that. But it's time to end this cycle. I am so glad that I did give up meat over a decade ago, and you will too. It helped me to give it up by thinking how when I ate meat, I was ingesting the fear and terror that the animal experienced when it was killed. If you still won't give up eating meat, please go and visit an abattoir, or look for videos on www.youtube.com, to see and feel what it is like for the animals to be killed, as well as to be kept in factories that are pure torture for their whole life.

A plant diet, without wheat and limited grains, will get you the body and health you want, while keeping you free of hunger. That is, a diet made of vegetables, fruits, nuts, seeds and soaked legumes (that are non-GMO). It is especially good for you the more you include *raw* fruit, vegetables, nuts, seeds and sprouted legumes, in your diet, as I will discuss in the chapter on raw food.

REFERENCES

1. *Woman's World*, 1/30/12, page 18

2. circ.ahajournals.org/content/105/25/e197.full

3. Young VR (1994). "Adult amino acid requirements: the case for a major revision in current recommendations". *J. Nutr.* 124 (8 Suppl): 1517S–1523S PMID 064412. jn.nutrition.org/cgi/reprint/124/8_Suppl/1517S.pdf.

4. Protein and Amino Acid Requirements in Human Nutrition (PDF), World Health Organization (2002). Recommendations on p. 126. Recommendations are an "average requirement" of 0.66 g of protein per kg of ideal body weight, and a "safe level" of 0.86 g/kg.

5. Dietary Reference Intakes for Energy, Carbohydrate, Fiber, Fat, Fatty Acids, Cholesterol, Protein, and Amino Acids, Food and Drug Administration, Institute of Medicine of the National Academies, 2005. (Protein Estimated Average Requirement and RDA for adults is 0.66 and 0.8g per kg of ideal body weight, respectively. These are married to the daily energy requirements listed in the same report for various genders, ages, heights, weights, and activity levels, to get the range of percentage of calories from protein.)

6. USDA National Nutrient Database for Standard Reference (accessed August to December 2009). FRUIT: Average of Apples, Pears, Grapes, Bananas, Plums, Oranges, Grapefruit, Watermelon, Strawberries, Peaches, Nectarines, Cantaloupe. VEGETABLES: Average of Broccoli 27.2%, Carrots 8.7%, Celery 17.3%, Corn 13.4%, Cucumber 17.3%, Green Beans 21.6%, Lettuce iceberg 25.7%, Mushrooms white 31%, Onions 12.4%, Peas 28.8%, Potato 10.8%, Spinach 49.7%, Tomato 19.6% (accessed December 2009). Analysis is for each individual food all supplying calorie needs (closest to the "low active" category for a 5'11" 181lb. 25BMI male, as per the FDA).

7. www.innovateus.net/health/how-many-proteins-exist-human-body

8. en.wikipedia.org/wiki/Amino_acid

9. www.libertyzone.com/hz-Amino-Acid.html *Forks Over Knives* documentary

10. www.living-foods.com/rawgourmet/newsnov99.htm Different texts offer different percentage numbers. These numbers are derived from lectures at Hippocrates Health Institute in Florida.

11. rawschool.com/raw-food-basics/#proteincalcium

12. *Wheat Belly*, William Davis M.D., 2011, page 160-164

13. michaelbluejay.com/veg/natural.html

14. www.seaworld.org/animal-info/info-books/gorilla/physical-characteristics.

htm

15. Fisher, Irving: "The influence of Flesh Eating on Endurance", *Yale Medical Journal*, 13(5):205-22,1907.

16. Senior Research Professor at the Chinese Center for Disease Control and Prevention

17. rawfoodsos.com/the-china-study/

18. www.jainworld.com/jainbooks/images/20/Recycling_of_Slaughterhouse. htm

19. www.bornfreeusa.org/articles.php?p=378&more=1

20. www.huffingtonpost.com/michael-greger-md/antibiotics-chicken_b_1470098.html

21. *New England Journal of Medicine* (quote from "Rainbow Green Live-Food Cuisine" by Gabriel Cousens, M.D.)

22. *The Magnesium Factor*, Midred Seeling M.D., page 108

23. articles.mercola.com/sites/articles/archive/2009/09/29/warning-new-ev-idence-shows-that-mercury-present-in-nearly-all-fish.aspx

24. www.activistpost.com/2013/03/voices-from-gulf-do-not-eat-our-food-pt. html

25. www.usatoday.com/story/news/nation/2013/02/20/fish-seafood-fraud-common-oceana-report/1927065/

CHAPTER 20

TOXIC FOOD #7
DAIRY:
DO YOU WANT TO LOOK LIKE A COW?

Did you know that cheese is addictive? If you have found it hard to give up cheese, you are not alone. Dr. Neal Barnard in the documentary *Super Size Me* explains how cheese is filled with substances called casomorphins, that act like opiates! That is, cheese affects you, and addicts you, as if it was a drug.

Here's one example of this; *Woman's world* magazine tells the story of Molly who lost 170 pounds and 12 dress sizes so that she could finally look good in a bikini. She made this comment about a time in her life after she lost the first 110 pounds from eating healthier meals,

> "I read in a book that eliminating dairy might be a good idea. I was hesitant, because I felt addicted to cheese. But I gave it a shot." Molly says her lifelong tummy troubles disappeared instantly. "And those last 60 pounds just flew off me."

We are told that it is good to drink milk, so long as we drink low-fat milk, if we have weight problems, because supposedly we need all that animal protein. Once again, I am sorry to say that you have been lied to by the Food Mafia.

The brilliant documentary *Forks Over Knives* showed two amazing discoveries by Dr. Campbell. First, from studies in the field in the Philippines, Dr. Campbell found that children from poorer families with less animal based protein were healthier than children from affluent families. He then studied the effect of the main protein in milk (casein) on rodents and found casein levels of 20% *turn cancer cells on.* 5% levels of casein turn cancer cells *off.*

Dr. Campbell was able to make these levels go up and down again, purely by changing diet, within three weeks. Most importantly, a 20% protein level from plants did *not* promote cancer.

He concluded that animal protein is really good at turning cancer on. While he was not looking directly at weight gain, this shows us how animal protein is toxic to our bodies. And since we know that it's toxins, not calories, which are the main cause of obesity, we can see why the growing consumption of dairy, whether or not it's low fat, goes along with increasing fat gain.

Year	Pounds of dairy products consumed per person
1909	294 lb.
2006	605 lb

DAIRY PROTEINS CAUSE DIABETES

Secondly, Dr. Campbell found that dairy products are a major cause of diabetes in the US. If your insulin is messed up, it's going to be easier to gain fat. Dr. Campbell says that while we have been conditioned to think that too much carbohydrate in the blood causes diabetes, in countries like China, Japan, Cambodia and Thailand, the people there have a very high carbohydrate and low fat diet, and they have the lowest diabetes rates in the world.

Dr. Campbell explains how the body recognizes the proteins in cow's milk as *foreign protein.* After all, cows are a different species from us. It's not human milk. And we are meant to be weaned in any case. The body makes antibodies to destroy the foreign proteins. These same antibodies then *destroy the insulin producing cells* in the pancreas, which means that person then has type II Diabetes.

Damaging insulin production can easily lead to fat gain, since insulin is central to regulating carbohydrate and fat metabolism. If you mess up the original design, you are going to have problems. Is a car going to run properly if part of the engine is faulty? No. For example, one way that diabetes could make a person fat is because excessive appetite is a symptom of diabetes. Instead, you want your body to function properly, to decrease your appetite.

We have been conditioned to thinking that milk is the "perfect food" by the dairy industry. That's because $180 million are spent each year in the U.S. to convince you of that[1]. They do that to sell 180 billion pounds of their product every year. How much money do you think is spent telling you that, say, fresh juice or raw spinach and carrots will make you thinner and healthier, without all the bad effects from drinking milk?

Fresh raw cows' milk, which is the healthiest to drink, is fairly toxic to adult humans. Pasteurized is more toxic. Homogenized ('ultra-pasteurized') milk is very toxic, *whether or not* it's organic. And homogenized milk from cows fed GMO corn, soy and alfalfa, which most are, is super toxic. And this is true, whether it's organic or not. As Dr. Campbell said in *Forks Over Knives;*

> "The protein is the same whether organic or not. It is not the difference in the quality of the food (that counts), it is the kind of food that it is."

How would you like to have a glass of nice cold camel milk? No? How about zebra milk? Maybe raccoon milk? You see, there is no particular reason why we chose cows to produce milk for us, other than that they are docile. We are the only animal that drinks milk from another species.

The chemical composition of milk is very different from species to species. Plus, we are the only animal that drinks milk way past weaning age. This has contributed to many problems, including obesity, diabetes and even lack of intelligence for several reasons.

You see, a cow's milk has everything in it to help a young calf grow into an adult within two years, that weighs around 1,000 pounds. Is that the kind of chemical messages you want in your food? Even if it's raw milk, which is the best choice, it is not going to help you to get thin. It's not even good for infants because it is very deficient in iron.

Human milk, on the other hand, has 6-10 times more essential fatty acids than cows' milk. Essential fatty acids are essential for brain development, and for keeping us thin. Before we had the fat-epidemic, humans used to breast feed most babies. I am not saying that non-human milk is the only cause of the obesity epidemic, but it is certainly one of the causes.

In five years after 1988, 2,700 articles about milk did not mention *any* health benefits. Instead they reported how it causes major health problems[2] including:

- Allergic reactions.
- Anemia.
- Arthritis.
- Asthma.
- Bed-wetting in children.
- Diabetes.
- Heart disease.
- Intestinal bleeding.
- Intestinal colic.
- Intestinal irritation.
- Leukemia & cancer.
- Tonsillitis.

Over 50 years ago, cows produced 2,000 pounds of milk a year. Now they produce up to 50,000 pounds a year! This was not done by natural means. Genetically Modified Bovine Growth Hormone (rBGH) was one of the causes of this increase. To learn how terrible this stuff is, see the excellent documentary *The World According to Monsanto*. Do you really want a *growth* hormone in your food? Organic milk won't have these extra hormones, but it still has natural growth hormones, telling the calf to grow *very large*, very quickly.

The USDA allows milk to contain up to 1/30 of an ounce of white blood cells. I am sorry to have to say this, but another word for white blood cells is pus.

Some people will say that you should drink goat's milk instead, but please note that no animal drinks milk once it is an adult, or from another species. Whatever the species, the body recognizes the milk proteins as foreign protein. So it makes antibodies to destroy the foreign proteins, but these same antibodies then also destroy its own insulin-producing cells.

ALLERGIES

Dr. Keith Scott-Mumby, author of *Diet Wise*, estimates that 80% of us are allergic to dairy and / or wheat. Anything that you are allergic to, will often cause weight gain.

In addition, if you have children who have any kind of negative behavior, because dairy allergies often affect the brain, I suggest that you have them go totally dairy-free for at least three weeks and note the results. (They should also give up the toxic foods discussed in this book, including meat, wheat, sugar, high fructose corn syrup, MSG, microwaved food, aspartame and caffeine. Please see the chapters on these to learn why). Write the results down so you remember them. If the results are really noticeable, then consider removing dairy completely from the family diet, to keep everyone calmer, as well as slim.

WHAT WOULD YOU DO WITH $20 MILLION?

Well, you could buy one million kidnapped children working as slaves in Africa to grow cocoa for chocolate companies, and set them free (www.FreeTheSlaves.net). Or you could give clean drinking water to 670,000 women and children who currently walk six miles a day to get really filthy water, which is all they have (donate to www.WaterAid.org / www.WaterAidAmerica.org).

Or, if you were the US government, you would use it for rent, to store dried milk powder that no one wants, but was purchased by tax-payers to bail out the dairy industry, and has to go somewhere[3].

If you don't think that the government brainwashes people into eating dairy products, consider what Dr. Neal Barnard has to say in *Forks over Knives*. After submitting a Freedom of Information request, he discovered that in the year 2000 there was a conference where the dairy industry and the US Federal government worked on how to produce a cheese *craving*. Another word for 'craving', is 'addiction'. Why would people in the government, who are meant to be our servants, purposely do that? (Follow the money). The conference was a success. A strategy was devised and put into effect whereby Wendy's fast food outlets (I cannot call them a restaurant) promoted the cheddar-lovers' bacon cheese burger. Similar promotions then followed at Pizza Hut, Subway, Taco Bell and Burger King.

One hundred years ago, when people were slim, the average American ate less than 4 pounds of cheese a year. In 2009 that average sky-rocketed to 32 pounds! And remember that averages don't mean much, because since people on a plant-based diet aren't eating cheese, someone else is getting their share.

Lactose, the main carbohydrate in milk, is toxic to most people. This is why even skim milk is fattening. Nature gives only babies the ability to metabolize lactose. We lose this ability around 4-5 years, which is the age that children should be weaned at, after they have all their teeth, which are an essential part of digestion. In my opinion, nature is telling us to not have any milk at all, even skimmed milk, after five years old.

WHAT ABOUT CALCIUM?

While there are literally hundreds of different vitamins, minerals, essential fatty acids and other nutrients that science is only just now starting to discover, all we ever hear about is calcium. That's because calcium is just about the only good thing in milk. So, if you don't get calcium from milk, where do you get it? From the same place that cows do, from plants. In fact, *all* whole foods contain calcium[4].

But did you know that excessive amounts of dairy food actually *interfere* with calcium absorption? This is because dairy foods contain a lot of phosphorus which combines with calcium in the intestines, and prevents you from absorbing it[5]. You can't determine how much calcium you are having, purely by how much you are eating or drinking. There are many other factors involved. Ultimately, it is not nature's design for children to drink non-human milk, or for adults to drink any milk, and things get messed up when we go against nature's design.

We have been told by the dairy industry that osteoporosis has been linked to a lack of calcium, in order to scare us into buying their products. If this is true, countries with a western diet and high dairy consumption should have low osteoporosis. But, according to a Harvard researcher, nations with the highest levels of calcium intake have the highest level of hip fractures[6]!

Daily Calcium Consumption	Countries	Number of hip fractures per 100,000 people / per year
Low (500 mg / day)	Singapore Hong Kong	Under 30
Medium	Holland, Finland	40 - 60
High (1000 mg / day)	USA, UK, NZ	60 - 100

How does more calcium create more osteoporosis? Dairy creates acid conditions in the body. To combat acid, the body calls upon an acid buffer to protect it. That buffer is calcium in our bones. So it removes the calcium in our bones to neutralize the acid condition (This would apply to other acid causing foods as well, such as meat, grains and caffeine).

A diet made of vegetables, fruits, nuts, seeds and soaked legumes, especially with a lot of raw food, on the other hand, creates alkaline conditions in the body, that the body likes. Therefore, the calcium is left where it belongs, in the bones.

WHAT ABOUT PROTEIN?

This is usually the first question that people ask. Most of us have been raised with the notion that a lot of protein is good for us, because money for the meat and dairy industries depend on you thinking that. But, think of this; if we need lots of protein, when should we need it the most? When we are a baby. There is no other time in the life of a person when growth is so dramatic. The infant will triple or quadruple in weight in its first year, and needs more protein to grow than at any other time in its entire life span. And just how much protein is in mothers' milk, the perfect food for the growing baby? The amount of protein in mothers' milk is 2.5 to 3.5 per cent[7] (Some people estimate this amount at 1-6%).

Compare that to the amount of protein in cow milk at 30%. A baby cow needs to gain hundreds of pounds of mass in its first year, while it's relatively small brain does not need to grow very much. If the amazing growth in the first year of life is beautifully served by the amount of protein in mothers' milk, why would any human being ever need more? The answer is, he/she does not need more protein than that.

In fact, most of us have too much protein. Balance is necessary for getting thin. Protein is acidic and your kidneys have to process the excess, rather than deal with the stored toxins in your fat cells.

In the *Forks Over Knives* documentary you will see Mac Danzig, a plant-based fighter champion. He gave up dairy when he was 18 years old, and after he gave up chicken and fish, he has more energy and recovers better between workouts.

PASTEURIZED MILK

Pasteurized milk is heated milk. Dairy producers started pasteurizing milk so that they could store it longer. We were told that this was to make us healthier, by destroying bacteria, but the more you cook something, and the hotter you cook it, the less healthy it gets. This is because cooking destroys 50% of protein, and damages vitamins and minerals[8].

What pasteurization really did was make farmers able to have less healthy cows, because it no longer mattered if the milk they produced contained a lot of bacteria.

HOMOGENIZED MILK

However, today's milk is not just pasteurized, it's also homogenized, which is a lot worse. If you can't see cream on the top of the bottle in a separate layer from the milk, it's homogenized. When milk is homogenized, it is passed through a fine filter at pressures equal to 4,000 pounds per square inch. How natural is that? This makes the fat globules at least ten times smaller[9]. This enables them to travel into areas of your body that they would not normally be able to get to!

GENETICALLY MODIFIED DAIRY

We now face two big added toxins in our dairy, in the form of genetically modified organisms:

- rBGH – Recombinant Bovine Growth Hormone.

- GMO corn, soy and alfalfa, which is fed to dairy cows. You get the poisons second hand.

BOVINE GROWTH HORMONE

In addition to getting fatter, girls in the U.S. are beginning to menstruate at younger and younger ages. According to the Cancer Prevention Coalition, some girls are now experiencing the effects of puberty as young as three years of age. Something is clearly wrong. Here's a major reason for this: Bovine Growth Hormone (BGH) occurs naturally in cows' milk. It tells the calf to *grow* big and quickly. BGH in milk has been shown to create a host of problems[10].

However, recombinant BGH (rBGH) is even worse. It is a genetically engineered hormone which is given to cows. It is produced by Monsanto, the same company that made DDT, Agent Orange and aspartame. 80-90% of U.S. dairy food is contaminated with rBGH. Since 1994, every industrialized country in the world except the U.S has banned rBGH milk.

GENETICALLY MODIFIED POISONS ARE IN DAIRY

Genetically Modified Organisms (GMOs) are food plants that are made to either *drink* poison, or *produce* poison, by inserting the genes from another species, often a bacteria, into the plant. They are rightly called frankenfoods.

Dairy cows are fed GMO corn, soy and alfalfa, as well as injected with dangerous genetically modified Bovine Growth Hormone (rBGH). Genetically modified alfalfa was introduced into the food supply in 2005[11]. You will be eating it second hand if you have non-organic dairy products. Even dairy will not be safe forever, because pollen from alfalfa goes everywhere.

If you must have some dairy, it must be organic, just to keep the GMOs out. Or from a country that does not feed GMOs to cows or give them rBGH.

ORGANIC YOGURT MIGHT BE OKAY

Having said all this, there is one dairy food that might possibly be slimming, so long as you make sure it's organic and that it doesn't have any sugar or artificial sweeteners in it. A 20 year Harvard study of 120,000 people said that yogurt was the most slimming food, followed by nuts, fruit, whole grains and vegetables. I believe that seeds would have been on this list, but were probably not considered, since so few people eat them. The most fattening foods were potato chips, potatoes, sugar-sweetened drinks, red meat and processed meat[12]. (A hamburger with French fries and a Coke have all of these). Just as I am saying in this book, they found that calories were not as important as what was eaten.

Add your own raw honey, fruit and seeds. However, I would not recommend organic yogurt if you know you are allergic to dairy. This is a strange anomaly which appears to be conflicting data, since it is the protein in milk which causes problems, and yogurt has protein in it. It is possible that the good bacteria in yogurt have changed the milk sufficiently that it becomes okay for us, and that the good bacteria in the yogurt replenishes the intestines with good bacteria so well that it makes up for the toxins from the animal protein. Taking a good probiotic supplement like iFlora could be a better alternative.

TAKE THE CHALLENGE - GO DAIRY FREE

On TV I saw videos of children at school drinking their homogenized milk, along with pizzas covered in embalmed meat (pepperoni). No wonder we have a growing problem with obesity, as well as emotional problems. Because a toxic body is not a happy body.

Do you want to look like a cow? If so, have more dairy. But if you would like to be thin, then give up dairy, including organic dairy. Be like many people who have had great reduction in fat and body size by going dairy free, by eating a whole-foods plant-based diet, that is free of wheat, soy and other toxins.

A good alternative to milk for adults and older children is almond milk. The only milk that babies should have is mother's breast milk, from a mother who eats healthy food, otherwise the toxins in the mother's food get passed on to the baby.

To learn more about how fattening and unhealthy dairy products are, I recommend the website www.NotMilk.com.

Remember what Dr. Campbell said in *Forks Over Knives*:

"Even plants with little protein, such as 8% in potatoes, have as much protein as we need. There is no one nutrient you need. Nutrition is a symphony of hundreds of thousands of chemicals, that must all work together."

LATEST NEWS: As of time of going to press in mid 2013, the dairy industry has shown how evil they truly are. They are currently asking the FDA to allow them to add the fattening poison, aspartame, to milk products *without labeling*[13].

REFERENCES

1. Not Milk: The USDA, Monsanto, and the U.S. Dairy Industry, 2002. www.alternet.org/story/13557
2. www.notmilk.com/kradjian.html
3. www.notmilk.com/forum/965.html
4. Forks Over Knives, documentary
5. Don't Drink Your Milk, 1996 by Dr Frank Oski, M.D.
6. Forks Over Knives documentary
7. www.living-foods.com/rawgourmet/newsnov99.htm. Different texts offer different percentage numbers. These numbers are derived from lectures at Hippocrates Health Institute in Florida.
8. Rainbow Green Live-Food Cuisine, 2003, by Dr Gabriel Cousens, M.D.
9. www.notmilk.com/deb/022199.html
10. www.alternet.org/story/13557/?page=3
11. www.naturalnews.com/036023_Monsanto_GM_alfalfa_USDA.html
12. Woman's World Magazine, 1/30/12, page 18
13. www.cnsenvironmentallaw.com/2013/02/22/1725.htm

CHAPTER 21

TOXIC FOOD #8
BAD FATS MAKE YOU FAT
GOOD FATS MAKE YOU THIN

Strange as it may seem, part of the reason why we have increasing obesity around the world is because of the "war on fat." By "fat" I mean "fats and oils". It is true that most of the fats we consume are very fattening, because most of the fats and oils we eat are toxic. But not all fats are fattening. We absolutely, positively *need* some fats, the good fats, for us to live and function and to *be thin*. For example:

- 60% of your brain is made of fats. Half of these are saturated fats. You must have fat or you die.

- Nerves need fats to function. Obviously, your body can't function or burn fat if your brain and nerves aren't working properly.

- The cell walls of the body are 50% made of saturated fats, and need fat to work properly[1].

In addition, fat is needed in other parts of the body to work properly, including your liver, heart, lungs and kidneys. You name it, your body needs good fats to work properly, and therefore, to make you thin and healthy. If you don't eat good fats, your body will keep telling you that you are hungry until you get some.

The very best source for quality, good fats is raw seeds and nuts. For example, California researchers found that those who snacked on almonds shrank their waistline 50% more than dieters who did not eat them, even though they ate the same number of calories[2]!

Keep a bowl of raw seeds and nuts handy, perhaps with a few dried berries or raisins to encourage others to eat them. Use more seeds than nuts, because muscle testing indicates that they are likely to be less toxic than nuts, as all plants have some toxins in at least tiny quantities. Put the bowl, with a small spoon, in front of each family member before most meals, and ask everyone to have a few spoonfuls before eating. Having a spoon makes it a lot easier to get a decent mouthful than just picking them up in your fingers.

Add raw nuts and seeds, ground or whole, to just about everything you eat. If you cook a meal, throw them on just before serving, either whole, or ground up, so that no one notices them.

To help you to not get an allergy to any particular seed or nut, totally avoid a particular type for a week every now and again. Avoid peanuts, which have toxins and in any case are not a nut, but a legume.

CHOLESTEROL IS GOOD FOR YOU

Cholesterol, a type of fat, is another good thing that you have been lied about. In fact, cholesterol is essential to keep you thin and healthy. You need cholesterol because it:

- Makes hormones.

- Makes Vitamin D, which is needed for bone growth, and to keep you thin.

- Is an antioxidant that protects your body against free radicals. These are super toxic. Think of free radicals as red hot particles that damage anything they touch[3].

- Makes you feel good, by maintaining serotonin levels.

- Gives you healthy intestines.

- Repairs damaged cells. This indicates that high cholesterol levels occur when there is cell damage (from toxins). Cholesterol is not the problem. Toxins are.

If you want to lower your cholesterol, magnesium supplementation has been found to lower cholesterol by up to 23%[4].

Basically, without good fats, you're dead. It's a miracle that people still look as normal as they do, since so many people have either given up on eating good fats, or eat only toxic fats. If you analyze the diets that have worked for people long term, you will see that they nearly always gave up on bad fats but also ate more good fats.

The growing awareness that there are two very different kinds of fats probably started with the publishing of the highly acclaimed book *Fats That Heal, Fats That Kill,* by Udo Erasmus[5].

Healing fats are essential for reversing obesity, as well as for so called "incurable diseases" such as heart disease, cancer and Type II diabetes. However, fats should not be subjected to heat. In the brilliant documentary *Forks Over Knives* it was shown how people who converted to a whole-foods plant-based diet, that eliminated bad fats, lost excess weight and became healthy and more energetic, as well as healing blood vessels and diabetes. (Note: They must also give up wheat).

The toxic fats and oils that make our bodies fat, and ruin health, are mostly the ones in margarine, most vegetable oils, shortenings and heated oils. The very worst thing is when oils are super-heated, as in deep-fried, as this creates a massive amount of toxins. The higher the heat, and the longer the cooking time, the more toxins are created.

OILS TO COOK WITH

An important rule is, no more deep-frying, because the higher the temperature, the more toxins you create, and the more dangerous they become. If you are going to cook, it should be only gentle sautés and stir-fries, where you need only a tablespoon or less of oil and the temperature is less.

It may be hard to give up French fries, because they cause addictions, just like drugs. Go cold turkey on them. If your cravings get too hard to bear, see my recipe for potato chips cooked with coconut oil. Like any addiction, once you have given them up for a period of time (three weeks or longer), your body will heal the addiction and the craving will reduce, and eventually totally disappear. Avoiding television, so you don't see commercials, will help.

There are just a few kinds of fats that you can have in the kitchen, because these are the ones that stay reasonably stable at high temperatures[6]. Use them in minute quantities, because cooking any oil will create toxins:

- Coconut oil. Coconut oil is the very best oil to eat and cook with, for health and to get thin. It is stable up to 170°F. It may seem weird at first to fry organic eggs in coconut oil, but you can get used to it.

- Sesame oil (unrefined, cold-pressed or expeller pressed, so chemicals weren't used).

- Almond or cashew oil (unrefined, cold-pressed or expeller pressed, so chemicals weren't used).

- Avocado oil.

You can cook with the oils listed above in small amounts, because they are less likely to go rancid when heated. That is, they don't create the highly toxic free radicals that other oils do when heated. However, as you will learn in the section on raw food, you will get thinner if you have food that is raw whenever possible. If you must cook your plants, do it as little as possible, with minimal and preferably zero oil, and on as low a heat as possible.

Every time you add heat you will be destroying some of the nutrition, and creating extra toxins, just less toxins than some other oils. So, whenever possible, eat the above oils raw, such as on salads. Instead of frying, bake or do more thick vegetable soups and stews.

At one time I had butter on this list, so long as it was salted, organic butter, so that the cows are not fed GMOs. It may be all right for you. (Unsalted butter is not as healthy). However, I removed it because most people are allergic to dairy foods. And allergies make you fat. I did not lose any weight for months until I cut out all butter. Some people suggest that you may be able to have ghee, so long as it's organic and from grass-fed cows, especially once you are close to your desired body size.

THE CON: MOST "EXTRA VIRGIN OLIVE OIL" IS HIGHLY TOXIC

Extra Virgin Olive oil is one oil that should be on the above list, as it is an oil that stays fairly stable when it is heated. Plus it is has amazing healing properties when eaten *raw*. However, there is a massive problem with using olive oil. You can not assume that anything that is labeled "extra virgin olive oil" is actually olive oil, let alone "extra virgin" olive oil.

Tom Mueller in his excellent book *Extra Virginity, the Sublime and Scandalous World of Olive Oil* tells us that 70% of the world's "extra virgin" olive oil contains a mixture of:

- "Lampante oil". That is, lamp oil. Lampante oil can only be legally sold as fuel, because it's not fit for eating[8]!

- All kinds of cheap and toxic oils, including genetically modified oils, such as cottonseed and soy oil.

If it's labeled only "olive oil" rather than "extra virgin olive oil", it's possible that it's pomace, which is even worse than lampante oil. Pomace is made from the left over olive skins, stems, pits and leaves, not the fruit itself, and at one time in its manufacturing it is black. This is the oil that is used in a lot of pizzas and pastas. So it's no wonder pizza is perhaps one of the most fattening foods in the world — it's got wheat and cheese – two toxic foods with opiate-like substances in them, that most people are allergic to, plus tomatoes, which a lot of people are allergic to, plus – for 'good' pizza – so-called olive oil, which may possibly be toxic pomace. Plus maybe some embalmed meat (pepperoni) for good measure!

Organized crime has been diluting "Extra Virgin Olive Oil" since before the Roman civilization[9]. They make tens of billions of dollars each year from fake oil, and the situation is getting worse. They are very clever at doing all kinds of things to make the oil taste okay and look the right color. In fact, organized crime in Italy has even been guilty of selling fake butter made from lard, petrochemicals and animal carcasses, and pasta was made from Canadian wheat infected with a carcinogenic mold. (Learning how to muscle test food accurately may be the best way to know what food is safe).

"Extra virgin" olive oil should come from healthy fruit that is not bruised when picked, that is processed immediately after harvest, in a clean facility, properly stored and bottled just before sale. Olive oil is the opposite of wine. Wine ages, but oil goes bad. The instant an oil is bottled, the decay accelerates.

You can't tell what you are getting from fancy labels, fancy awards or even high prices, because much of it is marketing lies. Although, if it *is* a low price you know for sure it's not extra virgin, because extra virgin olive oil costs a lot to produce.

Extra virgin olive oil has many very powerful healing abilities, but only when it is a first rate oil, and only when eaten *raw*[10]. Experts drink it straight, like wine, and can recognize hundreds of different flavors. Real extra virgin olive oil apparently tastes amazing (I haven't tasted any yet), and should have a pungent, bitter or peppery taste. Mueller says that people, even children, who have tasted real extra virgin olive oil, will never eat supermarket olive oil again, because it tastes, and is, literally rotten, even if it has not been adulterated with toxic oils. They compare it to cat urine.

When extra virgin olive oil is cooked, it all tastes the same. This tells us that the chemical composition has been changed. It's rather a waste to cook something that is so precious.

As far as I can tell, currently the only extra virgin olive oil that you can trust to be the real thing, and free of toxins and GMOs, is oil bought straight from the olive grove, and possibly oil grown in Australia. Be careful, because Australia imports a lot of olive oil. Australia has the advantage of having seasons six months out of sync with the northern hemisphere, so its oil is fresh when other oil is getting old.

You can't depend on the FDA to protect you. They only test 0.3% of American oil[11]. I guess they are too busy going after harmless natural health practices instead, because they hurt the profits of drug companies. I recommend that you never use any extra virgin olive oil, unless you truly, positively, know that all of it came directly from a reputable olive grove.

EAT COCONUT OIL TO GET THIN

There are many reports of people losing weight permanently by regularly eating coconut oil. Coconut oil has a lot of abilities to help you to reduce fat and get strong. For example, while it is a saturated fat, if you have a lot of saturated fats then your body needs a lot less essential fatty acids. Plus, we do need some saturated fats. I imagine that not all of the outstanding abilities of coconut oil to help our bodies have been fully discovered yet, or reported to the public, because there is nowhere near as much money in coconut oil research as there is in disease-causing drugs.

Researchers in Japan have found that when you consume a food rich in medium chain fatty acids such as coconut oil, *metabolism increases*[13]. This helps you to get thin. Researchers now know that weight loss associated with coconut oil is related to the length of the fatty acid chains[12]. Coconut oil contains what are called medium chain fatty acids, or medium chain triglycerides. Medium chain fatty acids are different from the longer chain fatty acids, or triglycerides, found in other plant-based oils. Triglycerides are typically stored in the body as fat, while medium chain fatty acids burn up quickly in the body.

People in the animal feed business have known this truth for quite some time. If you feed animals vegetable oils, they put on weight and produce more fatty meat. If you feed them coconut oil, they will be very lean. Coconut oil is nature's richest source of medium chain fatty acids.

Traditionally people in the Philippines ate a lot of coconut oil. Here is one comment from one of the creators of "The Coconut Diet"[14]:

> "I was astounded by the health of the older generation that lived in this rural farming community. There was one old man who was *over 100 years old* and still walked down the mountain to town and back once a week on market day."

More studies are coming out showing how great coconut oil is. Just one dose can tremendously boost brain function[15]. We discovered this for ourselves one day when my husband and I put virgin coconut oil on our scalps, for our hair. There was an immediate increase in energy and brain clarity which was quite marked. To give you an idea of how powerful coconut oil is, one product, monolaurin, which is made from coconut oil, has been found to be successful in healing even Lyme disease[16]!

Virgin coconut oil is best, and tastiest. The best way to consume it is raw by the spoonful. It melts in your mouth. Melt it, mix it with nuts and seeds and put it in the fridge (see my 'Power Balls' recipe). In addition, use coconut oil in place of butter and for cooking, and eat more meals made from coconut and coconut milk. Drink coconut juice as often as you can get it. Basically, include coconut into your diet as much as you can to burn off fat while you heal your body.

GOOD OILS ARE NEVER HEATED

A study at Tufts Medical School found that overweight people were deficient in lipase, which is an enzyme that digests fat[17]. I believe that this would be because their bodies are so toxic that they cannot make lipase as they should do. Therefore, fat was being stored instead of being broken down.

We can make lipase, and we can ingest it. But cooking and refining oils destroys lipase. Lipase is present in *raw* seeds, nuts and bean sprouts.

IF YOU EAT BUTTER, USE SALTED, CULTURED BUTTER (GMO FREE, OF COURSE)

I read a book that explored why the French are so thin, even though they eat scads of heavy cream and butter. I found out what I believe is part of the reason for this when we visited France a few years ago. I noticed that the ingredients of their butter listed something that is not in the ingredients for American butter. It was a bacterium, just as if the butter was yogurt. This means that the bacteria had digested the butter and made it easier for the body to use. I learned that this is called "cultured butter" in America. When I returned to the USA, I found butter in my supermarket that is from Europe, and listed "culture" among the other ingredients, which are only cream and salt. Try it and you will see that unlike other butters it is:

- Golden, not pale at all.
- Soft as margarine.
- Absolutely delicious.

I gave a cracker with some cultured butter to a lady in her 70s who grew up on a farm in the northeast. She exclaimed, "That's what grandmother's butter tasted like!" Ah ha! I had a clue. Back in those days, there were few problems with people being overweight. It does cost a little more, but I believe it's worth it.

Of course, whether your butter is cultured or plain salted butter, it is essential that it is GMO-free, such as organic butter, or grown in a country where the cows are not fed GMO feed. Be aware that many countries in Europe that don't grow GMOs, still import them.

However, since so many people are allergic to dairy, if you are not losing weight even with salted, cultured, non-gmo butter, don't eat any until you are at your ideal body size.

By the way, even the French are having a growing obesity problem these days. I could see some of the reasons why, from my short visit there. They eat wheat, which you will remember has been radically altered from the original wheat. Frozen puff pastry had hydrogenated oils in it, just like in the USA. Young people line up at McDonald's. And French women are using microwave ovens instead of conventional ones[18].

Here's something to consider. Since we have only just recently found out the importance of essential oils in the last few decades, and only found out in the last few years that fat cells, far from being 'inert', actually produce the most important hormone in the human body, namely leptin, what else don't we know?

ESSENTIAL FATS
DO NOT USE FOR COOKING

Essential fats are so-called polyunsaturated fats. These are the omega-3 and omega-6 essential fatty acids, that you may have heard so much about, because omega-3 especially is necessary to help you reduce fat. They are called "essential" because your body supposedly cannot make them, and so they must come directly from the food you eat. (I say "supposedly" because science continues to learn new things about the body). However, note that the more saturated fats you take (like coconut oil), the less essential fats you need. Your bones need saturated fats to absorb calcium[1].

A lot of heating makes them produce dangerous free radicals, so these oils should *never* be used for cooking. You need to consume them in the form of raw, whole-food nuts and seeds.

OMEGA-3 IS THE MOST IMPORTANT FAT TO GET THIN

Omega-3 is the fat most missing from people's diets, including vegetarians and vegans, because we don't eat enough raw seeds. Except for egg yolks, omega-3 sources should be eaten raw:

Sources of Omega-3 (raw)

- Chia seeds (Half a cup of chia seeds has as much Omega 3 as 30 oz. of wild Atlantic Salmon. Also as much iron as 9 cups of raw spinach. Add them to anything raw - smoothies, salads, sandwiches).

- Flax oil (must be cold-pressed and kept in the fridge at all times to make sure it's not rancid).

- Flax seeds, ground (Whole flax seeds are said to be indigestible). See breakfast recipes in the recipe chapter.

- Sunflower seeds[19] (add to smoothies, salads).

- Sesame seeds.

- Pumpkin seeds[20] (Also called "pepitas". Add to smoothies, salads. Wonderful by themselves).

- Brazil nuts.

We must have essential fatty acids. But when essential fatty acids are subjected to heat or oxygen, through cooking or processing, they produce highly toxic free radicals that can cause cancer, heart disease and obesity. That is why you must never cook with oils made from these.

This fact makes it so shocking that most of the chips and snacks at health food stores are now cooked in these oils. In fact, there are quite a number of foods sold in health food stores which are toxic. Health food stores these days seem, unfortunately, more interested in making money than making us healthy. And the people running them are mostly as addicted to some toxins as the rest of the population, so they don't see any harm in selling those products.

Corn and soy oils should be avoided altogether in any case because they contain GMOs (see more in my chapter on GMOs).

TRANS FATS - NEVER, EVER EAT THESE AT ANY TIME[21]

Trans-fats are found in:

- Margarine.
- Vegetable oil.
- Any fat where you see the word "hydrogenated".
- A lot of fast food & restaurant meals, where they don't have to label them.

These are the most dangerous, the most toxic and the most fattening of all, because they are totally artificial. They are so dangerous that New York has rightfully outlawed them[22].

Anything that has been made in a lab and not by nature, is going to make you fat, because it's very toxic. Trans fats were made in a lab to increase their shelf life, not their health benefits. The longer something takes to rot, the more toxic it is. (The only exception to this is plants which are still living, like fruit and vegetables, because it is life force, not chemicals, which prevents them from rotting).

Basically, with trans fats, scientists have taken a food and changed it so that they can last virtually forever, because no bacteria in its right mind will look at it. I am sure that you are smarter than bacteria! Also, they have made it go solid when it should be liquid. It's as though they turned it into *liquid plastic*. Best of all for the manufacturers, it saves the corporations millions of dollars, because they can use the cheapest oil they can lay their hands on. They didn't even have to identify trans fats in the ingredients until 2006.

For years the world was lied to, as usual, by the Food and Drug Administration (FDA) and medical organizations such as the American Heart Association (AHA), who told people to give up traditional saturated fats like butter, in favor of partially hydrogenated oils, supposedly to reduce the risk of heart disease. In fact, this caused an explosion in cases of heart disease. I read of a doctor who, back in the 1920s, travelled across the whole of the USA to have the chance to study the body of a man who had died of heart disease, because it was such a rare occurrence, he thought he would never get a chance to do so closer to home!

Trans fats hurt many body functions, including many that are directly connected to the ability to get thin, including the heart, hormones, insulin and tissue repair. In *Eat fat, lose fat* there is a sentence that repeats a theme that I will be repeating in this book, that it's not about calories, it's about toxins and nutrition:

> "In fact, a person whose dietary fats are mostly trans fats is likely to weigh more than a person who does not consume trans fats, *even if their caloric intake is the same.*"

SAY GOOD BYE TO DEEP FRIED FOODS - THEY ARE TOO TOXIC

The longer a food is heated, and the higher the temperature, the more toxic it becomes. This is why it is important to say good bye to deep fried foods. Instead, sauté them in a saucepan in coconut oil, or organic, grass-fed ghee (clarified butter, available at Indian food stores, health food stores and online).

MARGARINE. EVEN COCKROACHES WON'T EAT IT

Yes, margarine spreads ever so nicely. And, you can leave it lying around for months or even years and it won't `go off'. That's a clue. Anything that doesn't rot is not 'food'. Food has to be broken down by microbes in your gut. 'Food' that doesn't rot is more similar to plastic than food.

No animal, insect or microbe goes near margarine. And that should tell us something important. The animals, insects and microbes must know something we don't know. Even cockroaches won't eat margarine. And cockroaches can eat axle grease!

What animals know is that there's nothing good in margarine, nothing worth the trouble of eating. In fact it's toxic, to both humans and other life. It's especially bad for the human heart. But the Heart Foundation not only says it's okay, it recommends it.[23] Heart Foundations all over the world are misinformed or lying, and there is evidence that this misinformation has killed millions `before their time'. For example, the U.S. Surgeon General's report for 1988 (and similarly more recently), concluded that fifteen out of every 21 deaths (over two thirds) among Americans involve nutrition; that is deficiencies, excesses or imbalances[24].

NEVER USE CANOLA OIL

Canola oil is a Pesticide and Industrial lubricant. Canola oil is rapeseed oil, which is a type of mustard seed. The name "Canola" was developed as a marketing ploy, and comes from the words "**CAN**adian **O**il **L**ow **A**cid". It's so cheap that if the ingredients say "may contain canola", you know that is what they used. Never use canola, even if it's organic, because:

- Canola oil was originally developed as an industrial lubricant. It was not meant for humans to eat.

- It's used as a pesticide[25]. It is even more toxic than soy oil.

- According to *AgriAlternatives, The Online Innovation, and Technology Magazine for Farmers*, "By nature, these rapeseed oils, which have long been used to produce oils for industrial purposes, are... toxic to humans and other animals".

- Rapeseed oil is strongly related to symptoms of emphysema, respiratory distress, anemia, constipation, irritability, and blindness in animals and humans[26]. These symptoms may take ten or more years to show up.

- Rapeseed oil is also the source of the infamous chemical-warfare agent, mustard gas, which was banned after blistering the lungs and skin of hundreds of thousands of solders and civilians during World War One[27].

- It has a tendency to inhibit proper metabolism of foods and prohibits normal enzyme function. (That means, it will make you fat).

Eat LOTS of these RAW, to promote fat loss & health	Eat a LITTLE of these if desired, *raw only*	Use only these for cooking, and that in moderation	Don't ever eat
- Raw seeds, e.g. pumpkin, sunflower, sesame. - Raw nuts, e.g. walnuts, almonds, cashews, brazil. - Especially use raw chia and flax seeds in different meals. - Coconut oil. - Extra virgin olive oil, but only if you can totally trust the source. - Avocado.	- Flax oil. Must have been kept in the fridge. - Safflower oil, expeller or cold-pressed only. - Sunflower oil, expeller or cold-pressed only. - Organic or non-gmo salted butter, if you can eat it and still lose weight. Preferably cultured butter.	- Coconut oil. You can be generous with this. - Sesame oil, unrefined, cold-pressed or expeller pressed. - Peanut, almond or cashew oil (unrefined, cold-pressed or expeller pressed). - Avocado oil. - Extra virgin olive oil, but only if you can totally trust the source. - Organic or non-gmo salted butter or ghee, from grass-fed cows, if you can eat it and still lose weight. It's best if the butter is cultured.	- Anything deep fried. - Margarine. - Trans fats. - Hydrogenated fats. - Corn oil (It's gmo). - Soy oil (it's toxic and gmo). - Canola (it's toxic and gmo). - Cottonseed oil (it's super toxic and gmo). - Vegetable oil.

REFERENCES

1. *Eat Fat, Lose Fat*, by Dr. Mary Enig & Sally Fallon, 2005

2. *Prevention magazine*, Oct 2008, www.prevention.com

3. *Excitotoxins*, by Dr. Russell Blaylock, 1997, page 45

4. *The Magnesium Factor*, by Mildred Seelig, M.D., 2003, page 125

5. *Fats That Heal, Fats That Kill*, by Udo Erasmus, 1986

6. *Eat Fat, Lose Fat*, by Dr Enig, 2005, page 9

7. *Extra Virginity*, by Tom Mueller, 2011

8. *Extra Virginity*, by Tom Mueller, 2012, page 5

9. *Extra Virginity*, by Tom Mueller, 2012, page 10

10. *Extra Virginity*, by Tom Mueller, 2012, page 103-105

11. *Extra Virginity*, by Tom Mueller, 2012, page 48

12. www.coconutdiet.com/weight_loss.htm

13. Aoyama T, Nosaka N, Kasai M., "Research on the nutritional characteristics of medium-chain fatty acids." *J Med Invest*. 2007 Aug;54(3-4):385-8.

14. www.coconutdiet.com

15. www.naturalnews.com/039811_coconut_Alzheimers_dementia.html#ixzz2PmmɪtlnC

16. www.inspirednutrition.com/3/3_Step_Natural_Answer_for_Lyme_Disease.html

17. *Rawsome*, by Brigitte Mars, 1984

18. www.thelocal.fr/2774/20120308/

19. www.savvyvegetarian.com/articles/omega-3-vegetarians-vegans.php

20. www.savvyvegetarian.com/articles/omega-3-vegetarians-vegans.php

21. *Eat Fat, Lose Fat*, by Dr Mary Engi & Sally Fallon, 2005

22. www.nbcnews.com/id/16051436/

23. N.Z. Heart Foundation information leaflets, dated August 1996; received February, 1997

24. *Fats That Heal, Fats That Kill*, by Udo Erasmus, 1986

25. www.epa.gov/opp00001/chem_search/reg_actions/registration/fs_PC-011332_25-Nov-09.pdf

26. www.breathing.com/articles/canola-oil.htm

27. www.shirleys-wellness-cafe.com/canola.htm

CHAPTER 22

TOXIC FOOD #9
SOY IS DANGEROUS AND FATTENING

While I am recommending a whole-foods, plant-based diet with an accent on raw food, there is one plant you should virtually never eat (in addition to wheat), and that is soy, even if it isn't genetically modified, which most of it is.

A carcinogenic substance is one that causes cancer. Soy is carcinogenic. This is because processing of soy protein results in the formation of nitrosamines which are *highly carcinogenic* toxins[1] (and toxins cause fat gain). Food is not meant to cause cancer.

So can you think of a reason why it is highly subsidized by the government? (Hint....follow the $$$). A massive 70% of soybeans are paid for by the government[2]! That is, by taxpayers! Why does someone in the government want us to eat soybeans?

In addition, many of the foods we eat have too much estrogen, or chemicals that act as if they are estrogen, called phytoestrogens. Estrogen is primarily a female hormone, although men have some in smaller quantities. Excess estrogen causes an increase in fat tissue. Plus, the more fat you have, the more estrogen you make, which then makes you even fatter![3]. This is making both men and women fat. Of all the foods we eat, by far the worst for causing excess estrogen is soy[4].

In addition, because estrogen causes breasts to grow larger, it could be why some men are now growing breasts.

Here's a horrifying fact: Babies fed soy based formula have 13,000 - 22,000 times more estrogen compounds in their blood than babies fed milk-based formula. Infants fed only soy-based formula receive the equivalent amount of estrogen as *4 birth control pills a day!*[5] No wonder so many children are now obese. Children fed the perfect food for them, which is the milk of a mother who eats healthy food, will grow a natural slim body, just as wild animals do.

Any time you hear how 'good' soy is for you, find out who paid for that study. Most of the studies were paid for by soy product manufacturers, who are only looking at the good parts of soy, not the toxins in it. Compare it to rat poison, which is 95% good food.

Some more facts which show how toxic soy is, and which therefore show how it's fattening, are[6]:

- High levels of phytic acid in soy reduce assimilation of calcium, magnesium, copper, iron and zinc. All of these minerals are necessary for fat loss. (Phytic acid in soy is not neutralized by preparation methods such as soaking, sprouting or long, slow cooking).

- Soy interferes with protein digestion.

- Vitamin B12 analogs in soy are not absorbed and actually increase the body's requirement for B12.

- Soy foods increase the body's requirement for vitamin D (and Vitamin D is needed for fat loss).

- Processing of soy protein results in the formation of nitrosamines which are *highly carcinogenic* toxins (and toxins cause fat gain).

- MSG, a potent neurotoxin, is formed during soy food processing, and MSG makes people fat (see the chapter on excitotoxins).

- Soy foods contain high levels of aluminum which is toxic to the nervous system and the kidneys (and indirectly makes it harder for the body to reduce fat).

Never use soy milk. Use unsweetened almond milk instead. Years ago, before GMOs, I used a lot of soy milk. At that time, I used to get what felt like period cramps, but I got them in the *middle* of the month. It got so bad that I went to a gynecologist who told me some mumbo jumbo about it being caused from blood leaking into my muscles, when I ovulated. That was no help. Eventually, when I learned muscle testing, I found that the cause of my cramps was soy milk. I gave up soy milk, and never had the cramps again. Soy is very toxic!

I used to think that it was alright to eat a little tofu, as long as it was organic and therefore GMO free, because the worst toxins have been removed by fermentations, and soy sauce. But you still have the fact that soy is much higher in phytoestrogens than anything else, and estrogen makes us fat, whether we are male or female. I now try to avoid even these products.

On my suggested shopping list, you will see that I suggest you get a magnifying glass, because if you see the word "soy" listed *anywhere* on the ingredients, do not buy that product, even if it sold in a 'health food' store. And, of course, now virtually all soy is GMO, so even if you do eat tofu or soy sauce, you absolutely must make sure it's organic.

Until our government works for us, and not for the mega corporations which profit from fat, diseased people, you must take personal responsibility for what you eat.

REFERENCES

1. www.westonaprice.org/soy-alert
2. www.organicconsumers.org/gefood/govtsoyloans.cfm
3. *The Anti-estrogenic diet* by Ori Hofmekler, 2007, page 6
4. *The Anti-estrogenic diet* by Ori Hofmekler, 2007, page 9
5. www.westonaprice.org/soy-alert/soy-formula-birth-control-pills-for-babies
6. www.westonaprice.org/soy-alert

CHAPTER 23

TOXIC FOOD #10

SUGAR &

HIGH FRUCTOSE CORN SYRUP

Refined sugar almost always turns into fat, and starches can also turn into fat. While many people know that sugar is fattening, less people know that it is also very toxic. It is sugar's toxicity which makes it so very fattening.

Unfortunately, many people keep on consuming more and more sugar, probably because sweeteners are also very addictive. Somewhere, this addiction has to stop. Look at how US consumption of sweeteners has skyrocketed:

Processed Sweeteners (sugar, high fructose corn syrup etc[1].)

Year	Per person, per year
1913	40 lb.
1999	147 lb.

Virtually every time we process what God made, we make it more toxic. The more it's processed, the more toxic it becomes. Surprisingly, raw sugar cane is actually quite nutritious. Molasses, which is one of the steps towards making sugar, has some nutrition. But when we process sugar cane all the way to white sugar, we remove the good nutrition and change it, so much that it becomes what some people have called "white poison". I recommend that you read *Sugar Blues,* by William Dufty, for more incentive to give up sugar. Here is one testimonial for that book from www.Amazon.com:

"For weeks I walked to and from work, over one hour each way, to help drop through a weight plateau of 199 pounds. No matter what I did, including dieting, I was destined to be a 199-pounder for life! Then, one Sunday evening, I read the first few chapters of a book a friend lent me, *Sugar Blues* by Dufty. My first reaction to the information contained in it was entirely emotional: anger and disgust.

Until that moment I had never given sugar a moment's worth of thought. That Sunday evening, I felt my anger so intensely, that I promised myself that I immediately would stop my ingestion of sugar for *moral* reasons. As I read further, I wished that I had known this information years ago. I wished that I had used this information while raising my children. I am saddened that I didn't get to the profound wisdom in this book sooner than I did. But, life is full of important lessons. This book is but lesson number one. And learning this lesson later is better than not learning it at all.

While reading *Sugar Blues* I was also reading another book on the topic of meats. I decided to give up sugar and meats". (Note: Artificial sweeteners are more fattening than sugar. See the chapter on aspartame for more information).

"On Thursday of that week I spent time between the fetal position in bed and sprinting to the washroom. I thought I had the flu, but looking back, I now realize I had what I'd describe as, "withdrawal" symptoms. 24 hours later I was feeling better.

Seven days later, when I weighed myself, I received the first of many self-fulfilling rewards: I cracked my weight-loss plateau, was finally down to 190 pounds. Three weeks later, I lost another 6 pounds and was down to 184. Seven weeks later I was at 177. 10 weeks later 174.

I have had to tighten my belt 5 notches! I fit into pants that I had not fit into since 1978. As of this last week, I stabilized at a weight plateau of 174 pounds. I have lost a cool 25 pounds.

This book made me *think* about the quality of, and effect from, the "foods" I shoveled into my mouth. This book motivated me to read the labels before I bought. It is an absolute must have for your home library...a must show to friends who you care about...a book that you must dog-ear and underline, (use over and over again). It might be a good idea for you to think about buying several or more copies of this book... to either give away or circulate among your friends and relatives. If you do, you just might enhance your life and theirs."

Dr. Nancy Appleton, Ph.D., author of the book, *Lick The Sugar Habit*, has done extensive research and uncovered 76 ways that sugar can cause illness[2]. Here are few of them (comments in italics are by myself):

1. Sugar upsets the mineral relationships in your body: causes chromium and copper deficiencies and interferes with absorption of calcium and magnesium (*all of which are necessary for fat loss*).

2. Sugar can produce a significant rise in total cholesterol, triglycerides and bad cholesterol and a decrease in good cholesterol (*all of which make people fat*).

3. Sugar feeds cancer cells.

4. Sugar can cause many problems with the gastrointestinal tract (*which makes it harder to reduce fat*).

5. Sugar can cause premature aging. In fact, the single most

important factor that accelerates aging is insulin, which is triggered by sugar.

6. Sugar contributes to obesity.

7. Sugar can cause a decrease in your insulin sensitivity, thereby eventually causing diabetes.

8. Sugar can interfere with your absorption of protein.

9. Sugar causes food allergies.

10. Sugar lowers the ability of enzymes to function (*You will learn in the chapter on raw food how important enzymes are to fat loss*).

11. Sugar can increase your body's fluid retention (*so you will look fatter*).

12. Sugar can cause depression. (*Depressed people are more likely to eat fattening food*).

13. Sugar can cause hyperactivity, anxiety, difficulty concentrating, and crankiness in children.

14. Sugar can suppress your immune system, so that you get sick.

15. Sugar is an addictive substance. Sugar can be intoxicating, similar to alcohol.

Sugar is something that you need to give up for life. You are not fat, you are toxic. Sugar is not fattening just because it's concentrated calories. It's also because it's highly toxic, and does all kinds of damage to your body, so that the body cannot work properly. In fact, according to researchers at the University of California, San Francisco (UCSF)[3], sugar and other sweeteners are so toxic to the human body that they should be regulated as *strictly as alcohol*.

HIGH FRUCTOSE CORN SYRUP IS MORE FATTENING THAN SUGAR

Unfortunately, now we have something even worse in our food than sugar, and that is high fructose corn syrup. In 1973 the government started a massive corn subsidy, so companies started making high fructose corn syrup. That means, the government is using lots of taxpayers' money to make us fat and sick. This is great for the drug companies, but not for you. Corn is the most heavily subsidized of all foods grown with government subsidies[4]. It receives billions of dollars. That is why healthy vegetables and fruit cost as much as they do. Eating healthily would be easier if the government would not take from the taxpayers and then give it to farmers, so that they can grow toxic GMO corn, soybeans and wheat with it, and then meat and dairy, for much less than it should cost. To learn more about this, please watch the excellent documentary *Food, Inc.*

Corn is particularly toxic these days because it is genetically modified. But, even apart from that, high fructose corn syrup is super fattening. High fructose corn syrup began to be used in many foods in the 1990s. This is a major cause of obesity[5].

High fructose corn syrup is produced by processing corn starch to yield glucose, and then processing the glucose to produce a high percentage of fructose. It *sounds* rather simple. However, the process is actually very complicated. High fructose corn syrup has the exact same sweetness and taste as an equal amount of sugar from sugar cane or beets, but it is much more complicated to make, involving vats of murky fermenting liquid, fungus and chemical tweaking. Yet in spite of all the special enzymes required, two of which are *genetically modified*, which adds to toxicity, high fructose corn syrup is cheaper than sugar, which is the main reason why more and more products are switching to high fructose corn syrup.

You may think that because it contains fructose, which occurs naturally in fruit, which is good for you, that it is a natural food, and therefore healthier than sugar. But a team of investigators at the USDA, led by Dr. Meira Field, has discovered that this is not so.

Sugar is composed of glucose and fructose. When sugar is given to rats in high amounts, the rats develop multiple health problems. The researchers wanted to know whether it was the fructose or the glucose that was causing the problems. So they repeated their studies with two groups of rats, one given high amounts of glucose and one given high amounts of fructose.

Again, just like processed sugar is not the same as raw sugar from healthy raw sugar cane, processed fructose is different from healthy raw fructose in fruit. It is the processing which makes it so toxic.

The glucose group was unaffected but the fructose group had disastrous results.

The male rats did not reach adulthood. They had anemia, high cholesterol and heart hypertrophy. That means that their hearts enlarged until they exploded. They also had delayed testicular development.

Dr. Field explains that fructose in combination with copper deficiency in the growing animal interferes with collagen production. (Copper deficiency, like most mineral deficiencies, is widespread in America.). In a nutshell, the little bodies of the rats just fell apart.

"The medical profession thinks fructose is better for diabetics than sugar," says Dr. Field, "but every cell in the body can metabolize glucose. However, all fructose must be *metabolized in the liver*". The livers of the rats on the high fructose diet looked like the livers of alcoholics, *plugged with fat*."

SUGAR & HIGH FRUCTOSE CORN SYRUP KILL PEOPLE

Sugar and high fructose corn syrup are one of the major causes of Type II Diabetes[6], which kills people. (Wheat, caffeine and dairy are also major causes. Please see chapters 16, 20 & 25). They do this by exhausting the body's ability to produce enough insulin.

Here's a shocking quote from the documentary *Super Size Me* by Dr. William Klish M.D., Head of Dept. of Medicine, Texas Children's Hospital:

"If diabetes starts before age 15, a person *loses between 17 and 27 years* of life span."

What a bonanza for the government! No wonder they are in bed with corporations that sell junk food. Think of all the social security payments that they will not have to pay.

DO NOT EVER USE:

• Sugar.

• Any corn syrup (Because it's genetically modified).

• High fructose corn syrup, because it's a lot worse than sugar.

• Fructose, because only the liver can deal with processed fructose.

• Aspartame, AminoSweet, NutraSweet, Neotame (as was discussed in the Aspartame chapter).

• All artificial sweeteners and anything that is a chemical rather than a plant, such as Sucralose, Splenda, Saccharin. They cause similar problems to Aspartame.

• Unnatural sugar substitutes like xylitol, maltitol, sorbitol.

• Stevia. While many in the health industry think this is okay because it is 'natural', we must remember that poisons like hemlock are also natural. Stevia is 300 times sweeter than sugar[7]. Therefore it still *acts the same* as an artificial sweetener, in that it tricks your brain into what it is getting. If you eat this, your brain will be *craving more sweet things later on.* It's better to get your taste buds to adapt to *less* sweetness.

• Agave nectar. It's worse than high fructose corn syrup[8]! It's so highly processed that it has little resemblance to the agave plant.

Nearly everyone needs to cut down on the amount of sweet things they eat and drink, especially if they have unwanted fat. However, you don't need to totally give up all sweet things. You can still have *raw* fruit, and some fresh-squeezed fruit in your vegetable juice. Here are a few alternatives to sugar and high fructose corn syrup to use in your dishes:

SWEETENERS TO USE
Use only in tiny amounts, like 1/4 teaspoon at a time.

- Raw honey. It should be grown away from GMO farms.

- Maple Syrup (must be 100% maple syrup).

- Organic molasses, so it is GMO free (beet molasses are mostly genetically modified, and they are starting to genetically modify cane sugar).

- Coconut sugar (for very occasional treats, or maintenance, only).

- Plus you can use raw or dried fruit in moderation. For example, add some apple or raisins.

REFERENCES
1. *Forks Over Knives* documentary
2. *Lick The Sugar Habit,* by Dr. Nancy Appleton, Ph.D., 1988
3. www.livescience.com/18244-sugar-toxic-regulations.html
4. articles.mercola.com/sites/articles/archive/2011/08/03/the-9-foods-the-us-government-is-paying-you-to-eat.aspx
5. *Forks Over Knives* documentary
6. www.naturalnews.com/009333_diabetes_sugar.html#ixzz2DjOafZqx
7. *Diet Wise,* by Dr. Keith Scott-Mumby, 1985, page 215
8. articles.mercola.com/sites/articles/archive/2010/03/30/beware-of-the-agave-nectar-health-food.aspx

CHAPTER 24

TOXIC FOOD #11
PROCESSED FOOD

When we process foods, we change them, from natural to unnatural. When we do that, we add toxins. Cooking is just one part of processing. Other parts of processing include super high temperatures, adding chemicals, doing strange things to the molecular structure like when milk is homogenized, and removing the nutritious parts of food. Our genes were not made for processed food. Wild animals don't eat processed food.

If you look at diets that worked for some people, you will see that they nearly always contain mostly unprocessed foods. They use fresh ingredients that they prepare themselves, and include a certain quantity of raw plants, usually in the form of salads without dressing, plus nuts and seeds. That means that when you go shopping, you stay out of the 'middle' of the supermarket and mostly just shop around the edges. Probably 80% or more of the items in a supermarket are processed, because that's where the profits are.

For example, *Woman's World* magazine told the story of Miss South Carolina who went from 234 pounds and size 18 to Beauty Queen and 122 pounds. She lost 7 pounds a week without going hungry when a nutritionist taught her to switch from processed foods to whole foods.

She also walked at first and did more exercise later on[1].

This doesn't work just because "it takes the body longer to process it". It's because our bodies were *designed* to eat unprocessed foods. Plus there's more nutrition in them, and less toxins.

The more we cook and process food, and the higher the temperature, the more we destroy nutrients and create dangerous toxins. Lack of nutrition and extra toxins are making us fat.

Research done at Stockholm University, in cooperation with Sweden's Natural Food Association, showed that the heating of carbohydrate-rich foods, such as bread, potatoes, rice, and breakfast cereals, create *acrylamide*, a human carcinogen. The researchers found that a bag of potato chips may contain up to *500 times* more acrylamide than allowed in drinking water by the World Health Organization (WHO). French fries sold at McDonald's and Burger King in Sweden showed 100 times the level permitted by WHO in drinking water[2]. The research was deemed so important that the scientists decided on the unusual step of going public with their findings before the research had been officially published in an academic journal.

Acrylamide has been found to cause benign and malignant stomach tumors, and to cause damage to the central and peripheral nervous systems. Acrylamide occurs in baked potatoes, French fries, biscuits, and bread, as well as other high-carbohydrate foods. You are not fat, you're toxic. This is yet another reason why people who change to eating vegetables, fruit, nuts, seeds and legumes, as raw as often as possible, get slim and gain health and energy.

BREAKFAST CEREALS ARE DEADLY

That may sound like a wild statement, but please consider the results of two more studies that were never published. If you, like me, have found that you never reduce weight when eating any breakfast cereals, the following two pieces of information will explain why. It's not because they are high in carbohydrates, but because they are highly toxic.

I was told of these studies years ago by my naturopathic teacher around 1996. With the internet I was able to find details of the studies, from an article by Sally Fallon, founding president of the Weston

A. Price Foundation.

PUFFED GRAINS KILL FASTER THAN STARVATION

Paul Stitt wrote about an experiment conducted by a cereal company in which four sets of rats were given special diets[3].

#1 – Received plain whole wheat, water and synthetic vitamins and minerals.

#2 - Received puffed wheat, water and the same nutrients.

#3 - Given only water.

#4 - Given only water and the same nutrients.

The #1 rats that received the whole wheat lived over a year on this diet. The #4 rats that got nothing but water and vitamins lived about two months. The #3 rats on water alone lived about a month. But the #2 rats given the vitamins, water and all the puffed wheat they wanted died within two weeks! They died before the rats that got no food at all! It wasn't a matter of the rats dying of malnutrition. Autopsy revealed dysfunction of the pancreas, liver and kidneys and degeneration of the nerves of the spine, all signs of insulin shock.

Presumably, the pressure of the puffing process produces chemical changes, which turn a nutritious grain into a poisonous substance. Do not eat anything that is puffed, even if it is sold by a 'health food' store. This includes pop corn.

RATS DO BETTER EATING THE BOX, THAN THE CORN FLAKES

Another unpublished experiment was carried out in the 1960s. Researchers at Ann Arbor University were given 18 laboratory rats[4]. They were divided into three groups:

#1 - Received corn flakes and water. (This was in the days before corn was made poisonous through genetic modification).

#2 - Was given the cardboard box that the corn flakes came in, and water.

#3 - The control group received normal rat food and water.

The group #3 rats in the control group remained in good health throughout the experiment. The #2 rats eating the box became lethargic and eventually died of malnutrition. But the #1 rats receiving the corn flakes and water died before the rats that were eating the box! The last corn flake rat died the day the first box rat died. Before death, the corn flake rats developed schizophrenic behavior, threw fits, bit each other and finally went into convulsions. (Does this sound like some children you know?).

This experiment was actually designed as a joke, but the results were far from funny. The startling conclusion of this study is that there was **more nourishment in the box than there was in the corn flakes.** Naturally, in this crazy world we live on, where profits rule almost everything, the results were never published and similar studies have not been conducted as of time of printing. The famous American Buckminster Fuller once said something that, while not totally accurate, nevertheless holds a lot of truth:

"You have to decide whether you want to make money or make sense, because the two are mutually exclusive."

EMBALMED MEAT IS THE MOST FATTENING KIND OF MEAT

What I call "embalmed meat" are those meats which have had so many toxins added to them, that they hardly ever rot, similar to Egyptian mummies. Bacon, pepperoni, hot dogs and beef jerky are examples. They have so many preservatives, which are toxins, added that they don't rot much, if at all. That is, bacteria won't eat it. Bacteria are smarter than us in some cases. You need bacteria to break down your food. Basically, the longer a food takes to rot, the worse it is for you. (The exception to this is plants, which are *alive*. With plants, the longer they live, the better for you they are).

The new study of AGEs (which age you and cause a massive range of serious health problems) backs this up. Cured meat like bacon, pepperoni and hot dogs are highest of all in AGEs[5].

Now you know another reason why McDonald's food was shown to be so fattening in the excellent documentary, *Super Size Me*. People have left McDonald's fries and burgers on the shelf for months, and they still look much as they did on the first day! No bacteria in it's right mind would eat at McDonald's.

My teacher David Bridgman said that owners of morgues report that bodies now last three or four times longer than they used to. This is because of all the preservatives in them, just like Egyptian mummies. Now you know why I call pepperoni "embalmed meat". This is why it's harder for people to reduce fat, because they are full of preservatives. Basically, except for living plants which are kept alive by live force rather than chemicals, the longer a food will take to rot, the more toxic it is, and the more fat it will cause, because the body has to store it until it can, hopefully, get rid of the toxins later on when you improve your eating habits.

NATURAL FLAVORS

There is absolutely no legal meaning to the word "natural", so profit-hungry companies use it for virtually everything. Note that poisons like coal tar and mercury are natural. An example of how "natural" a natural flavoring is, is "Strawberry flavor", which is made of 50 chemicals, such as benzyl isobutyrate[6]. You will remember from the chapter on excitotoxins that "natural flavor" can mean fat-causing excitotoxins.

Further evidence that natural flavors are highly toxic comes from studies of workers in factories that make, or use, natural flavors. It was found that natural flavors caused lung disease[7], whether or not they were 'natural' or manmade. Food should not do that.

Get out your magnifying glass and avoid 'natural flavorings' wherever possible. Better yet, whatever you want to buy, find a recipe for it on the internet and make it yourself.

ARTIFICIAL COLORINGS

Words like "Red 3" and "Yellow 2" might sound cute and safe, but these are not grown in a garden like real food. They are dangerous chemicals that are made in a lab with raw materials derived from petroleum[8].

For example, the real name for "Red40" is - 6-hydroxy-5-[(2-methoxy-5-methyl-4-sulfophenyl)azo]-2-naphthalenesulfonic acid[9]. Doesn't sound quite as healthy as, for example, "beet juice", does it?

Some children eat as much as *three pounds* of these chemicals by the time they are 12 years old[10]! The amount of additives in food continues to grow, so we won't see the full results of this until these children grow up.

Current food colorings have been founds to produce DNA damage, allergies, thyroid tumors, lymph tumors, brain tumors, bladder tumors and kidney tumors[11]. That lets you know they are toxic for everyone. We can therefore assume that they are contributing to obesity, especially in children. There is no need to ever eat anything with these in them. Get out your magnifying glass and read the label before purchasing.

If it says a color (like 'blue 1'), 'artificial coloring' or 'US Certified Colors', do not buy it or consume it, even if someone offers it to you for free.

CANNED FOODS

Frederick vom Saal, Ph.D., professor of biological sciences at the University of Missouri[12] said that the problem with tin cans is the resin lining. It contains BPA (bisphenol-A), a synthetic estrogen that, like other substances that mimic estrogen, has been linked to health problems including obesity as well as heart disease, diabetes and others. You can get 50 micrograms of BPA per liter out of a tomato can, and that's a level that is going to impact people, particularly children, says vom Saal.

Instead use products in glass bottles, which do not need resin linings. Better yet, make your own food. See my recipe for spaghetti. The raw tomato sauce tastes as good as cooked sauce and is more slimming because raw is more slimming than cooked.

REFERENCES

1. *Woman's World* magazine, 1/9/12
2. April 24, 2002 11:20 AM ET - Reuters.com/news
3. Excerpted from a presentation at the conference of Consumer Health of Canada, March, 2002, given by Sally Fallon, Nutrition Researcher
4. Excerpted from a presentation at the conference of Consumer Health of Canada, March, 2002, given by Sally Fallon, Nutrition Researcher
5. *Wheat Belly*, William Davis M.D., 2011, pages 140-141
6. naturalsociety.com/strawberry-flavor-consists-of-50-different-chemicals
7. www.osha.gov/SLTC/flavoringlung/
8. www.npr.org/2011/03/30/134962888/fda-probes-link-between-food-dyes-kids-behavior
9. www.red40.com/pages/chemistry.html
10. www.feingold.org/Research/dyesinfood.html
11. www.feingold.org/Research/dyesinfood.html
12. health.yahoo.net/articles/nutrition/photos/14-foods-you-should-cut-your-diet#5

CHAPTER 25

TOXIC FOOD #12
CAFFEINE
26 WAYS COFFEE MAKES YOU FAT

Do you have fat, especially on the belly, that 'nothing' else has worked for? Are you committed to health and getting rid of that fat? Then read on, because, painful though the truth may be, I am going to explain why giving up coffee, and any other drink or food that contains caffeine, may be the most important thing you ever do.

This will probably be the most unpopular chapter in this book. After all, when 'everyone' drinks it, it must be okay, right? And it makes you feel so GOOOOODDDD. The trouble is that caffeine is so addictive, that nearly everyone, including most doctors and scientists, have blinded themselves to the truth about how fattening this drug is. Understanding how you have been conned about caffeine may be the missing key to reducing fat, that you have been looking for. It doesn't matter what form the caffeine is in, whether it's from coffee, tea, green tea, sodas, chocolate, energy drinks or herbal substitutes like guarana, it's the same drug. Even so-called 'de-caf' has caffeine in it.

In addition, caffeine is a major cause of stroke, which affects someone in the USA every 40 seconds, and can cause untold suffering for themselves and their family for the rest of their life.

Because I knew that toxins made you fat, and caffeine is so very toxic, I knew that caffeine was fattening, especially long-term. The first clues I found are in the brilliant book *Caffeine Blues*, by Stephen Cherniske, Clinical Nutritionist and Researcher, which has *forty pages* of references.

CAFFEINE RAISES CORTISOL. CORTISOL GIVES YOU A FAT BELLY

Cherniske explains how caffeine tells your body to go into "fight or flight" mode. That is, caffeine gets you ready to fight a tiger, or to run away from a tiger. One way that caffeine does this is by raising cortisol levels. Cortisol is a stress hormone. That is, caffeine stresses your body. Most people's bodies are in *constant stress* from cortisol from caffeine. Our bodies were not made to be in constant stress. An article in *First* magazine explained[1]:

- *Cortisol triggers fat deposition*, especially in the *belly* region.

- High levels of cortisol also *damage insulin* receptors on cells to make them insulin-resistant (which leads to fat gain & diabetes)

Yale University found that when cortisol levels are raised, even for just a few hours, the body stores more fat, especially around the belly. Dr. Dean explains: "Cortisol causes fat cells in the belly area to store ... fat because the body perceives almost any stress as starvation stress[2]."

Like most people, I used to be addicted to caffeine. It is a drug after all, and a highly addictive one at that. Caffeine is a "psycho-active" drug[3], which means that it is a chemical substance that forces the brain and central nervous system to do things it would not normally do. That's why people get addicted to it. It alters one's state of mind, similar to the way morphine, nicotine and cocaine do! Does that sound harmless? Why are children drinking this stuff?

If you think, like most people, that you aren't addicted to caffeine, then just think about the difference between giving up caffeine and, say, apple juice, for two months, and you might perceive the difference.

You won't hear the truth about a drug from a drug addict. And you won't hear the truth about caffeine from anyone who takes any caffeine. That includes most doctors and scientists. Any drug addict will do anything to justify why they should continue to stay with their addiction. And there are plenty of caffeine-addicts and companies making billions from it to keep them company. The only people who have the will to tell you the truth about caffeine are those who have managed to totally give it up themselves.

The companies that sell caffeine products invest billions to keep you a customer for life.

CAFFEINE STEALS ENERGY FROM YOU. THE APPARENT EFFECT OF ENERGY IS SIMPLY A HALT TO DRUG WITHDRAWAL SYMPTOMS.

Caffeine "gives you energy", right? Wrong. Caffeine does not give you energy. Just like any drug, it stimulates you chemically. In fact, caffeine *steals* energy from you. It does this by driving your adrenals and putting your body into stress. It uses chemicals to tell your body that there is a tiger in the room, just about to kill you, every minute of the day. Taking caffeine, in any form, is like going to a bank for a loan of energy of $100 worth, but you have to pay back $150 worth afterwards. **You borrow with your lifespan, and pay back with interest.**

Caffeine gives you a 'lift', right? Wrong again. Like any drug, it gives you a little lift in the short term, but a major downer in the long term. What goes up chemically, must come down, and the 'down' will always be a lot stronger than the 'up'.

26 WAYS THAT CAFFEINE CAUSES FAT

Here are 26 ways that caffeine causes fat gain, especially *long-term*:

1. Caffeine raises *cortisol levels*[4]. Cortisol triggers fat deposition, especially in the *belly*.

2. High levels of cortisol damage insulin receptors on cells to make them *insulin-resistant*, which leads to diabetes and fat gain.

3. Caffeine causes *leptin resitance*, because caffeine stresses the body. Leptin resistance is a major cause of obesity. (see the chapter on leptin).

4. Caffeine stops people from getting to *sleep*. The only time this does not occur is when they have a massive sleep debt, because lack of sleep is accumulative. Sleep is the most important time for burning fat.

5. When there is *any* caffeine in your blood stream, you are unlikely to get any *deep sleep*[5]. One of the first things to go when proper sleep is affected is motivation. You need to maintain motivation to do what you have to do to get a thin body. Caffeine tolerance may allow you to fall asleep, but if your deep sleep is disturbed, you will wake up tired instead of renewed. Tired people are more likely to reach for more caffeine as well as something sugary to gain fake energy.

6. Because caffeine prevents deep sleep, it *decreases or prevents growth hormone production*. Extra growth hormone is released during the night's first period of deep sleep[6]. Growth hormone is needed for repair, muscle growth, correct metabolism and helps with fat loss. This also means that caffeine is an *aging drug*.

7. The half-life of a substance is the time that it takes the body to remove half of the substance. The half-life of a single dose of caffeine is a shocking *3 - 12 hours*. That means that many people who have just *one* caffeinated drink in the morning still have plenty of caffeine in their body when they go to bed.

8. Caffeine increases stress hormone levels. It can take *three weeks* or more for levels of stress hormones of a habitual caffeine drinker to return to normal. More and more studies are finding that stress causes fat gain. Chemical stress is as much a stress as emotional stress.

9. Caffeine is not the only toxin in coffee. There are over *seven hundred* (700) volatile substances in coffee, including 200 acids[7] as well as pesticides. A body dealing with lots of toxins has more important things to do than to burn fat.

10. *Malnutrition* is one of the most well-defined effects of habitual caffeine intake[8]. Malnutrition is also a major cause of fat gain, since the body can't work as well, and people suffering malnutrition get hungrier, because the body urges its owner to find the minerals it needs. A single cup of coffee can reduce iron absorption from a meal by as much as 75%[9]! A mere 50 mg of caffeine (a half cup) depletes the body of calcium and magnesium. Bigger doses deplete even more. Just 300 mg increases potassium loss by one third. Caffeine also depletes the body of other substances including zinc, folic acid and B vitamins.

(Note: Most blood tests for iron deficiency are useless, because levels will look normal as long as you have some iron. They measure only how much iron is travelling in the *blood*, not how much is in the *body cells*. However, Stephen Cherniske says that a "serum ferritin" test *is* accurate[10]).

11. Caffeine causes *magnesium deficiency*[11]. Lack of magnesium makes people fat (see the chapter on magnesium).

12. Caffeine causes gas (giving you a big tummy) and other digestive problems. When your body is under stress, all kinds of maintenance and repair activities stop. As David Morgan, director of the University of South Florida's Institute on Aging says, "There's no reason to digest your breakfast if you are about to become lunch." (There's that tiger again).

13. The vascular resistance which is part of the stress response of caffeine naturally *reduces metabolic efficiency*. How can your body burn fat if it can't even move blood around the body properly? (Note: This means that the people who tell you that caffeine

raises your metabolism (common with "weight loss" scams) are uninformed or lying).

14. Caffeine *damages your adrenal glands*, by making them continually produce stress hormones that should only be produced very occasionally. Your adrenals are needed to produce about 150 hormones that your body needs to function efficiently and keep you thin[12].

15. Constant caffeine intake causes *adrenaline resistance*[13]. Adrenaline should make fat cells release energy. But because this has happened too many times, the fat cells go into *hibernation mode* and stop releasing energy.

16. Caffeine causes *DHEA deficiency*, by raising cortisol levels[14]. Natural DHEA, rather than DHEA from pills, is what gives you real vitality, energy and optimism, all of which you need to burn fat. People with higher levels of fat have less DHEA than thinner people.[6]

17. Caffeine directly *suppresses melatonin* production. This accelerates aging. In addition, several studies have shown that melatonin deficiency is associated with weight gain, because melatonin has control over fat accumulation[15],[16]. (This is also why you should not look at a computer screen before going to bed, and why you should sleep in total darkness, with no night lights whatsoever).

18. Caffeine's flight or fight response cuts you off from the brain's higher centers of reason and evaluation (because you are forcing the brain into defensive, emergency overdrive).

This makes it harder to shop and prepare food for healthy habits, and increases the chance that you buy and gobble down "whatever you feel like".

19. Moderate caffeine intake can more than double the stress

response, whether a person is a light or habitual user. (So studies of caffeine often remove anyone who is under significant stress from the study, because this would make their results a lot worse). If you don't handle stress well, when a stressful situation arrives, it is possible that will be the time when you break your good habits and put on extra fat. Many people are surprised at how much their moods improve after going two months with zero caffeine. As one man said, "I was less aggressive but far more *effective*".

20. Caffeine causes *depression*[17]. When you first have caffeine, or do anything exciting, you feel great because your brain fires off all the dopamine it has stored. But several hours later there will be a 'let-down' feeling because you have run out of dopamine. This feeling will continue until your brain stocks up on more dopamine. In addition, caffeine causes lack of deep sleep, which also causes depression. Depressed people are more likely to take pharmaceutical drugs (which cause fat gain) and to eat toxic food. If you feel any depression, try going caffeine free for two months. You may be shocked to learn that was all that was required to heal your depression, and to feel optimistic and powerful again. Even if you never feel depressed, you won't know how much happier you can be, until you try zero caffeine for two months.

21. Digestion is a highly complicated process. Caffeine interferes with digestion in many ways. For example, it makes the amount of hydrochloric acid in your stomach either too high or too low[18]. Anything that interferes with the body's natural processes can indirectly cause fat gain.

22. Commercially grown coffee is heavily sprayed with poisons. In fact, Brazilian coffee has DDT among other poisons, even after roasting[19]. Tea leaves are sprayed with a whole lot of poisons immediately before harvesting[20]. More toxins make your body need more fat cells to store them.

23. Caffeine affects children even worse than adults. Unhealthy, fat

children will likely grow up to be even bigger adults, even bigger than we are seeing now.

24. Caffeine affects women much more than men (and yet about 75% of all human caffeine research has been done on men)[21].

25. Animal experiments showed that coffee and tea decreased the availability of protein[22].

26. Caffeine, one of the main components of most soft drinks, is a drug. It dehydrates. This is one reason why a person is forced to drink so many cans of soda every day and never be satisfied. The water does not stay in the body long enough, so the person is still thirsty. People confuse messages of thirst for hunger (see the chapter on water). Thinking they have consumed enough 'water', the person then assumes they are hungry and begin to eat more[23].

Here's a piece of evidence that proves that caffeine makes you fat. Factory farmers feed caffeine to chickens "to keep the chickens awake so that they eat more and grow faster"[24]. Apparently, farmers know more about caffeine than most doctors!

SUBSTANCES THAT CONTAIN CAFFEINE INCLUDE:

- Coffee.

- Tea – black, green, pu-erh or oolong.

- Soft drinks – read the label.

- "Energy" drinks – the very worst of all. These are killing teen-agers. Visit www.energyfiend.com/death-by-caffeine to see how many containers of your favorite "energy drink" will kill you.

- Chocolate, cocoa and cacao (even if it is raw).

- Medications.

- De-caffeinated drinks – still contains quite a bit of caffeine! And it's more acidic than ordinary coffee (and acidity is fattening).

- Guarana.

- Kola nuts.

- Yerba mate.

- Ma huang (ephedra).

- Diet products.

CAFFEINE IS A MAJOR CAUSE OF STROKE

While the fact that caffeine is a major cause of stroke is not related directly to weight loss, I felt that knowing this might give you the extra push you need to give up caffeine totally. This information is so vital for everyone who consumes caffeine to know, that I felt I must include it here. Please study this information before you regret not taking action right now.

The stress responses caused by caffeine make it harder for blood to flow. This significantly increases risk of heart attack or stroke. A stroke is caused by a blockage or rupture of a blood vessel in or surrounding the brain. People who suffer stroke can suffer severe brain damage. Caffeine causes stroke in two ways:

1. Caffeine *decreases blood flow* in the brain, by constricting blood vessels. It does this with even small doses[25]. This happens at the same time that -

2. Caffeine *increases blood pressure* in the brain.

Stroke is a truly terrible thing to have, for both the sufferer and the family who may have to look after the person for the rest of their life. Unfortunately, according to the Centers for Disease Control and Prevention, "no national surveillance of stroke incidence exists in the United States"[26]. That is a really strange thing for a government body to say. It looks like someone doesn't want us to make the connection between caffeine and stroke. However, we do know that about 800,000 people get stroke each year in the USA[27], every 40 seconds! And that stroke can occur at any age.

Of the approximately 800,000 people who get stroke, only about 140,000 die. They might be the lucky ones. Of the 660,000 who survive, there can be untold suffering for themselves and their families, because the after effects can include the following, and these are often for the rest of their lives:

- Paralysis of arms and legs, one side of the body.

- Paralysis of face on one side of the body.

- Paralysis of the ability to swallow.

- Blindness.

- Memory loss.

- Speech problems.

- Incontinence.

- Loss of bowel control.

- Constant pain.

- Inability to think and reason.

Further more, caffeine should not be given to children, since it has been shown that caffeine inhibits a most important enzyme system (phospho-diesterase) that is involved in the process of learning and memory development[28].

The strange truth is that the things you want to get from caffeine, you will have by getting totally off it for two months!

The only people who can face the truth of how dangerous this drug is are those who have given it up totally themselves. I can tell when I read a health book, whether or not the author has managed to kick this drug habit by their attitude towards caffeine. It will help you to give up caffeine if you understand how addictive it is. You will need to use some extra will power for a while until you get the benefits of being drug-free. I still find it hard to walk past the coffee aisle, without feeling the smell of coffee trying to draw me back for a drug-fix, so I do my best to not go near where I can smell it.

To reduce unpleasant withdrawal symptoms like headaches, it may be best to take several weeks to give up caffeine. Drink extra, good water to assist with the detox. Gradually replace parts of your caffeinated drink with caffeine-free substitutes, available from your health-food store. In addition, improve your nutrition with simple things like fresh-squeezed vegetable and fruit juices (see recipe chapter).

You may notice a difference within weeks of having zero caffeine. Or, you might have to wait two months to feel and see a difference.

I finally harnessed the will power to totally quit caffeine in all forms after reading *Caffeine Blues*. By then I had cut down to one coffee every three days and two cups a day of green tea, which has a lot less caffeine than coffee. But since even green tea and decaf contain caffeine, I did what Cherniske recommended everyone tries, which is zero caffeine for two months. Within three weeks I was surprised to see that I had a lot more energy than when I was drinking caffeine. I can also see now that I am a lot calmer. Hundreds of other people who have had zero caffeine for two months have discovered similar changes, once they got over the initial detox period. From *Caffeine Blues*:

> "The caffeine industry has generated a tremendous amount of propaganda and disseminated it successfully throughout the scientific, medical and public arenas. But you won't see "sponsored by the caffeine industry" stamped across the top. This material is

invariably published by foundations and institutes with very academic sounding names."

Please remember the story about my professor who taught me how any scientist can make just about any scientific study prove what they want it to, if they keep blinkers on. For example, you will note that when a study says something like "green tea is good for you" – it usually isn't green tea they are studying, but something good that is in green tea. Rat poison is 95% good food. Plants with good nutrition produce caffeine, which is poison, to protect the rest of the plant. Wild animals have the sense to stay away from it.

Shockingly enough, there have even been scientific studies where scientists were found to have *lied* about their results.

In another study I saw, it claimed that chocolate was good for you, but the study looked only at healthy people. The effects of caffeine are much, much greater when people have health problems, so that was why they were not included in the study. Remember, as the saying goes, there are three kinds of lies - lies, damned lies and statistics.

Reducing caffeine consumption greatly threatens not just the billions of dollars yearly from caffeine products, but also the profits from the $2.2 trillion a year the Medical Mafia receives for so-called 'health' care in the United States of America (five times more than the defense budget[29]). That buys the services of a lot of scientists and marketing campaigns. Even many health-food stores like to profit from this addiction. The truth is the truth, and does not change with time.

There are now ridiculous studies out which try to show that drinking coffee reduces one's risk of death. How that can be true when other studies show, for example, that "Even in moderate doses, caffeine can raise blood pressure in healthy young men and women to the level of borderline hypertension."[30,31] Before you believe any article telling you that anything that contains caffeine is good for you, find out who paid for both the study and the article.

But it's not just about money. A major problem is that caffeine is a highly addictive drug, and almost everyone is addicted to it, including doctors and scientists. It's easy to tell what particular toxins a lot of weight-loss authors are addicted to – just look at what they tell you to eat and drink. They won't be telling you to give up something that they have not yet themselves been able to give up. If they are addicted to a toxin, they will not want to, or think about, researching how bad it is, because then they will have to give up their addiction themselves.

The addictive quality of caffeine is why they put it in sodas, and in Australia, they even add it to lollipops for children! Corporations had to find something that was almost as addictive as cocaine, once they were no longer allowed to use cocaine in sodas. (Plus they add 9 teaspoons of sugar, which is also addictive, to one can of soft drink to mask the bitter taste of caffeine).

> "A survey at the campus of Pennsylvania State University has shown that some students drank 14 cans of soda a day. .... If deprived, these persons would develop withdrawal symptoms, very much like those addicted to drugs. .... *Caffeine is addictive.*"[32]

Now there are even fraudulent studies that look as though they are showing how caffeine helps all kinds of health problems, including weight problems, because, as one TV doctor likes to say, it "raises your metabolism". What a joke. I will quote from "Caffeine Blues":

> "Is caffeine a "fat-burner"? Only in so far as stress accelerates the conversion of fat to fatty acids. Remember, this reaction is part of the fight-or-flight response. But *unless* that conversion is followed by *strenuous exercise*, the fatty acids will simply be redeposited in fat tissue when the caffeine wears off.

> What about the claim that caffeine raises metabolic rate? Once again, caffeine promoters are using half-truths to push their product. Caffeine will increase metabolic rate, but only to the extent of burning an extra 50 – 75 calories a day. And even that effect requires more caffeine than most people would normally consume."

This mild apparent gain is more than destroyed by all the other negative side effects of taking a drug that puts your body into chemical stress. For example, remember that caffeine reduces metabolic efficiency by constricting blood vessels. So again, it's a scam, designed to make money.

Some people will say that "moderate" amounts are okay. But the problem is that no scientist has been able to work out what 'moderate' amounts are. And, since the effects of caffeine are cumulative over time, and most scientific studies are short term, we may never know the truth. A toxin is a toxin no matter what. We have enough toxins in our environment without drinking extra ones. And caffeine is not an ordinary toxin. It is a drug that puts your body into stress, for a long time. The chapter on drugs shows how drugs are fattening. Dr. Dement M.D., Ph.D. in *The Promise of Sleep* says of caffeine:

> "Most of my colleagues agree that if caffeine were a new drug, it would never get approved for human use from the Food and Drug Administration because its side effects outweigh its benefits as a stimulant."

CHOCOLATE IS BAD NEWS

We are now being told that it is great to eat dark chocolate if you want to get thin, but the truth is, I am sorry to say, the opposite. Perhaps you always knew this deep down inside? Please keep an open mind about what I am about to say, no matter how unpleasant this information may be to you. Unfortunately, chocolate contains caffeine, which is fattening because it's a dangerous drug which puts your body into stress. But chocolate also has other fattening toxins.

Anything that is as addictive as chocolate is, is very toxic, and therefore messes up your body's ability to function properly, and therefore makes people fat. The harder it is for you to give it up, the more important it is that you should do so.

Like a lot of women, I got suckered in for a while that a little dark chocolate was okay, maybe even slimming. HA! At first it made no difference to my weight – wonderful! But before long the toxins got to my body so that it could not work so well. Kinesiology and muscle testing showed that chocolate was continually putting my body out of balance, and before I knew it, I put on an extra ten pounds. It took me months and zero chocolate to get those pounds back off me. Some people would say that is just because "I am allergic to chocolate". I would say to them that chocolate is so toxic, that it will affect everyone in some way or other, even if the effects will not show up until the long term.

Unfortunately, even though the chocolate industry keeps putting out articles which supposedly show that chocolate is 'good' for you, the truth is that if you are eating any chocolate, and have fat to lose, or health problems to heal, then you should give up the chocolate for at least three months to see what it does for you. This is because chocolate contains the following.

1. Theobromine. This is an alkaloid, which means it has similarities to morphine, nicotine, cocaine, strychnine. No wonder chocolate is so addictive! This is why dogs often die if fed chocolate, because they can't survive doses of theobromine as large as we can. (Hint: If it kills dogs, it's not something you should have either).

2. Phenylethylamine (PEA) (Pronounced Phenyl-ethyl-amine). I was told this by a naturopath I know and respect, who is very well read and knows all kinds of interesting facts about natural health, that phenylethylamine is something that your body produces when you are happily in love.

"If it could really make two hearts as one, the Arrow of Love may have been spiked with phenylethylamine, the same organic compound contained in chocolates that causes you to walk on Cloud 9 similar to the feeling when you are crazy in love. The delightful intoxicating feeling that is accompanied by the accelerated pounding of the heart is not simply a sign of being mushy, after all. It is the response of your body to the increase of the concentration of this compound in parts of the brain.[33]"

I have an intuitive feeling that is a main reason why people, especially females, are addicted to chocolate. They are getting a chemical replacement for love. The problem with any chemical replacement is that your body then *stops producing* that chemical naturally, since your eating the substance saves your body the trouble of making it. Then you will feel the desire to keep getting more fixes, just like with any drug addict.

3. Very high oxalate content, especially in cocoa. This means more toxins. High oxalate can also cause kidney stones.

4. Anandamide. This substance *mimics marijuana!* (Note: Unknown to many people, marijuana can cause anger). Is this something that children should have?

5. Dangerous levels of *lead*[34]. Interestingly, while cocoa beans tested had an average lead concentration of less than 0.5 ng/g, manufactured cocoa and chocolate products were as high as 230 and 70 ng/g.

6. Sugar. Sugar is so toxic that any sugar can make a person fat, but it is the least of your problems with chocolate.

7. Caffeine. Caffeine raises cortisol levels, which give you a fat belly, in addition to a whole host of other fattening reactions.

It may help you to get the willpower to give up chocolate if you know that 50% of all chocolate, cocoa and chocolate flavoring is farmed by **real slaves**, many of them **children**. For more information on this, please see the excellent and horrifying documentaries *Slavery: A Global Investigation* and *The Dark Side of Chocolate.* If you must eat chocolate or chocolate flavorings, please eat only organic or fair trade products, which are free of slave labor (see www.FreeTheSlaves.net).

If you have children, do you think they should have chocolate which has dangerous levels of deadly lead, as well as caffeine which puts their body into stress, anandamide which mimics marijuana, and theobromine which is similar to strychnine?

Muscle testing and kinesiology show that many health problems are partly caused by toxins from chocolate. To do this test, one needs to know how to do a test for "emotional over-ride". When a kinesiologist does a normal muscle test for a food that is weakening to the body, the arm being tested goes weak. This doesn't happen a lot of the time with chocolate, because the body has become so addicted to chocolate and the "high" that it gives, that it does an extra effort called "emotional over-ride" to make the test appear to be positive.

When one does the emotional over-ride technique, some substances that previously appeared to test positive will then test negative. This often happens with chocolate. In fact, this happens with many foods that people are addicted to, including caffeine, bread and French fries, and explains why some people believe that muscle testing for negative foods is not okay.

I have been in balance and out of balance so many times, and found that the cause was chocolate so many times, that I have actually given up chocolate. Most people find it very hard to believe that I never eat chocolate, and haven't for years. On the occasions when someone has sent me chocolate, I have either given it away or (horrors!) put it in the trash. That's where it belongs.

Just because something is 'natural' does not mean that it is good for you! Deadly nightshade and mercury are natural. In any case, chocolate is highly processed, which is not natural. The more a food is processed, the less the body likes it. In fact, in the days around 1999 when I was still eating chocolate, but at the same time starting to get more sensitive and in tune with my body, I found that the chocolate that seemed to affect me worst was the more delicious and more expensive (i.e. more processed) chocolate.

However, even raw cacao has caffeine and other toxins, so that you should not have even that, especially if you have fat or health problems.

The fact that some people now think that chocolate is a food rather than a super treat meant to be saved for special occasions is evidence that the marketing program for chocolate has been very successful. It has nothing to do with the truth. Note that many studies that are done always look at things that are in chocolate, not at chocolate as a whole. A scientific study can be made to 'prove' just about anything, especially when there is big money to fund it. Remember, each cancer victim gives the medical industry an average of $300,000 to $1.3 million[35].

I recommend going cold turkey on chocolate and cocoa and never go back. It's a drug, and like any addictive drug, the only safe way to stay off it is to never go back. Giving up chocolate was a lot harder for me than giving up caffeine in the form of coffee and green tea. But it was sure worth it. Amazingly, if you can stay off chocolate long enough (say 3 months), you will begin to forget that it ever existed.

You can substitute carob on occasion, because at least it does not have caffeine in it. But unfortunately, carob seems to have its own set of toxins (after all, it looks and tastes rather like chocolate), and is not something that you should have often, if at all.

TIP FOR WAKING UP IN THE MORNING

If you need caffeine to get going in the morning, try this. Have a shower and get your head wet. Running water has negative ions which help to wake you up. And, most importantly, just before you get out, for one or two seconds, make the water as cool or even as cold as you can bare. The colder it is, the more you will wake up!

TAKE THE CHALLENGE

Most people have no idea what life would be like without the background of caffeine and other chemicals coursing through their veins.

Please re-read the 26 ways that caffeine makes people fat. Then, if you have tried many ways to get rid of fat, and you have been taking any caffeine, it just may be that one of these facts that show how caffeine makes people fat is the one that has been affecting you. Go two months without all caffeine. Note the difference and write it down, so later on if you feel the addiction again, you will have the strength to resist it.

REFERENCES

1. *First for women*, 2/12/12 – quoting "Cracking the Metabolic Code" by James LaValle NC.
2. *First for women* magazine, 7/9/12.
3. *Caffeine Blues*, by Stephen Cherniske, MS, page 17.
4. W. Lovallo, M. Al'Absi, K. Blick et al. "Stress-like Adreno-corticotropin Responses to Caffeine in Young Healthy Men, *Pharmacology, Biochemistry*

and Behavior, Nov 1996:55(3):365-69.

5. *Caffeine Blues* by Stephen Cherniske, M.S., Page 80.

6. *The Promise of Sleep,* William Dement M.D., Ph.D., 1999, page 269.

7. *Caffeine Blues,* by Stephen Cherniske, M.S., page 16.

8. *Caffeine Blues* by Stephen Cherniske, M.S., Page 89.

9. *Caffeine Blues* by Stephen Cherniske, M.S., Page 91.

10. *Caffeine Blues* by Stephen Cherniske, M.S., Page 237.

11. *Caffeine Blues* by Stephen Cherniske, M.S., Page 149.

12. *Caffeine Blues* by Stephen Cherniske, M.S., Page 203.

13. *Mastering Leptin,* by Byron Richards CCN, 2002, 3rd edition 2009, pg 41.

14. *Caffeine Blues* by Stephen Cherniske, M.S., Page 68.

15. www.naturalnews.com/032285_melatonin_weight_gain.html

16. www.expert-weight-loss-tips.com/melatonin-supplement.html

17. *Caffeine Blues* by Stephen Cherniske, M.S., page 110.

18. *Caffeine Blues* by Stephen Cherniske, M.S., page 171.

19. *Caffeine Blues* by Stephen Cherniske, M.S., page 268.

20. *Caffeine Blues* by Stephen Cherniske, M.S., page 314.

21. *Caffeine Blues* by Stephen Cherniske, M.S., page 225.

22. *Caffeine Blues* by Stephen Cherniske, M.S., page 172.

23. *Your Body's Many Cries for Water,* by F. Batmanghelidj M.D., 1992, pg 106

24. www.huffingtonpost.com/michael-greger-md/antibiotics-chicken_b_1470098.html

25. R.J. Matthew and W.H. Wilson, :"Substance Abuse and Cerebral Blood Flow," *American Journal of Psychiatry,* March 1991;148(3):292-305.

26. www.cdc.gov/mmwr/preview/mmwrhtml/mm6120a5.htm

27. www.strokecenter.org/patients/about-stroke/stroke-statistics/

28. *Your Body's Many Cries for Water* by F. Batmanghelidj M.D., 1992, pg 69

29. *Forks Over Knives* Documentary.

30. W.R. Lovallo, G.A. Incomb, B.H. Sung el Al, "Hypertension Risk and Caffeine's Effect on Cardiovascular Activity during Mental Stress in Young Men," *Health Psychology* 1991;10(4):236-43.

31. J.M.MacDougal, L. Musante, S. Castillo et al, "Smoking, Caffeine, and Stress: Effects on Blood Pressure and Heart Rate in Male and Female College Students", *Health Psychology,* 1977: 7(5):461-78.

32. *Your Body's Many Cries for Water,* page 105.

33. phenylethylamine.wikidot.com/example-item-1

34. www.wellsphere.com/healthy-eating-article/processed-chocolate-contains-dangerous-lead-concentrations-study-says/533819 quoting a study done by Environmental Health Perspectives

35. www.beating-cancer-gently.com/index.html

CHAPTER 26

TOXIC FOOD #13
MICROWAVED FOOD IS FATTENING

This is possibly the most contentious issue that I am going to raise. Some people really go ballistic when I tell them that microwaved food is fattening, as well as seriously harming them. So, even if you think I'm crazy, please hear me out.

I have known for years that microwaved food harmed people's health greatly. This was the subject of one of my first articles for my website "Health, Wealth & Happiness" at www.Relfe.com, back in 1998. When I began to realize that toxins were the main cause of the growing epidemic of obesity, I knew that microwave ovens were part of the problem. So, I went looking for evidence to back up my theory that microwaved food is fattening. Thanks to the internet, it was easy to find. This was reported by BBC Online:

"Professor Jane Wardle says obesity rates started to rise soon after 1984 - around the time of the rapid spread of microwave owner-ship. In 1980, 8% of women and 6% of men were classified as obese. By 2004 this had increased to 24% of men and women....Professor Wardle who is professor of clinical psychology at University College London said: 'I looked at the figures showing rates of obesity in the population over many years and it seems *very clear it began between 1984 and 1987*. So then we looked at what changes were going on in the food and activity world at that time and one of the striking changes was there were differences in the speed with which we could prepare a meal as a consequence of the *introduction of microwaves.*'"

By 2001 obesity rates in the UK had risen to 34% in men and 39% in women[2]. (Which showed an opposite trend to figures from the USA, where men were shown to be have a higher percentage).

The Professor did not suggest how microwaved food caused obesity. She just noticed that obesity went up suddenly when microwave oven sales went up. You will now learn why this is the case. Much of the following information was first published in an article in the 1994 edition of *Acres Magazine.*

There was a lawsuit in 1991 in Oklahoma. A woman named Norma Levitt had hip surgery, but was killed by a simple blood transfusion when a nurse "warmed the blood for the transfusion in a microwave oven.[3]" Logic suggests that if heating is all there is to microwave cooking, then it doesn't matter how something is heated. Blood for transfusions is routinely warmed, but not in microwave ovens. Therefore, microwaving must be *different* from normal heating.

There have been very few scientific studies done on the effect of eating food cooked in a microwave oven. This is rather surprising when you think about the fact that microwave ovens have been with us for only a few decades, and in that time the incidence of many diseases, as well as obesity, has continued to increase.

MICROWAVES DENATURE FOOD

Two researchers, Blanc and Hertel, confirmed that microwave cooking *significantly* changes food nutrients. Hertel previously worked as a food scientist for several years with one of the major Swiss food companies. He was fired from his job for questioning procedures in processing food because they *denatured it.* He got together with Blanc of the Swiss Federal Institute of Biochemistry and the University Institute for Biochemistry.

They studied the effect that microwaved food had on eight individuals, by taking blood samples immediately after eating. They found that after eating microwaved food, *hemoglobin levels decreased.* "These results show anemic tendencies. The situation became *even more pronounced* during the second month of the study".

That is shocking. Food is meant to strengthen the body, not make it anemic! Who knows what results they would have found if they had studied people who ate microwaved food for a year or more?

The violent change that microwaving causes to the food molecules forms new forms called *radiolytic compounds.* These are mutations that are unknown in the natural world. Ordinary cooking also causes the formation of some radiolytic compounds (which is no doubt one reason why it is better to eat plenty of *raw* food), but microwaving cooking causes a *much* greater number. This causes deterioration in your blood and immune system.

Lymphocytes (white blood cells) also showed a more distinct short-term decrease, following the intake of microwaved food, than after the intake of all the other variants.

Another change was a decrease in the ratio of HDL (good cholesterol) and LDL (bad cholesterol) values. More good fats and less bad fats is a key to getting thin. Each of these indicators pointed to degeneration.

The results were published in *Search for Health* in the Spring of 1992. How was this research greeted? A powerful trade organization, the Swiss Association of Dealers for Electroapparatuses for Households and Industry somehow made the President of the Court of Seftigen issue a `gag order'. Hertel and Blanc were told that if they published their findings they would face hefty fines or up to one year in prison. In response to this, Blanc recanted his findings. Hertel, on the other hand, went on a lecture tour and demanded a jury trial.

Finally, in 1998 the Court `Gag Order' was removed. In a judgment delivered at Strasbourg on 25 August 1998 in the case of Hertel v. Switzerland, the European Court of Human Rights held that there had been a violation of Hertel's rights in the 1993 decision. The Court decided that the `gag order' prohibiting him from declaring that microwaved food is dangerous to health was contrary to the right to freedom of expression. In addition, Switzerland was sentenced to pay compensation of 40,000 Francs.

Sometime after I published my article about microwaved food on the internet, I was approached by Richard Patterson, the author of the *Lawyers Medical Cyclopedia*. The Lawyers Cyclopedia is used by lawyers who sue in medical cases. At that time it was eight volumes, and it has now grown to ten volumes. Because Mr. Patterson was able to verify the court proceedings, he published my information about microwaved food and the results of Hertel in the Cyclopedia. Here is some additional information about the *Lawyers Medical Cyclopedia.*

"Lawyers' Medical Cyclopedia authoritative reference for attorneys involved in personal injury, medical malpractice, workers' compensation, social security, disability income, and health insurance cases. First published 40 years ago, this 10-volume reference is now in its fourth edition.

Lawyers' Medical Cyclopedia offers in-depth information and case law on hundreds of medical and surgical specialties. It includes an extensive bibliography of references to medical journals, law review articles, and American Law Reports, as well as summaries of state and federal appellate opinions. Written by physicians skilled at translating complex anatomy, physiology, and medical treatment into clear language that is easy for you to understand, it provides quick, accurate insight into medical issues.

Lawyers' Medical Cyclopedia keeps you up-to-date on the latest medical and legal developments with annual supplementation written by specialists in both medicine and the law. It saves you valuable research time by emphasizing medical and medicolegal issues most likely to be the subject of litigation and focusing on information most useful to busy practitioners."

Lawyers' Medical Cyclopedia
of
Personal Injuries and
Allied Specialties

SIXTH EDITION

LexisNexis

MICROWAVED FOOD CAUSES CANCER

After World War II, the Russians also experimented with microwave ovens. From 1957 up to recently, their research was carried out mainly at the Institute of Radio Technology at Klinsk, Byelorussia. According to US researcher William Kopp, who gathered much of the results of Russian and German research, and was apparently prosecuted for doing so[4], the following effects were observed by Russian forensic teams:

1. Heating prepared meats or plants in a microwave oven created a number of *cancer-causing* agents.

2. Microwave emissions caused alteration in the breakdown behavior of elements within frozen fruits when thawed in a microwave oven.

3. Microwaves altered the behavior of plant-alkaloids when raw, cooked or frozen vegetables were exposed for even very short periods.

4. Ingestion of micro-waved foods caused a higher percentage of *cancerous cells* in blood.

5. After eating microwaved food, malfunctions occurred in the *immune system*.

6. Micro-waved foods altered food substances, leading to *disorders in the digestive system*.

7. Those ingesting micro-waved foods showed a statistically higher incidence of stomach and intestinal *cancers*, plus a general degeneration of digestive and excretory system function.

8. Microwave exposure caused significant decreases in the nutritional value of all foods studied, including a decrease in B vitamins, vitamin C, vitamin E and essential minerals.

As a result microwave ovens were banned in Russia in 1976. Unfortunately, the ban was lifted a number of years later.

MICROWAVING FOOD CREATES TRANS FATS

In 1989, the Lancet medical journal reported that heating baby formula in a microwave changed its chemistry. Dr. Lita Lee found that microwaving converts some trans-amino acids into synthetic substances similar to unhealthy trans-fatty acids. No wonder obesity started to sky rocket when microwaved ovens were introduced![5]

MUSCLE TESTING VERIFIES THAT MICROWAVED FOOD IS TOXIC

During my kinesiology training, I was told that it was important for people to stop eating microwaved food, but initially I did not pay too much attention to this because I had been using a microwave oven for years. I never thought much about it. I suppose that I figured that if something was so bad for us, then there wouldn't be so many people using it. Little did I know.

When I first began seeing clients for sessions of kinesiology in 1993, I did not tell them to give up eating microwaved food. However, I kept a record of all of the corrections that were needed for each client when they came in. Now, once a correction is made, it is to be hoped that the correction will stay in place for a long time to come, hopefully months if not years. People often ask me "How long will it last?" My answer to them is "That depends on your lifestyle".

Most of my clients came back to see me after about two weeks. In the early days I found that many who came back were not much better. I found that they still had most of their symptoms and they were again `out of balance'. That is, their electrical circuits were not working correctly, which is common for many people. It was therefore not surprising that their symptoms had not improved, because the body does not fix itself fully until the electrical circuits are in balance.

The question was, why did their electrical circuits go out of balance? The answer had to be something that was *highly* stressful, to affect the body in such a short space of time.

Once that answer was remedied, the client would begin to get better. Using muscle testing, I went through the process of 'talking' to the body, and testing to see if the cause was electrical, chemical, nutritional, emotional or structural. Again and again the same answer would come up - electrical. When I then went through a range of possible electrical causes, the same answer again came up again and again - the person had eaten microwaved food! Incidentally, this answer never came up when a person had *not* eaten microwaved food.

I began to tell all of my clients on their first visit that under no circumstances were they ever to eat microwaved food again. That includes heating up food, or even water, in a microwave oven. (Microwaves work on the water in the food). I gave this a higher priority than any of things that are normally considered as health risks, such as cigarettes or alcohol. Immediately I began to get a marked improvement in the results I was getting. Long term problems such as headaches, back aches and emotional instability went away within a few weeks.

Other kinesiologists can confirm these results. David Bridgman, who has years of experience as a kinesiologist, said "Of all the people I test for allergies, 99.9% so far show *severe sensitivity* to any microwaved food".

I experienced the effect of eating microwaved food for myself one time. I had been doing quite a lot of kinesiology and was feeling on top of the world, when for no apparent reason I began to feel rather `grey' and rather low. I realized that I needed a balance from a kinesiologist. Sure enough, I was out of balance. When the kinesiologist used muscle testing to see why my body had gone out of balance, the answer that came up was microwaved food. The trouble was, I couldn't remember eating any, until I remembered a particular vegetarian restaurant I had been to. When I went back to the restaurant and asked them if they microwaved their food, they told me that they did. The 'steamed' vegetables were in fact microwaved!

So be warned! Many restaurants use microwave cooking, even `health' restaurants. Ask if anything is microwaved.

MICROWAVED PLASTIC WRAP HAS 10,000 TIMES FDA LIMITS OF CARCINOGENS!

As a seventh grade student, Claire Nelson learned that there is a carcinogen called DEHA, in plastic wrap. She also learned that the FDA had never studied the effect of microwave cooking on plastic-wrapped food. Three years later Claire set out to test what the FDA had not.

Dr. Jon Wilkes at the National Center for Toxicological Research agreed to help her. The research center, which is affiliated with the FDA, let her use its facilities to perform her experiments, which involved microwaving plastic wrap in virgin olive oil.

She found that DEHA was migrating into the oil at between 200 parts and 500 parts per million[6]. The FDA standard is only 0.05 parts per billion. Claire tested four different plastic wraps and found that not only were carcinogens migrating into the oil, but also Xenoestrogens which are linked to obesity, as well as low sperm counts in men and to breast cancer in women.

ALTERNATIVES TO MICROWAVES

You can easily and quickly heat up food, even frozen pasta, by using a stainless steel saucepan with a lid and a little water, to moisten it from the steam. If someone is coming home late, and you want to give them warm food when they arrive, put a saucepan lid over the food while it is on a plate. Put the plate of food on a simmering saucepan of water. It will stay warm without drying up, for ages. You can also heat food quickly in a convection oven. It's just an ordinary oven with a fan.

If you want to cook food, do it the old fashioned way. It tastes much better that way!

Microwave cooking is adding dangerous toxins to your body, plus destroying nutrition, thereby hurting your body and causing you to be more hungry. Put the microwaved oven in the garage, or throw it out. Make these simple changes to your life and see if you don't feel better, and reduce fat.

REFERENCES

1. *BBC Online*, 6 June 2007
2. www.nhs.uk/news/2013/02February/Pages/Latest-obesity-stats-for-England-are-alarming-reading.aspx
3. *Acres Magazine*, USA, 1994, article by Tom Valentine
4. *J. Nat. Sci*, 1998; 1:42-3
5. www.pccnaturalmarkets.com/sc/0601/sc0601-microwave.html
6. *Carcinogens --At 10,000 Times FDA Limits* Options, May 2000. Published by *People Against Cancer*, 515-972-4444

CHAPTER 27

TOXIC FOOD #14
JUNK FOOD = JUNK BODY

Fast food is part of junk food, but it's not the only source of it, because supermarkets are full of junk food. Since so many people know that junk food is fattening and unhealthy, one would think that all fast food outlets would have closed down by now. However, since so many people still give their money to junk food companies, and because junk food is a major cause of obesity, I thought I would include information on it, not because it's high in calories, but because it is so toxic, in the hope that this will encourage you to never give them another dollar of your money, until they change their ways. Fast food does not have to be so toxic and fattening.

Why do people keep eating fast food when obviously everyone wants to be slim, so that they can look and feel great? Why do we have to have organizations like "Overeaters Anonymous" for people who believe, as they say on the website, *"Our symptoms may vary, but we share a common bond: we are powerless over food and our lives are unmanageable[i]."*

It's because junk food works *like drugs*. That is, junk food is *addictive*. People who can't control their eating are not addicted to food. It's just that the particular foods that they eat are addictive. When these people make the switch to a diet made of vegetables, fruit, nuts, seeds and legumes, with a few other foods such as organic eggs and millet bread, they will see their hunger and cravings go down.

Nature programmed us to want to get the most energy-dense foods. This was designed to help us to stay alive when food was scarce, so that we could pack maximum energy into a small stomach. Therefore, nature gave us *pleasure-circuits* in our brain that cause feelings of euphoria and excitement when we eat foods that have lots of energy in a small volume[2]. The trouble is that now we can increase calorie density artificially, by processing and adding sugar and fats.

The junk food companies know this, but they don't care, because it makes them rich. I like to think of them as a part of the Food Mafia. They are little more than drug pushers. To make matters worse, companies such as McDonald's add *emotional* addiction to the chemical addiction. Why else do they continue to sell so-called "Happy meals" to children, and advertise on children's programs, if not to addict people at a young age and keep them customers for life? Other methods used include free toys, selling toys in toy stores that are designed by them, and providing play centers.

Every time you think of McDonalds, they want you to have feelings that are based on happy, fun times. Since most people don't think about where their feelings come from, these people will have false urges to eat McDonalds to relive those feelings, until they recognize and refuse those urges.

In the brilliant documentary *Forks Over Knives*, Dr. Terry Mason M.D., Commissioner of Health for the City of Chicago, tells us that unfortunately, it's often poor people who eat fast food. This is particularly sad when you work out that fast food these days is expensive, especially if you work out how much actual nutrition you get dollar for dollar. Five dollars buys one fast food hamburger, or a large amount of nutritious lentils and carrots. Dr. Mason says that unfortunately poor people are poor in everything, not just money, but they are also poor in health and poor in their *choices*.

If you eat any junk food, or smoke cigarettes, realize that you are a slave to the multinational companies. They are living off your work and your body so that they can be rich. And, of course, they are killing you while they do it.

I was shocked with what I saw on a TV show run by a doctor, that was meant to be about health. This same doctor had done some good work previously telling people to avoid GMOs, and therefore to not eat any dairy that was not organic. But on this particular show, the doctor asked two other doctors to go and find a healthy fast food meal. (Is that possible?) Strangely, only three fast food outfits were chosen for this task; McDonald's, Domino's Pizza and Subway. Nothing else was considered. I wonder if those companies paid for the privilege, just as most authors have to pay tens of thousands of dollars to appear on all the top talk shows?

The overweight heart surgeon picked chicken McNuggets. That was unbelievable! There are few things as toxic as McDonald's chicken McNuggets. First of all, there is little chicken in them. They are 56% corn, mostly GMO corn[3], and the chickens are also fed GMOs and other toxic stuff, including their own manure. Then the McNuggets are super heated in toxic oils, so that they are full of trans fats and AGEs. Worst of all, there are a massive total of 38 *ingredients*, including tertiary butylhydroquinone, a *lighter fluid*[4]. Are chicken McNuggets really *food*?

Moral of this story: Keep an eye on who is benefiting financially when watching any so-called 'health show'.

The other doctor chose pizza with pepperoni. Pepperoni is embalmed meat. And this piece came just after a part where the doctor had restaurant insiders admit that pizzas have sugar added to them.

If you ever eat any fast food at all, please watch the fabulous movie *Super Size Me*. While it's mostly about McDonald's, many of the lessons learned in this movie apply to all fast food outlets. Even if you have seen this documentary, you may have missed some of the more important points, as I did on first viewing the movie. So I will outline some of them here.

In the documentary Morgan Spurlock, writer and director, begins with a court case where two overweight girls, one 14 years old, 4'10" and 170 pounds and the other 19 years old, 5'6" and 270 pounds, sued McDonalds in 2002, for making them fat. The girls ended up losing the court case. But, just in case something like this happened again, in 2004 congress passed the 'cheeseburger bill' which made it illegal for people to sue food companies for making them obese. You see, congress currently works to protect corporations, not you.

The judge said the lawsuit was "frivolous" because "the dangers of eating its food is universally known." Yet, despite this, McDonalds has 30,000 outlets in over 100 countries. 46 million people are served daily, even in hospitals! No wonder obesity is global.

The judge further said that if the plaintiffs could show that McDonalds intend for people to eat McDonald's every meal of every day, and that doing so would be reasonably dangerous, they may be able to state a claim.

So Morgan decided to go on a diet of nothing but McDonald's food and drink, three times a day, for one month. During the month, he ate everything on the menu. In addition, since most Americans don't get any exercise, he got very little exercise as well. This was ground breaking research because it was being done on a real human in a real-life situation, not just a few rats in a lab. And the research was independent of any large organization that might interfere with the conclusions. Morgan definitely showed that, for him, it was *very* dangerous.

First he visited three medical professionals, including a cardiologist and General Practitioner, as well as an exercise physiologist. His blood pressure was normal and his blood tests were excellent. His general health was determined to be outstanding. The doctors thought that the McDonalds' diet would be no big deal. The cardiologist thought that his triglycerides would go up but nothing else would change. The M.D. thought his cholesterol and weight would 'probably' go up. They were all in for a massive shock, because it did not occur to any of them how bad this diet would be for him, or that it would prove to be incredibly toxic. In fact, it became so toxic that it became life-threatening! Here are some of the results for Morgan after only 30 days:

- He gained 25 pounds (185 to 210).

- Body fat percentage (BMI) went from 11% to 18%.

- Cholesterol went from 65 points to 230.

- At day 14, two different liver enzymes skyrocketed. One enzyme went from 21 to 130, the other went from 20 to 290. The massive increase in liver enzyme activity showed that the diet was *highly toxic*. The M.D. said after just day 14, "If someone was doing this with alcohol, they could theoretically wipe out their liver". (Note: If you don't have a functioning liver, you are not going to get rid of fat, assuming you stay alive).

- At day 21 the M.D. said after a blood test, "For the first time we're seeing uric acid elevated. The danger of this is gout and kidney stones". (Note: Gout, a very painful disease 'of the past' is now on the rise). "The results for your liver are obscene beyond anything I would have thought....My advice to you, as a physician, is that you've got to stop. You're pickling your liver. And you're kicking it while it's down...If you were an alcoholic, I'd say, *"You are going to die."*

I guess the doctor did not want to say the obvious on video: That means that McDonald's can kill you.

Despite this warning, and feeling chest pains and depressed and moody most of the time, which was unusual for him, Morgan completed the 30 day McDonalds' diet. Perhaps most importantly of all for anyone who wants to get thin, he noticed that he got hungry soon after eating. Whereas, when you go on a wheat-free, soy-free, whole-foods plant-based diet, with lots of raw plant food, you will notice that you seldom get hungry. The more totally raw meals you have, the less hungry you will get.

In just 30 days, Morgan ate 30 pounds of sugar from the food alone, not counting drinks. That's one pound a day, because nearly everything on the menu has sugar added to it, even the salads. You see, sugar is addictive, and cheap, so that makes good financial sense. During the month, Morgan craved the food more and more, and got massive headaches when he did not eat it. Those are signs of addiction.

After the McDonald's diet, Morgan went on a vegan diet to detox[5]. It took 8 weeks for his cholesterol and liver to go back to normal. Then he gave up being vegan. It took him 5 months to lose 20 pounds, and another 8 months to lose the last 5 pounds.

It was truly amazing and sad that after this fantastic documentary came out, it barely made a difference to any fast food outlets, except that they made a little effort to *appear* as though they were offering healthier food, by adding a few salads with toxic dressing, but they did little if anything to alter the basic toxic menu items.

We have to break the addiction to junk food. Addictive food is high in calories and toxins. Unfortunately, there are two kinds of addiction that we get from fast food.

TWO KINDS OF ADDICTION FROM JUNK FOOD

1. Chemical addiction

Dr. Neal Barnard M.D., of the Physicians Committee for Responsible Medicine, has this to say[6],

"There is a drug used in emergency rooms called naloxone. It's used for heroin overdose. A guy comes in overdosed on heroin, comatose, he's going to die. If you inject him with this drug and it blocks the opiate receptors in the brain, heroin doesn't work, he wakes up. If I give that same drug to a real chocolate addict, a person who just shovels it in, you find the most amazing thing. They lose much of their interest in chocolate. They take a bite, they set it back down.

In other words, it's not the "taste in the mouth" feel, it's the drug effect of the food in the brain which keeps us coming back".

Dr. Barnard further explains –

"If you look at the menu at a fast food restaurant, they use all of the addicting components. They'll take a slab of meat, cover it with cheese – cheese, of course, which is filled with casomorphins, the opiates that are found in cheese protein. And then they serve it with a sugary soda, which has the addictive power of sugar, with plenty of added caffeine" (Caffeine is a highly addictive drug. Plus, you learned in the chapter on wheat that wheat also has opiate-like substances in it).

This chemical addiction is so bad, that scientists found that rats fed nothing but junk food from the supermarket (bacon, sausage, cheese cake etc) for long enough, not only got obese – they voluntarily *starved themselves* when later offered nothing but healthy food. It got so bad, that after 40 days of addiction, the rats were willing to put up with painful electric shocks to the feet, just so they could get hold of more junk food! [7]

We need to make new laws where addictive food is concerned. As Pediatric Endocrinologist Dr. Robert Lustig says, free speech does not work with addictive substances, especially where children are concerned[8].

2. Emotional addiction

Banzhaf III, Law Professor, George Washington University[9] has this to say:

"A secret study by one of the tobacco companies had the ominous title of something like *'Brand Imprinting for later actuation in life'* ".

You can bet that the junk food companies have something similar. That's why junk food companies spend so much on advertising to children. They want you to have commands in your brain to eat their food, combined with good feelings from childhood, buried in your mind. For example, the average American child sees a whopping 10,000 ads per year for things to eat and drink. 95% of these ads are for fast food, candy, soft drinks and cereals, none of which are nutritious.

Don't go thinking it's just McDonalds, either. All junk food and pre-packaged food is contributing to fat gain, because of the toxins and excess calories which they contain.

Any food outlet which does not give you a list of all their ingredients is suspect. I am not talking about a chart that says how many calories or grams of fat are in the food, but *what* is in the food. In fact, even with the list of ingredients, you still don't get to know the quantity of each ingredient. Listen to a quote from the lawsuit against McDonalds:

"McDonald's claims that ...it is... a matter of common knowledge that any processing that its foods undergo serve to make them *more harmful* than unprocessed foods."

DON'T LISTEN TO THE MOUTHPIECES FOR THE CORPORATIONS

Be very, very wary of anyone who has a story of getting thin from a fast food outlet, rather than preparing their own fresh food at home. Subway is a case in point. They have this guy Jared who says he lost hundreds of pounds from eating their food. Note that he went from doing no exercise to doing quite a bit of walking[10]. I wonder how much? Subway had nothing to do with that.

It broke my heart to watch a young, very overweight 14 year old girl say about Subway, on *Super Size Me*, after listening to a speech by Jared;

"It's kind of hard. I can't afford to go there every single day and buy a sandwich two times a day. And that's what he's talking about. That's the only solution....But I can't do it."

The only solution? Telling people that eating a whole lot of baked wheat and meat will work for them? This is terrible. So many people have big guts from the many toxins in wheat, and whatever else they add to the bread that makes it so fluffy.

However, pictures of Jared in 2009 show the weight coming back on[11]. That was no surprise to me, since he said he had caffeine and diet drinks, and anyone who lives off a diet of food that is not prepared at home will end up getting toxic, and therefore putting on weight, in the long run. (See my chapter "Health is like a bank account").

Please, anytime you hear anyone saying that they lost weight from eating a particular brand of food, ask yourself how much money that person makes from telling you that.

MOST SCHOOL FOOD IS JUNK FOOD

It's no wonder that, for the first time in history, children are getting obese. When you watch *Super Size Me* you will see that schools now serve up cakes, chips, fries, Gatorade (which is toxic sugar plus other toxins), sugared drinks, candy bars and pizza. For many students, that's all they eat. Filtered water and fresh fruit cannot be seen, and even if healthy food is offered as an alternative, when children have been addicted to junk food, the changes are not going to happen by themselves.

Who profits from junk food? *Super Size Me* shows an example of one such company, Sodexho, which serves 400 school districts, as well as prisoners.

There is one public school in the USA where this is not the case. The Appleton Central High School, Wisconsin, used to have children who were out of control. Children even brought weapons to school. But in 1997. a private group called Natural Ovens installed a healthy lunch program. Fast-food burgers, fries, candy and sodas were replaced with fresh fruit and salads, baked rather than fried meat and whole grain bread and good drinking water arrived. The teachers saw a major change in the children. As reported in a newsletter called Pure Facts, "Grades are up, truancy is no longer a problem, arguments are rare, and teachers are able to spend their time teaching." And while they did not mention it, you can bet that these children are not going to have weight problems as serious as those where junk food is the norm.

Surprisingly, the cost is about the same. So why aren't all schools doing this? Paul Stitt M.S., Founder of Natural Ovens Bakery, explains:

"There's an awful lot of resistance from the junk food companies that are making huge profits off the school system at this time. They don't want to be kicked out of the school system. They want to be there to addict the children for life."

What a great scam! Get taxpayers to pay for their companies to addict children to their cheap, toxic and fattening junk food, for the rest of the children's lives! It sure beats advertising.

If only accurate muscle testing was taught in all schools. I have found that when I show children, especially small children, how junk food is weakening, rather than just 'bad' for them, they become very committed to not consuming that product any more. Some children like being bad, but no child wants to be weak. (Please see Chapter 12 on kinesiology and muscle testing, for more information).

The food industry is an 1.8 trillion dollar business in the United States[12]. It therefore employs very well-paid lobbyists, who work with the government to make you eat more of their product. I strongly believe that one of the best ways to counteract the effects of the wrong messages we are being sent from big corporations and government, as well as from the addictive toxins in our food, is for each and every person to learn how to do accurate muscle testing of food. Even children as young as 12 years old or less can learn how to do this. Children as young as six years old can be muscle tested. When a person has experienced for themselves how just *thinking* of a toxic food makes their arms and legs go weak, their brain often finds the extra willpower that is needed to take personal responsibility, and to eat and drink only healthy food instead.

Remember, wild animals keep slim by eating the food that nature designed them to eat. That's what you need to do. You are a herbivore. Eat plants. That is, fruit, vegetables, nuts, seeds and legumes, as unprocessed as possible. And also have as much raw food as possible. People need to learn new ways of shopping and preparing food. Please see my shopping list in this book. Learn how to prepare food by going to the internet and searching for a vegan and/or raw recipe for the food you bought. The recipes in this book will give you a good place to start. And boycott the Food Mafia whenever you can.

REFERENCES
1. www.oa.org/newcomers/about-oa/
2. *Forks Over Knives* documentary
3. www.alnyethelawyerguy.com/al_nye_the_lawyer_guy/2007/03/so_what_really_.html
4. *The Omnivore's Dilemma*, by Michael Pollan, 2007
5. www.HealthyChefAlex.com

6. *Super Size Me* documentary
7. www.cbsnews.com/2100-204_162-6343889.html
8. www.psmag.com/health/robert-lustig-sugar-obesity-diet-50948/
9. *Super Size Me* documentary
10. en.wikipedia.org/wiki/Jared_Fogle
11. www.thatsfit.com/2009/12/02/subway-guy-falls-off-the-diet-wagon/
12. en.wikipedia.org/wiki/Food_industry

CHAPTER 28

TOXIC FOOD #15
RESTAURANT FOOD

Many people believe that eating out is fattening because you eat a lot, and you eat more fattening food than you would normally. But have you ever had the experience of eating out and putting on two or more pounds, even though you ate a normal amount of what should have been reasonably healthy food, the same kind of food that, if you cooked it yourself, would not have put on weight?

I sure have. I grew up in Australia and ate out at many restaurants in Sydney. Sydney has the some of the best restaurants in the world, both cheap and five star. There are literally hundreds of delicious "mom and pop" restaurants, of many different ethnic backgrounds, and very few chains. I believe that generally, the quality of food in these restaurants is higher than in chain restaurants, probably because they are run by a chef instead of by an accountant.

When I married my American husband Michael in 1997 and we moved to the USA, I began to learn about chain restaurants. Over the years, I started to notice that I would put on at least 2 pounds every time we ate out. It seemed to be mostly 'just' from fluid, as it came off fairly easily. And I could not see how such an ordinary amount of food could put on so much weight in just one day.

As I became more and more concerned about this, I noticed that I put on the two pounds even if I had no appetizer, no bread, no desert and ate just something that would not make me put on weight if I ate it at home, such as broiled fish with a green salad and vegetables, or a black bean burger without the bun plus a caesar salad.

I then began to notice how some chain restaurants seemed to have more than their fair share of customers with really big bottoms.

All these realizations helped me come to the realization that it is not calories that makes us fat, so much as toxins. Unlike supermarkets, restaurants don't have to tell us what ingredients go in the dishes. Unless you are eating at 5 star restaurants, you are bound to be eating food that is made from toxic substances such as vegetable oil, margarine, monosodium glutamate (MSG) and just plain-old chemicals - those words with six syllables that no one has ever heard of. Plus, we have the added problem of genetically modified food in nearly everything, even secretly being used to dilute olive oil.

When you realize the truth to this theory, you will see one reason why people have grown so huge over the last few decades. People used to prepare their own food at home, from real ingredients. Now the average American eats out nearly five times every week[1].

I had more verification of this theory when a particular restaurant chain started selling some of its food in supermarkets, and I was able to read the ingredients. The list of ingredients read more like a science experiment than a list of real food that was grown on a farm.

Probably the worst ingredient in nearly all restaurants is excitotoxins, such as MSG and autolyzed yeast extract. As I said in the chapter on excitotoxins, these are substances which stimulate brain cells into making you think that the food tastes good, even if it's tasteless. They addict you to that food.

JUST ONE RESTAURANT MEAL CAN CAUSE BRAIN LESIONS

Excitotoxins stimulate brain cells so much that just *one dose* is enough to kill brain cells, within hours. Many restaurant meals contain very high doses of MSG, the same doses that regularly produce brain lesions in animals.

Cajun, Chinese and some other Asian restaurants have the most. To make matters worse, humans are much more sensitive to MSG than animals[2]! This kind of damage leads not just to obesity, but also to diseases such as Alzheimer's in old age[3].

The effect of excitoxins is cumulative, so the person may not notice signs of brain damage until they are old, and then probably no one will realize that the dementia and senility that sets in then was the end result of lots of doses of excitotoxins. But, before senility sets in, the person could be getting fatter because of them.

This situation has gotten so bad with the advent of GMOs that we personally don't eat out now. Have a look at the menu of supposedly top restaurants that list their menu on the internet. Without knowing how the food was raised, and where it came from, it's quite likely that you would be much better off finding a way to eat without eating out.

I dream of the day when someone creates a chain restaurant where they do things like:

• Tell you what all the ingredients are. And where they were raised.

• Use only non-GMO food.

• Use only free-range eggs and meat, to prevent cruelty.

• Use only healthy oils. But now that we know that 70% of extra virgin olive oil is toxic, and possibly even genetically modified, this gets difficult (see the chapter on oils).

• Guarantee that MSG and other excitotoxins, wheat, homogenized milk and microwave ovens are never used.

One day on a TV doctor's television show, a restaurant insider admitted that they add tons of butter to meals. I was thinking – butter? - there's nothing wrong with that (except that it could be from cows fed genetically modified food), but it's way too expensive, and I bet they use something else in most restaurants. And then one of the insiders agreed with that thought of mine, by saying something along the lines of, "But, of course, that's in the *good* restaurants. The cheaper ones are more likely to use frankenfoods." Ah ha! As I said, it's accountants that design the meals in most US restaurants, not chefs, and certainly not lovers of health.

REFERENCES

1. www.upi.com/Health_News/2011/09/19/Americans-eat-out-about-5-times-a-week/UPI-54241316490172/
2. *Excitotoxins*, by Dr. Russell Blaylock, 1997, page 117
3. *Excitotoxins*, by Dr. Russell Blaylock, 1997, page 156

CHAPTER 29

TOXIC FOOD #16
FOOD ALLERGIES MAKE YOU FAT

If you eat a food that you are allergic to, it can cause weight gain. Even some doctors agree to this. Whether or not a food causes an allergic reaction, depends on at least four different things:

1. How toxic the food is to begin with.

2. How *often* you have the food (rather than how much you have it).

3. How toxic and out of balance your body is to begin with.

4. Your genetic makeup.

If you have done everything that this book suggests, and you are not yet at your ideal body size, it is quite possible that there is something that you are eating that you are allergic to. If it is not a full-blown allergy, your body could be temporarily negatively affected by a particular food. This usually happens because you have had the food too frequently.

If you ever put on a pound or more overnight, even though you ate sensible sized portions, of what you thought was healthy food, it is quite possible that you ate something that was toxic, or that you were allergic to.

I believe that this is the main reason why people find that last 20 pounds so much harder to reduce than the rest of the weight was. It's not the high calorie foods or the amount they eat. It's just that they are eating something they are allergic to, even if it's just a tiny amount of it, like one tomato or one bite of bread.

Dr. Keith Scott-Mumby wrote a very good book, *Diet Wise*, about allergies, which has some amazing case histories[1]. While I don't agree with everything in his book (for example, he pays very little attention to the vital importance of eliminating GMOs, seems to thinks that any oil is okay, and does not realize that there *is* a physiological reason why kinesiology and muscle testing work), he does have some very important points to make and has had some fantastic results. Until I read his book I was not fully aware of just how strongly an allergy-causing food could affect the *brain*. Anything that affects the brain, can affect your ability to reduce fat, since it's the brain that is going to decide what needs to be done.

If you remove the foods you are allergic to completely from the diet, the over-all burden on the body is reduced so much that the body can heal itself of many symptoms, even 'incurable' ones.

Here are some wonderful case histories from his book. Although they don't relate directly to fat loss, you get an idea of how powerful this can be:

- 39 year old Susan was definitely mentally handicapped, with the mind of a child. After giving up all beef, dairy, wheat and tomatoes for a few weeks, she said, "*I just woke up one day and I was here*". Now she is learning to read, write, count and she can even shop on her own!

- One woman got more drunk on orange juice than on vodka.

- An older youth was so violent that he was charged with attempted murder of his stepfather. Even the judge came to see that his violence was caused by food allergies, particularly potato, but also beef and strawberries. The boy was given a conditional discharge after Scott-Mumby healed him.

- 6-year-old Ryan had muscular dystrophy, which causes a boy to be unable to use his legs, and later on his whole body. It is supposedly 'incurable'. After just two weeks on Scott-Mumby's allergy-food-free program, Ryan was able to run, and later climbed a 200 foot high monument!

- An 8 month old baby had eczema so bad that he was swollen and red, with nearly all his skin cracked and weeping. Skin even came off with his diaper. After two days with no potato, many lesions healed and he peed himself back to his normal size.

- Maxine was moody with temper tantrums, had few friends and was the bottom of her class. After she was taken off a wide variety of foods including wheat, corn, egg, tea, beef, pork, yeast and onions, she became calm, made friends easily and went to the top of the class in a number of subjects. Consider food allergies if children are hyperactive or are having any mental problems.

The foods that you are allergic to are most likely something that you eat or drink every day, or nearly every day. They are especially likely to be something that you do not want to give up. So, to heal allergies and to make sure they don't occur, it's a good idea to make sure that there is no particular food that you eat every day. Unfortunately, you can be allergic to more than one food at a time.

Dr. Scott-Mumby says that it takes a minimum of 4-5 days for all of the food you ate to be removed from your body. If you react to it after 5 days without the food, you are allergic to that food at least for now.

There are a small amount of toxins in most things we eat, even if they are very mild and in tiny concentrations. Plants produce toxins to stop animals eating them. That is why wild animals eat a wide *variety* of plants. They have only a little bit of toxin of one particular plant, and then move on to eat another plant with a different kind of toxin, so that their body can deal with each toxin as it arrives. Whether a toxin becomes a poison or not, depends on the quantity, as well as the strength of the toxin. Only humans consume a vast amount of the same toxin, day in and day out.

Wild animals also have the advantage that by eating a lot of raw, natural plants picked while still living, they are eating food that has a lot more nutrition and life force, which helps them to combat the toxins they eat.

All of the foods that we have discussed so far are toxic to most people, and particularly to anyone who is overweight, whether or not they react obviously to them or not. If they don't appear to have any reactions to the food, it's just that so far their body is managing to cope with it externally, but there could be all kinds of bad things going on inside. Have another look at them when they are 90 years old to see how slim and healthy they look then.

Allergies differ from person to person, and even from time to time, depending on a person's lifestyle, and what kind of balance their body is in. Kinesiologists like myself believe that there are three main kinds of allergies which are specific for each person:

1. Those that can be healed with *three weeks* without that particular food, as long as the person later on does not eat it as frequently as before.

2. Those that can be healed with *three months* without that particular food, as long as the person later on does not eat it as frequently as before.

3. Those that may be a permanent allergy for your body no matter what you do.

Accurate muscle testing shows that food can be classified as positive, neutral or negative. Positive food is strengthening, and will help you get slim. Neutral food does little and you can have some of it for the fun of it. Negative food is weakening and is most likely to cause fat gain.

However, food that a person is allergic to, may appear to muscle test as positive, because the person's emotional attachment to the food interferes with the test. In this case, it is necessary to apply a special technique, called the "emotional over-ride test", when testing, to identify the truth and see that the food actually weakens the person.

Accurate muscle testing shows that the more often you eat a food that is positive for you, the more likely it is that it will eventually become neutral for you. And the more often you eat a food that is neutral for you, the more likely it is that it will become negative for you.

Fortunately, the converse is also true. If you totally give up a negative food, after enough time has elapsed, it may become neutral for you. And if you give up a neutral food for long enough, it may become positive for you, as long as it wasn't too toxic to begin with. This is why variety is so important. If you give up some foods, you end up eating more of other foods, so you could then become allergic to the replacement foods.

You can't always tell by symptoms alone if a food is causing an allergy, because if one develops negative symptoms after eating a particular food, such as being tired, it *may* be from an allergy, but it could also be from a cleansing reaction, as we discussed in the chapter on cleansing reactions. While toxins are being removed from the body, unpleasant symptoms may occur. However, I believe that a cleansing reaction will never cause an overnight weight gain of one or two pounds the way that a food that you are allergic to will.

MAIN ALLERGY-CAUSING FOODS

Dr. Scott-Mumby says that 80% of people are allergic to wheat and dairy, and a lot of people are allergic to different meats, sugar and caffeine. Well, we have already dispensed with these, by showing how they are too toxic for anyone to eat.

While any food can cause an allergy, even lettuce, onions or cinnamon, the following are the foods that cause most allergies. Note that these are also foods that most people eat very frequently.

- Tomatoes, especially cooked tomatoes.

- Potatoes.

- Eggs (it's possible that people are reacting to the toxins fed to the chickens, and that organic, free range eggs are okay).
- Bananas.

- Peanuts (Swap peanut butter for home made nut butters made from almonds, sunflower seeds etc. See the recipe chapter)

- Grains.

- Oranges and pineapple.

- Red plants, particularly red peppers, chili, strawberries, watermelon.

- Yeast (which is in many foods, including vinegar and bread).

- Corn (even if it's not GMO).

- 'Hot' peppery spices, including red pepper, black pepper, chili pepper and mustard.

- Onions, green onions / shallots.

- Garlic.

BANANAS

While a lot of people muscle test negative for bananas, some of these people do not muscle test negative for organic bananas. This is probably because they are not negative for bananas, but for the toxic gas that is used to force early ripening. The gas is ethylene, which is used in blowtorches. I suggest that if you can't afford organic bananas, that you don't eat them at all. This gas is also used on a lot of tomatoes and apples, which is why it is worth going organic at least every now and again, if you can't afford to do it all the time.

EGGS & CHICKENS

Dr. Scott-Mumby in his book *Diet Wise* mentions a number of people who found that they were allergic to eggs. However, it is a pity that at no time does Dr. Scott-Mumby discern between normal factory-farmed toxic eggs and organic, free-range eggs, because there is a world of difference between the two.

I mentioned in the chapter on meat how chickens are fed animal waste from rendering plants. Here's another gross story: I once saw a documentary that showed how factory chickens (which live permanently on wire (ouch), and can't ever stretch their wings) live in wire cages so that their feces can drop below. Once the chicken manure is about 3' high, the cages are removed and a bulldozer brought in. The chicken manure is then put back into chicken feed! (ugh) – with the thought that all the bugs that the chickens have been eating will provide protein. That is the kind of toxin that you might possibly be eating when you eat factory eggs. In addition, you are guaranteed to be eating poisons second-hand, from genetically modified (GMO) soy and corn that is fed to the chickens.

Because chicken parts from chicken factories go back into chicken feed, chickens have gone from being vegetarians to vultures, and it's never a good idea to eat carnivores, because toxins get concentrated the higher up the food chain you go.

One ingredient of some chicken feed is *tannery waste*[2]! And in 2011 the FDA even admitted that chickens are fed *arsenic* – on purpose[3]! To give you an idea of how toxic the food chain has become, chicken litter that contains arsenic is fed to cows to make beef! The cows have become vultures as well. And then they feed the left over parts back to the chickens, over and over.

There will be some people who are allergic to eggs and chicken, and this could be contributing to their body weight. I have already talked about why people should give up meat if they want to get slim and healthy. But I believe that it is quite possible that if these people went three weeks without any eggs at all, and then switched to only organic, free-range eggs, only once or twice a week, then fat loss and an improvement in health are possible while still having eggs.

PEANUTS

So many people are allergic to these, that you know they have more than their fair share of toxins, especially since they can kill people. At one time I had a pain in my hip which was stopping me from doing the 5 minute muscle resistance exercises that I will tell you about later, which indirectly was keeping me from getting slim. Eventually I realized that the cause was peanuts. I left out all peanuts from my home made nut butter, made from almonds, sunflower seeds and other nuts and seeds, and my pain went away, and I started getting a smaller waist again.

BEANS & LENTILS

There are substances in beans and lentils which can cause allergies. However, a lot of the time, these substances become safe if the beans or lentils are soaked for at least 8 hours before using. This 'sprouts' them, so that harmful substances get broken down into safe and easier-to-digest substances. Always soak all beans and lentils for 8 hours, outside a fridge, before using them. You can store them in the fridge after they have soaked.

REFERENCES
1. *Diet Wise*, by Dr. Keith Scott-Mumby, M.B., Ch.B., M.D., Ph.D. 1984, 2012
2. www.thedailystar.net/newDesign/news-details.php?nid=147986
3. www.naturalnews.com/032659_arsenic_chicken.html

CHAPTER 30

TOXIC FOOD #17
OTHER TOXIC FOODS

FOODS HIGH IN ESTROGEN

Excess estrogen causes an increase in fat tissue. Even worse, the more fat you have, the more estrogen you make, which then makes you fatter![1]

In addition, the more estrogen you have, the higher your chance of having blood sugar problems and high blood pressure[2]. Unfortunately, much of the food we eat and many of the toxins in our environment have xenoestrogens, which are chemicals that act as if they are estrogen. Although estrogen is thought of as a female hormone, xenoestrogens are making both men and women fat. Excess estrogen or xenoestrogens are in the following, with the worst offenders mentioned first:

- Soy (the very worst source of all, even if it isn't genetically modified).
- Hops (which explains why people get a 'beer belly').
- Meat. It is deliberately given to livestock to make them fatter. (Hint: These 'fatness' chemicals then make you fatter).

- Dairy.
- Pesticides (on non-organic produce).
- Flexible plastic (food containers, water bottles, toys).
- Perfume, nail polish.
- 100,000 chemicals.
- Licorice.

The best way to get your estrogen levels down is to (1) not eat foods that have excess estrogen, and to (2) eat more foods that are anti-estrogenic. The best anti-estrogenic foods are what are called cruciferous vegetables. Have some raw whenever possible for maximum effect (except for Brussels sprouts). They are:

- Broccoli (organic is best).
- Brussels sprouts.
- Cabbage.
- Cauliflower.

Other Anti-estrogenic foods are:
- Green vegetables (e.g. Italian parsley, spinach).
- Oranges.
- Lemons.
- Pineapple.
- Onions.
- Nuts, raw.
- Seeds, raw.
- Avocado.
- Olives.
- Berries.
- Apples.
- Red grapes.
- Raw honey.
- Chamomile tea.
- Oregano, thyme.

You will see from the above lists that if basically you eat more raw fruit, vegetables, nuts and seeds, that you will automatically get your estrogen levels down, especially if you have some cabbage, cauliflower, Brussels sprouts and broccoli as often as possible, preferably raw.

You probably already know that fiber helps fill you up, and helps keep your bowels efficient. But fiber does much more than that. The fiber from plants soaks up excess estrogen. Fiber also has plant estrogens, which crowd out the bad estrogens, which cause fat.

So, in the long run, it's best to eat whole, raw vegetables, fruits, nuts and seeds. That means, don't just juice everything. Eat *whole*, raw vegetables, fruit, nuts and seeds. This is because many of us gained fat from having too much estrogen.

In addition, do gentle exercise daily, as this also reduces estrogen a lot. Please see the chapter on walking.

ALCOHOL

By now you should know that anything that is toxic is fattening in some way or other. That means that alcohol is fattening, even if it is from wine. But don't expect to see too many well-funded papers proving this. The alcohol industry makes so much money that it's easy to find scientists who design papers that supposedly prove that drinking red wine is good for you. And since alcohol is addictive, it's easy for people to believe this. If that is the case, then it's because red grapes have nutrition, especially red ones, so drink some fresh-squeezed red grape juice instead. But alcohol is toxic and is never good for you.

It is true that there are people who drink wine and are thin, just like there are people who eat donuts and are thin. I am not talking about them. If you have fat you don't want, and you drink any alcohol, it's quite possible that alcohol is what is keeping that fat on you. After all, alcohol is not a food. It's pure toxin. Several of the ways that alcohol can make you fat are:

- Alcohol raises cortisol levels[3], which make you fat, especially in the belly.

- Alcohol depletes the body of magnesium, which is necessary for fat loss.

- Your liver has to detox alcohol, so it doesn't have resources left for handling the toxins stored in your fat cells.

- Alcohol dehydrates you, and you need water to stay slim (see the chapter on water).

- And, perhaps most importantly of all, alcohol *messes up leptin levels* and sensitivity. That means, alcohol makes you hungry[4]. But it gets worse. The more alcohol you have, the more chances there are of causing *leptin resistance*, which as you remember from the chapter on leptin, means you don't just get hungrier, you also store more fat.

SHELLFISH

Oysters, muscles, clams etc. are the garbage eaters of the sea. They are full of toxins. Shrimp do the same, and to make matters worse, most of them are now farm raised. You will have read in the chapter on meat some of the horrific things that are fed to farm animals, like GMOs and euthanized pets. Whatever the source, ultimately, it will not be something that is going to add to your health and if it's toxic enough, it could be adding to your waistline. Plus, it's still animal protein, that's acidic to your body.

NANOPARTICLES

As if genetically modified food wasn't bad enough, we are having something called nanoparticles added to food and other products, without any labeling or even a notice to the public. Nanoparticles are made as part of a process called nanotechnology. Even less people know about nanotechnology than genetically modified food. But at least with genetically modified food, we know which foods could be involved. With nanoparticles, no one has a clue which companies are using them or not.

Nanoparticles are sub-microscopic-sized particles which are super unnatural. They are super toxic because of their size: "If a nanoparticle were the size of a football, a red blood cell would be the size of the field." Therefore, they may be able to travel anywhere in the body that they want to. This is evil, because normally the body sets up barriers to control what goes in where. Some people have likened nanoparticles to being as toxic as asbestos[6].

No one has a clue how much they will harm us, especially in the long term, but you can be sure that they are helping contribute to obesity.

At time of printing, CNN reported that one organization decided to test donuts, and sure enough found that some contained titanium dioxide nanoparticles. One can only guess why they need to do that, since they did not used to. It's really scary that no one knows how many and which food products contain them. Companies are not telling us whether they are using nanoparticles or not. To further complicate the issue, some companies may not even be aware that they are selling products containing them.

I am sorry that I don't know how to avoid this one so far, except to prepare as much of your own food as possible, research nanotechnology and keep up with what's happening, and be wary of things like plastic wrap and beauty products.

REFERENCES
1. *The Anti-estrogenic diet* by Ori Hofmekler, 2007, page 6
2. *The Anti-estrogenic diet* by Ori Hofmekler, 2007, page 7
3. www.myhealthnewsdaily.com/121-chronic-drinking-increases-stress-hormone-cortisol-levels-100907.html
4. *Mastering Leptin*, 2002 by Byron Richard, page 59.
5. edition.cnn.com/2013/02/14/opinion/behar-food-nanoparticles/index.html?hpt=hp_t4
6. www.foodfirst.org/en/node/2862

CHAPTER 31

TOXIC SUBSTANCES THAT CAUSE OBESITY

HEAVY METALS

Of all the other toxins that are affecting our weight and health, heavy metals are one of the worst, because they are so poisonous. In addition to contributing to fat gain indirectly by damaging the body, they cause many serious health and mental problems. You don't have to work around heavy metals to have them inside you. Toxic heavy metals include, but are not limited to, mercury, lead, arsenic and aluminum.

We need enzymes to live and to lose fat. Dr. Hulda Clark, author of *The Cure for All diseases*, explains one way that metals harm us so much, and make us fat:

"Biochemists know that a mineral in raw element form always inhibits the enzyme(s) using that mineral"[1].

Another example of the harm that metals do is from a recent article in *The Journal of the American Medical Association* which linked arsenic exposure to increases in the risk of type 2 diabetes.[2]

Other data links mercury from eating fish, dental amalgams, and vaccines to obesity by damaging many mechanisms, including enzymes, glucose transport and mitochondria (the parts of each cell in the body, which produce energy for the body).[3]

MERCURY: THE MOST POISONOUS METAL

Mercury is one of the most toxic elements on the planet, probably second only to plutonium[4]. It's more toxic than lead or arsenic. Yet worldwide people have it in all tissues of their bodies, and it continues to be dumped into our waterways and soil, placed into our teeth (mercury dental amalgam contains about 50% mercury), and injected into our bodies in vaccines. There is no safe level of mercury[5]. It's truly a testimony to the healing power of the body that we are still alive with the amount that we contain.

Like a lot of toxins, mercury levels in the body can *not* be assessed by blood or urine levels[6]. For many people starting on a natural health plan, replacing mercury fillings with safe alternatives like porcelain is an important step. Eating healthily can remove the need for fillings altogether, because it is the blood that nourishes the teeth. While brushing is still necessary, sugar and other toxins rot teeth *from the inside out*[7], more than from the outside in.

Sources of mercury include air pollution, dental silver amalgam fillings, freshwater fish (bass & trout) & saltwater fish (especially carnivorous tuna & swordfish), insecticides, laxatives, paints, pesticides, tap and well water (drink reverse osmosis) and vaccines[8].

ALUMINUM IS POISONOUS[9]

Aluminum is a poison which particularly affects the nerves, but also digestion. Anything which affects your nerves and digestion can affect your ability to burn fat. Recent studies suggest that aluminum also contributes to neurological disorders such as Alzheimer's disease, Parkinson's disease, dementia, inappropriate behavior, clumsiness and inability to pronounce words properly[10].

Sources include: Aluminum foil, antacids, aspirin, auto exhaust, food additives especially baked goods, processed cheese and pickles, treated water, salt, beef, tobacco smoke, deodorants (try an aluminum-free deodorant from the health food store - and sometimes, don't use it at all. You will smell much nicer once you give up on toxic food and eat more plants), cans, saucepans and toothpaste[11].

It is very important to replace aluminum utensils with stainless steel or copper ones.

LEAD IS IN ALL OF US

Lead is practically everywhere in today's environment. It enters our bodies from many sources. We still do not know the long-term effects of lead exposure[12]. Lead poisoning symptoms are commonly overlooked by doctors and are not properly diagnosed as lead poisoning, since they are vague.

Dr. Claire Patterson of the California Institute of Technology did a study in 1965 called "Contaminated and Natural Lead Environments of Man," which offered first hand proof that high lead levels in industrial nations are man-made and endemic. The study showed that the average bone lead level of a deceased person today averages approximately *1000 times higher* than that of deceased people who lived 400-500 years ago.

After phasing out lead in gasoline, reducing lead levels in food should be our greatest health priority. Lead intake from fresh vegetables and fruits can be reduced by thorough washing and by peeling root vegetables. There are estimates that 13 to 22 % of our dietary lead intake is from lead-soldered food cans. Unfortunately, the U.S. does not regulate and test for lead in all canned foods. Food in cans with lead-soldered seams can be dangerous. Imported canned goods are more likely to have soldered seams. Cans with round bottoms (extruded cans) are safe and do not have a seam or use lead.

Sources include: Air pollution, auto exhaust, batteries, contaminated soil, cosmetics, fertilizers, foods (if grown in lead contaminated soil), processed foods, hair dyes, insecticides, lead based paint & pottery, pesticides, solder, tobacco smoke, water (if transported via lead pipes)[13].

ARSENIC

Arsenic can be inhaled, ingested or absorbed through contact. Arsenic poisoning is difficult to pin down because most of the arsenic leaves the body within three days of exposure. The arsenic that remains is stored in the brain, bones, and tissue and continues to do serious damage. Some people have no immediate symptoms, but the exposure can cause many types of cancer or diabetes later on. It may cause long term liver, kidney, and central nervous system damage, all of which contribute to obesity.

Sources: Coal combustion, paints, beer, pesticides, table salt, seafood from coastal waters (oysters, shrimp, muscles), drinking water[14].

COBALT

Cobalt used to be illegal. That was why you couldn't buy blue candy when I was growing up. Cobalt can be in anything that has *blue* coloring added to it, including candy. Never eat or drink anything that has blue coloring added to it. It's also in laundry & dishwasher detergent. I once had a client with stomach pain. Muscle testing indicated that she should change her brand of laundry detergent. She ignored me for several weeks and then one day decided to try my advice. Her stomach pain stopped immediately. Possibly, the laundry detergent contained cobalt.

HOW TO REMOVE HEAVY METALS

1. CHELATION

Chelation (pronounced key-lay-shun) therapy is a safe, effective, non-surgical method that has successfully been used to remove heavy metals and to prevent and heal hardening of the arteries since 1948, in the United States. It uses a chemical called EDTA, which safely removes heavy metals, as long as one's kidneys are working correctly. Much evidence indicates that chelation can also reverse the effects of many other degenerative diseases, such as heart disease, stroke, osteoporosis and senility.

Dr. Morton Walker says in his book *The Chelation Answer*, that EDTA chelation therapy has been used around the world for almost half a century for cardiovascular disease[15]. In his words:

> "In the last twenty-eight years of my experience with EDTA chelation, I would say conservatively…. I have given at least 100,000 to 120,000 infusions of EDTA and seen nobody harmed…I've never seen any serious toxicity whatsoever. I've seen only benefits."

I consider chelation is essential if you have life-threateningly high levels of metals. There are numerous books which report many lives being saved by chelation, as it appears to assist in removal of plaque as well as heavy metals. Unfortunately, chelation is a fairly expensive procedure that is done by an I.V. drip by a doctor (although a lot cheaper, more effective and safer than surgery).

We used to supply inexpensive methods (Detoxamin® and Kelatox®) whereby EDTA could be absorbed by suppository. It was wonderful! But once again, the U.S. government intervened to save the profits of the drug companies, and wrote us a letter telling us to stop selling these, even though many had benefited and no one had ever been hurt from these products. They can still be purchased from Canadian websites. The two other products the government told us to stop selling, at different times, were the Hulda Clark zapper (see *The Cure for All Diseases* by Hulda Clark) and ear candles (which helped people heal blocked ears, ear pain, sinus pain and sometimes even improved hearing). When the government doesn't like something to do with natural health, you *know* it's got to be really good.

2. EAT FRESH CILANTRO / CORIANDER.

I was told by a very knowledgeable naturopath that a hospital in Japan was doing a study on heavy metal poisoning, with 100 patients. Suddenly, for no apparent reason, one day the patients started to pass heavy metals in their urine. The doctors looked around for the cause of this. It turned out there was a new cook, who served soup before all meals. In every bowl of soup he added "Vietnamese parsley" - that is, *Coriandrum sativum* / cilantro in the USA / coriander in Europe & Australia. All metals were removed with the cilantro, including mercury and lead! The cilantro must be fresh. Add it to fresh-squeezed juice, salads and at the last second to hot meals.

FREON

Dr. Hulda Clark considered freon the top health hazard in the home[16]. Freon affects the nervous system[17]. Turn in your fridge for a non-CFC variety. Do not use more than one fridge. Do not use spray cans.

ANYTHING THAT IS NON-STICK OR NON-STAINING

1. Teflon coatings are toxic. Never, ever use non-stick cooking pans. Use steel woks or stainless steel pains instead.

2. Where possible, avoid clothing and carpeting that is super good at repelling stains. Fluorocarbon compounds are toxic and cumulative.

3. Don't eat food off wrappings that repel grease. Use a plate instead[18].

FLUORIDE

Most of us have been so programmed to think that fluoride is good for us, that it is hard to believe that fluoride is, in fact, a very strong poison that affects us in many ways, including making us fat.

FLUORIDE INTERFERES WITH HORMONES

The endocrine system is a system of glands which produce hormones. That means that fluoride interferes with hormones. Dr. Mercola reports[19]:

"According to a 2006 report by the National Research Council of the National Academies[1], fluoride is "an endocrine disruptor in the broad sense of altering normal endocrine function." This altered function can involve your thyroid, parathyroid, and pineal glands, as well as your adrenals, pancreas, and pituitary.

Your thyroid gland and its associated hormones are responsible for maintaining your body's *overall metabolic rate*, and for regulating normal growth and development. As all metabolically active cells require thyroid hormone for proper functioning, disruption of this system can have a wide range of effects on virtually every system of your body. Thyroid dysfunction is considered among the most prevalent of endocrine diseases in the United States".

Even tiny amounts can do this. Dr. Robert Carton Ph.D., who was with the EPA for 20 years, and a Risk Assessment Scientist with the Office of Toxic Substance, says:

"The government cannot prove its claims of safety. It is clear that fluoride is mutagenic (causes mutations). And that it may well cause cancer. The EPA has attempted to silence scientists who do not follow the party line."[20]

Studies have shown no reduction in tooth decay between fluoridated and unfluoridated cities. Dr. Carton says that the safe level of fluoride is zero.

The excellent book and documentary *The Fluoride Deception* show how much of the pro-fluoride information was created to protect the government from being sued for fluoride pollution, which resulted from the atom bomb project. However, it's hard to see why the government is still *so* insistent on fluoridating our water. Fluoride in water is not pharmaceutical grade. Today it comes as toxic industrial waste from the aluminum & phosphate industries.

FLUORIDE REDUCES I.Q.

Perhaps the research of Phyllis Mullenix, a leading neurotoxicologist, gives us a clue. She found that, just like other toxins that damage nerves, fluoride reduces I.Q[21]. Like other researchers who discover the truth, she was fired within days of publishing her discovery. Keep that in mind as you read the following:

NAZIS LOVED FLUORIDE

In an "Address in reply to the Governor's Speech to Parliament[22]," Mr. Harley Rivers Dickinson, Member of the Victorian Parliament, Australia, made a statement on the historical use of fluoride for behavior control:

> "At the end of the Second World War, the United States Government sent Charles Elliot Perkins, a research worker in chemistry, biochemistry, physiology and pathology, to take charge of the vast Farben chemical plants in Germany. While there, he was told by German chemists of a scheme which had been worked out by them during the war and adopted by the German General Staff. This scheme was to control the population in any given area through mass medication of drinking water.
>
> In this scheme, sodium fluoride will, in time, *reduce an individual's power to resist domination* by slowly poisoning and narcotizing a certain area of the brain, and will thus make him *submissive to the will* of those who wish to govern him. Both the Germans and the Russians added fluoride to the drinking water of prisoners of war to make them *stupid and docile.*"[23]

Ask yourself, if fluoride is so safe, why do all toothpaste manufacturers advise parents to "contact a Poison Control Center right away" if more than is used for brushing is "accidentally swallowed". Visit any store that sells toothpaste and you will see the following warning listed on the product:

"Warnings - Keep out of reach of children under 6 years of age. If more than used for brushing is accidentally swallowed, get medical help or contact a Poison Control Center right away."

You don't want this stuff in your body. Get fluoride-free toothpaste from your health food store. To get rid of fluoride from your water, use reverse osmosis filters. Carbon filters do not remove fluoride. Since we also absorb through our skin, it is best to have your bath and shower water treated as well. Ultimately, we need to get the government to stop putting fluoride into the water. Please support the Fluoride Action Network, www.fluoridealert.org.

WHAT YOU DON'T KNOW ABOUT VACCINES WILL SHOCK YOU (HOW VACCINES MAKE PEOPLE FAT!)

Few things make people more emotional than the subject of vaccines. And to suggest that they are contributing to obesity probably seems crazy. But, please, read on. You will learn how understanding vaccine damage from ingredients as well as from contaminants can not just help solve obesity, but also save your life and that of your family.

Consider that for the first time in history, *infants* have become regularly obese. In 2006, scientists at the Harvard School of Public Health found that rates of obesity in infants less than 6 months old have risen 73% since 1980.[24] This epidemic of obesity in 6-month-olds is not related to lack of exercise. It's probably not related just to diet either. While formula instead of breastfeeding contributes to this, babies do not drink sodas or eat fast food.

I will give you a clue as to a major cause for this. Be warned that this will likely shock you. Please look at the list on the next page to see how the number of vaccinations have increased over time.

It's pretty weird that we vaccinate babies, since it supposedly works by stressing the immune system to produce antibodies, and babies don't have a well developed immune system yet. In fact, studies have shown that a child's immune system doesn't completely mature until about 6 years of age[25]. Plus, germs are given a free ride into the bloodstream, without having to fight their way through the immune system.

Two of the worst ingredients in vaccines are mercury and formaldehyde. There is no safe level for either of these poisons. Other vaccine ingredients that are related to obesity as well as major health problems include, but are not limited to, poisonous aluminum and MSG.

1940	1980	2012
DTP Smallpox Some children got 4 shots before the age of 2. Never with more than 1 shot per visit.	DTP (2 months) Polio (2 months) DTP (4 months) Polio (4 months) DTP (6 months) Polio (6 months) MMR (12 months) DTP (18 months) DTP (5 years)	Flu / H1N1 (prenatal) HepB (birth) Dtap (2 months) Polio (2 months) Hib (2 months) Pneu (2 months) Rotavirus (2 months) HepB (2 months) Dtap (4 months) Polio (4 months) Hib (4 months) Pneu (4 months) Rotavirus (4 months) Dtap (6 months) Polio (6 months) Hib (6 months) Flu/H1N1 (6 months) Flu/H1N1 (7 months) Pneu (12 months) MMR (12 months) Varicella (15 months) HepA (15 months) Dtap (18 months) Polio (18 months) Hib (18 months) HepA (18 months) Flu/H1N1 (18 months) Flu/H1N1 (2.5 years) Dtap (4-6 years) Polio (4-6 years) MMR (4-6 years) Varicella (4-6 years) Flu/H1N1 (4-6 years) **49 Doses, just by the age of 6!**

You don't want these poisons in food, so why do we put them into perfect little babies? Since the truth to this answer is so shocking I will get an expert, Dr. Leonard Horowitz, to tell you what the mainstream media will not.

Dr. Len Horowitz, D.M.D., M.A., M.P.H. is a Harvard graduate, an internationally recognized authority in public health and a powerful public speaker. He was awarded "Author of the Year" award by the World Natural Health Organization. His best selling book, *Emerging Viruses: AIDS & Ebola - Nature, Accident or Intentional?* is a must-read. This work is largely responsible for public health and vaccine policy changes in at least three Third World nations.

The following is just a very little of the essential information from the excellent CD by Dr. Horowitz that I cannot recommend more highly to absolutely everyone, *Horowitz on Vaccines: The risks of following your doctor's advice may be deadly*, available from www.Tetrahedron.org.

In 1986 Dr. Maurice Hilleman, Chief of the Merck Pharmaceutical Company's vaccine division, and the world's leading vaccine developer, was interviewed by WGBH, Boston's famed public broadcasting station. The interview was never aired.

On the CD you will actually hear Hilleman discuss the fact that the Salk and Sabin polio vaccines in the late 50s and early 60s were both *hideously contaminated* with monkey viruses, much like they are *today*. The really weird thing about this interview is the laughter from those present at the shocking news. These people are not like you and me. Here are some brief, direct quotes from the radio interview:

Dr. Maurice Hilleman: ... so we brought African Greens (monkeys) in and I didn't know we were importing the AIDS virus at the time.

Miscellaneous background voices:...(loud laughter)... it was you who introduced the AIDS virus into the country. Now we know! (laughter) This is the real story! (laughter) What Merck won't do to develop a vaccine! (laughter) ...

Dr. Maurice Hilleman: So now I got to have something (to discuss at a conference).... And I thought.... That virus has got to be in vaccines...So I quick tested it (laughter) and sure enough it was in there.

Dr. Edward Shorter (Harvard's famous medical historian): I'll be damned.

Dr. Maurice Hilleman:... So I go down and I talked about the detection of non detectable viruses and told Albert, I said, "Listen Albert you know you and I are good friends but I'm going to go down there and you're going to get upset, because I'm going to talk about the detection of virus that it's in your vaccine...well he said basically, that this is just another obfuscation that's going to upset vaccines...

Dr. Maurice Hilleman: Well there are 40 different viruses in these vaccines, anyway, that we were inactivating ...

Dr. Edward Shorter: But you weren't inactivating his though...

Dr. Maurice Hilleman: No that's right, but yellow fever vaccine had *leukemia virus* in it ...

...So then the next thing you know is, three, four weeks after that we found that there were *tumors popping up in these hamsters.*

Dr. Guylaine Lanctot wrote the recommended book, *The Medical Mafia,* in Canada. She is a pediatric physician who refused to vaccinate her patients. So the Canadian Medical Association and the Canadian government brought her before a kangaroo court where she called as witnesses Dr. Horowitz and W. John Martin, one of the world's leading vaccine contamination analysts, in charge of testing human vaccines for contamination between 1976 and 1980 at the FDA Bureau of Biologics.

John Martin gave testimony saying that these vaccines carry major contaminants, and the fact is that they may or may not cause cancer or other illnesses in your lifetime, but they may be passed in the gene line to your children or your children's children, or even environmentally and they may cause cancer or other illnesses in their lifetimes.

The judge then came back after the first break and pounded his gavel and said, "Case dismissed." They do not want this information made public.

It helps to study the history of medicine that we were never taught in school. The Rockefeller led military-medical-industrial complex, which literally had a partnership with I.G. Farben and the Nazi Third Reich, is working to control the world's pharmaceutical and chemical industries, because they realized that they could literally eliminate humans silently and covertly through drugs and chemicals, promoted by propaganda.

Dr. Horowitz makes the valid proposition that vaccines today are being used like the gas chambers of World War 2, and that the health officials who offer you free vaccines are like the concentration camps of yesteryear. It's the same people, or their heirs and the same money, who believe in genocide (the murder of large numbers of people), at the same time that they make vast fortunes off of human suffering.

There is a good book called *The Science of Coercion*, by Christopher Simpson. Simpson studied psychological warfare methods used on scientists and physicians from 1945 to virtually the present. Simpson concludes virtually the same thing that Dr. Horowitz concluded in *Emerging Viruses, AIDS & Ebola*, that the Rockefellers established the agenda for science throughout the world. If you were a scientist or a health professional that did not go along with the agenda then you were, and still are, demoted, defunded, and ostracized or persecuted. This included alternative health professionals as well as independent doctors not under their control.

A man named Flexner was paid by John D. Rockefeller from his Standard Oil fortune, to get rid of competition in health care. To this end, he made a bogus scientific report which allegedly said that alternative therapies were quackery. The Flexner report also took a lot of power away from independent doctors, and centralized it into the hands of the big corporations[26]. With the help of the Flexner report, the Rockefellers and their associates established a monopoly of American medicine in the 1920s, when they also established the cancer industry.

Ernest Rudin became the director of the Rockefeller-built Kaiser Wilhelm Institute for Eugenics in pre-Nazi Germany. (Eugenics is the study of improving people by selective breeding). Today physicians and public health nurses tell you that vaccines are for your own good, because they've been persuaded by the Rockefeller-directed military-medical-industrial complex propaganda. The only difference between health care professionals that tell you these vaccines are safe and effective, and any other cult follower, is that most cult followers know who their leaders are. In health care, most physicians and public health nurses have no clue that they are puppets for the Rockefeller family.

The following is almost a direct quote from Dr. Horowitz's excellent, life-saving CD which I again strongly urge you to listen to. Dr. Horowitz proves that vaccines are for the purpose of depopulating earth. He does this with the vaccine company's *own literature*, that comes with the Hepatitis B vaccine.

As you read this, please note that Hepatitis B kills only 5,000 people in the U.S. each year[27], and that it is normally spread by drug addicts with infected needles, or from sexual contact. That is not something that a baby is going to do.[28]

If you look at the Merck literature and the Hepatitis B vaccine, just read the package insert to see what it says about side effects:

- It starts at 15%, with a little redness and swelling around the site of injection. (Okay, no big deal).

- Then it says 14% develop a little fever, some flu-like symptoms. It goes away in a few days.

- Then 12-13% develop more sustained fevers, longer duration, more flu-like symptoms. (Now we parents start getting a little worried now, don't we?)

- It goes on to say that 9-10% have more severe flu symptoms, potentially long-term chronic illnesses, 7-8% worse, 3-5% even worse than that!

- Finally it gets down to where they say – "Less than 1% of the people who get this vaccine sustain *serious injury*."

What does that mean – *"serious injury"*? Serious injury means "Brain damage, chronic crippling rheumatoid arthritis, or Sudden Infant Death".

Death.

Now, they say "less than 1%". Let's be conservative. Let's just cut the 1% in half. They want to inoculate 90% of approximately 50 million infants and children. So let's take half of that. Instead of 50 million, let's take 25 million. What's 1% of 25 million children?

That's 250,000! That's 250,000 of our children, over the next seven years, who will likely develop brain damage, chronic crippling arthritis or be dead. From that *one* vaccine! One out of over twenty vaccines that they want to give us and our children today!

All this for a disease that kills only 5,000 people in the U.S. each year[29], and that is normally spread only by drug addicts with infected needles, or from sexual contact.

250,000 over seven years, means approximately 35,000 children a year. And this is from just one vaccine. Every time a child receives another shot, they get another chance at death.

Dr. Horowitz expands this further to the other vaccines, using the Center for Disease control's *own* data. The CDC reported two publications in 1995 and 1996: Between 1990 and 1995 there were over 45,000 vaccine-injured people. And that, they said, represented – quote – "*less than 1%* of the actual injuries due to gross underreporting" – end quote.

Now you know what that means, because of what we read above about the literature that comes with the Hepatitis B vaccine. You have to take 45,000 over five years and multiply it by at least 100 to see how many children got injured. It could be 200, but let's take 100. What is 100 times 45,000? That is *4.5 million* vaccine induced injuries, according to the federal government statistics, over five years. And you don't read a word about it in the media.

That is an ongoing holocaust of vaccine injuries in the United States today! And you don't read one word about it. You only read wonderful praise about vaccines.

It was the evil Adolph Hitler who said that if you tell a lie long enough, eventually it will be believed as truth. And the greater the lie, the more people will believe it. Well, you know, the phrase that comes to mind with this is the phrase "vaccines are safe and effective".

In fact, they don't know whether they are killing and maiming more people than they are helping and saving, because they have no definitive long-term studies that show that most plausibly the entire gamut of autoimmune related disorders and weird cancers with no family history, including lupus, MS, fibromyalgia, Guillain-Barre, Attention Deficit Disorders, Hyperactivity disorders, AIDS, Chronic Fatigue, Gulf War Syndrome, chronic crippling rheumatoid arthritis, adult onset diabetes, Lou Gehrig's disease and asthma, all have now been scientifically linked to an immune system that is not functioning correctly.

This is what happens: As you get injected by contaminants and even the ingredients of the vaccines, you get foreign RNA and DNA. That is, carcinogens. Because what is foreign RNA when it gets injected into your blood? The cells in your immune system surround those, they take them into the genes, they can recombine with your own genes and then it becomes a pre-cancer cell. That is, cancer in an adult may be from viruses that they were given in vaccines as a child. For example, on the CD you hear Dr. Hilleman tell you how hideously contaminated the Yellow Fever vaccine was with leukemia virus.

The American Cancer Society and the Center for Diseases Control for decades tell you some ways to prevent cancer, but never discuss *viruses* related to cancer. Dr. Horowitz talks about how documentation shows how Litton Biomedics Labs was fooling around with *prostate cancer viruses* (and prostate cancer is exploding) and that after they studied mouse *mammary tumor viruses*, mouse mammary tumor viruses started turning up in mothers' breast milk!

Many people believe that vaccines have wiped many of the infectious diseases off the planet. To make people believe this, the CDC officials show a chart starting in 1960, when they initiated a vaccine program. The chart shows a drastic reduction in infectious diseases. But if they just extend their slide from 1960 back to the early 1900s, you would see that the vast majority of infectious diseases were well on their way out *before* the vaccines were administered. This was probably due to improvements in hygiene and clean drinking water.

On his CD, Dr. Horowitz tells the story of how a hospital took custody of their baby for four days, and they went through living hell, when they went to the hospital for an injury, and his wife said that they did not believe in vaccines. Dr. Horowitz then suggests some advice to people who are ever in a similar situation. I strongly urge you to get this CD to hear the full advice for yourself. Naturally, you must investigate this for yourself, but consider something such as:

"We'll get vaccinated under one condition. You provide me with a bonded, notarized affidavit that swears that you will assume all medical, legal and *financial* risks in the event that I or my child is injured from the vaccine".

Plus, many people do not vaccinate because it is against their religion. They do not want to defile the body, the Temple of the Holy Spirit. Others research home births, home schooling, the advantages of living in friendlier states and the excellent book *Vaccine Legal Exceptions* by Alan Phillips available at wwwVaccineRights.com.

While obesity is made worse from vaccine poisons such as mercury, aluminum, MSG and formaldehyde and others, that is only a small part of the problems you could easily be faced with over the years from vaccination.

If you have vaccinated, do not beat yourself up. Forgive yourself, and forgive your parents if they vaccinated you. You are a victim of the Medical Mafia. There are ways to overcome any health challenge, such as removing heavy metals through chelation, and using juicing and natural health to boost the immune system. As I said before, there is no 'magic pill'. It takes a wholistic approach. But please realize that it is time to change the system and what we do, now, for the sake of your grandchildren and great grandchildren.

Educate yourself fully before you take any vaccine. Read Dr. Horowitz' book and listen to the CD. Read *Vaccine Legal Exemptions*, by Alan Phillips JD (ebook). Visit websites created by people who had children die or made autistic from vaccines *before* you vaccinate. I talked on the phone once with a woman whose baby died shortly after vaccinating. It was beyond heart breaking. It still brings tears to my eyes just remembering that conversation.

Alternatives: I highly recommend you get these two books: *How to raise a healthy child, in spite of your doctor* by Dr. Robert Mendelsohn MD, and *Smart Medicine for a Healthier child* by Janet Zand.

REFERENCES

1. *The Cure for All Diseases*, by Dr. Hulda Clark, 1995, page 37
2. Navas-Acien A, Silbergeld EK, Pastor-Barriuso R., Guallar E. Arsenic exposure and prevalence of type 2 diabetes in US adults. *JAMA.* 2008;300(7):814-822.
3. Windham B. *Diabetes: The Mercury and Vaccine Factor. Scientific Research Collated and Summarized.* Tallahassee, FL: Dental Amalgam Mercury Syndrome, Inc; 2008.
4. Detoxamin brochure. www.Detoxamin.com
5. www.relfe.com/mercury.html
6. Lorscheider & Vimy. *The Lancet* Vol 337, May 4 1991
7. www.drjomd.com/highways/nutrition/sugar/sugar-rots-your-body-from-the-inside-out/
8. Detoxamin brochure. www.Detoxamin.com
9. www.drpepi.com/aluminum-poisoning.php
10. Detoxamin brochure. www.Detoxamin.com
11. Detoxamin brochure. www.Detoxamin.com
12. Detoxamin brochure. www.Detoxamin.com
13. Detoxamin brochure. www.Detoxamin.com
14. Detoxamin brochure. www.Detoxamin.com
15. *The Chelation Answer* by Dr. Morton Walker (1982), Chapter 5.
16. *The Cure for All Diseases*, by Dr. Hulda Clark, 1995, page 446
17. www.epa.gov/chemfact/f_freon.txt
18. www.ewg.org/news/safety-concerns-adhere-nonstick-chemicals
19. articles.mercola.com/sites/articles/archive/2011/08/13/fluoride-and-thyroid-dysfunction.aspx
20. www.doctoryourself.com/carton.html
21. *The Fluoride Deception*, book and documentary
22. Victorian Hanstard, August 12, 1987, *Nexus*, Aug/Sept 1995
23. www.newswithviews.com/Devvy/kidd102.htm

24. Kim J, Peterson KE, Scanlon KS, et al. Trends in overweight from 1980 through 2001 among preschool-aged children enrolled in a health maintenance organization. *Obesity (Silver Spring)*. 2006;14(7):1107-1112.
25. *Breastfeeding, Biocultural Perspectives*, Dr. Katherine Dettwyler, Ph.D.
26. en.wikipedia.org/wiki/Flexner_Report
27. www.hepb.org/patients/general_information.htm
28. en.wikipedia.org/wiki/Hepatitis_B
29. www.hepb.org/patients/general_information.htm

CHAPTER 32

WHAT CAN I EAT?

The basic rule is to eat vegetables, fruit, nuts, seeds, lentils, beans and some grains other than wheat. You may be able to add some organic , salted butter and organic, free-range eggs (so they are not GMO). That might not sound like much, but once you buy the food in the shopping list chapter, and learn new ways to prepare food, you will find that it is a lot.

Flours, beans and lentils should be soaked for 8 hours to sprout them and to break down toxins and make them more digestible.

There is no one single way of eating that is best for everyone, or for anyone all the time. However, there are some rules for everybody, such as, everyone should avoid the highly toxic and acidic foods that are discussed in the early parts of this book. Some of them are not really even "food", in that they don't exist in nature. An important rule is that everyone will benefit from a lot more *raw* plant food, with as many totally raw plant meals as possible. I will talk more about raw plant food in its own chapter. An additional rule while you are extra serious about getting thin, is to have very little sugary fruit, because high sugar in your blood stream can still make you hungry and mess up your leptin.

When it comes to working out exactly what each person should eat, muscle testing shows that different foods are negative, neutral or positive for different people, at different times. This is confirmed by science which has discovered that there are at least 1.4 million variations in human DNA[1].

This is partly why some diets get glowing testimonials from some people, while the same diet does not work for others. Another reason is because the people who did lose weight were probably those who were more in balance to start with, and were not having so much of the main toxins we talk about earlier in this book.

However, most of these testimonials are from people who lost weight in the short term only. I don't want you to do that. I want you to get thin for life, while being happy with what you are doing (after the initial detoxifying and when your taste buds change). This is why I am not going to tell you what to eat, but to teach the basic principles to discover what works for *you*.

A major key to staying thin is to add more *variety* to your diet. By that, I don't mean a different kind of breakfast cereal. Start to try new raw seeds, nuts, vegetables, fruits and herbs that you have not eaten before. Any one of these could contain the missing nutrients or taste that your body has been craving all these years, and that is why your body has been telling you that you are hungry, just to get more of that particular nutrient. Our bodies are unbelievably, highly, complex. There are thousands of different chemical reactions, in different balance, in each body at each time.

I know from my years of looking into people's shopping baskets in towns all over the USA, that most people have very little variety in their diet. If you look in people's shopping carts, you will see that there is very little variety at all. It is mainly just lots of different ways of packaging processed wheat, toxic fats, flesh and GMOs. In addition, you will see that most people purchase very little fresh produce, and virtually no raw seeds or healthy oils.

Start to talk to your body when scanning different items of food, or creating a meal, and ask your body what it wants. Learn to listen to your body. Because it's not just what you eat, but what balance of each food that you should eat that is important.

If you would like to take this ability to communicate with your body to a whole new level, I strongly urge you to learn muscle testing.

Unfortunately, you can't do it on yourself accurately, but you can be tested by a kinesiologist, or have people close to you learn with you. If you do this, you will be amazed at what the body tells you. And you will probably get some "a-ha!" moments, from your discoveries. Because basically, to get thinner you should eat none of the foods that your body muscle tests as negative, and more of the foods that your body tests as positive. Remember, when you muscle test a food, clarify whether the food is to be consumed raw or cooked in a particular way.

For a full listing of foods to eat, please see the chapter titled "Your new shopping list".

REFERENCES

1.   www.ornl.gov/sci/techresources/Human_Genome/project/info.shtml

CHAPTER 33

DROP 40-80 POUNDS IN A MONTH WITH JUICING & RAW PLANTS

"Drop 47 pounds by Memorial Day," which was one month later, proclaimed *First for Women* magazine on their front page[1]. Sounds a bit crazy, right? But this article is not crazy, and it's not about some fad diet. Women who switched from a diet filled with cooked, processed, and therefore toxic food to a food plan filled with fresh, raw juices and raw dairy-free smoothies lost up to 11 pounds a week. At the same time 91% reported feeling a greater sense of wellbeing.

WILD ANIMALS EAT ONLY RAW FOOD

Without knowing it or saying it, the article mentioned above is really about what I said at the beginning of this book, that if we look at what wild animals do, which regularly stay slim except when getting ready to hibernate, then we will know more about what we need to do. The article is about eating *only raw* food. (I am talking about eating only plant food, not meat).

COOKING DESTROYS ALL ENZYMES & 50% OF PROTEIN. IT ALSO DAMAGES MINERALS & VITAMINS

The article went on to explain how this is an "Enzyme break-through", because our body absolutely, positively must have enzymes. Our bodies have thousands of them![2] . But cooking destroys enzymes, as well as 50% of protein, and damages minerals and vitamins.

In one study, dieters who boosted their enzyme intake lost 2½ times more body fat than those who did not have more enzymes! Why don't you hear more about the benefits of enzymes? Partly because there are a lot of people in the field of nutritional medicine who are still relying on science they learned in school years ago. And probably because no one makes a fortune when someone makes their own juices at home, and thereby gets so healthy that they throw away their bottles of pills.

ENZYMES ARE ESSENTIAL FOR YOUR BODY TO WORK CORRECTLY

Enzymes are special chemical helpers that your body must have to do all of the thousands of different chemical reactions that your body does to turn food, air and water into all of the different parts of your body. Enzymes are totally necessary for the proper functioning of every part of your body. They direct and modify all body functions. Enzymes are the labor force for every single function of the body[3].

Enzymes are everywhere in all living things. They are in people, animals and plants. Our body has about 3,000 different kinds of en-zymes. It can make these, with difficulty, and at *great expense* to the body, from what you eat, but how much easier is it to *ingest* them in a perfect form through raw plant food? Enzymes are needed for every-thing, including:

- Digestion.
- Moving.
- Energy.
- The blood system.
- Heart.
- Kidneys.
- Liver.
- Elimination of toxins.

- Seeing, hearing, smelling, tasting.
- Breathing.
- Thinking.
- Reproduction
- Living.

COOKED FOOD IS DEAD FOOD

You can see from this list that enzymes are a key to getting thin. Since cooking destroys *all* enzymes, that's one reason why traditional diets don't work in the long run. Your body has to work out how to *make* the 3,000 different kinds of enzymes it needs from what you eat, rather than just absorb perfect enzymes from raw plants. Your body does not want to be fat, and will do all it can to be thin, as long as you give it what it needs, which must include lots of enzymes. In fact, since cooking destroys enzymes, it's a miracle that most of us are alive at all.

In addition, *lack* of digestive enzymes produces an overgrowth of the wrong bacteria in the gut, and a lack of good bacteria. Raw food corrects this imbalance.

There is a myth that many people hold that cooking helps with digestion. Actually, the reverse is true. *First for women* and other people have reported that heat kills the natural digestive enzymes, so it is cooking that makes digestion more difficult. When you cook vegetables, the less you cook them and the lower the temperature, the better. When steaming or stir-frying, basically just warm them up a bit before serving. Never boil, always steam vegetables, so that valuable nutrients are not washed away in the water.

POLYPHENOLS IN RAW FOOD CAUSE FAT CELLS TO SELF DESTRUCT

Here's another way that raw food helps you get thin. Plants contain compounds called polyphenols. Polyphenols stop cells from filling with fat. Best of all, polyphenols cause fat cells to *self-destruct*. There are plenty of polyphenols in plant food, but you won't absorb them properly if you don't have plenty of good bacteria. Once you stop eating cooked food and eat raw food, you get much less bad bacteria and more good bacteria, so you absorb more polyphenols from your raw food, and voila! Fat cells self-destruct.

Another reason why eating raw plant food will get you thin is that it's not just about what you are eating, but about what you are *not* eating, not because they are high in calories but because you are allergic to them. Since a lot of people are allergic to wheat, meat, eggs and dairy, it's hard for them to work out what to eat when they realize they have to give these up. But when you eat lots of different raw plants, you naturally give up all of these toxic foods, without ever going hungry.

For example, when I went totally raw for 3 weeks, I reduced the most weight I had done in years, fitted into paints I had not worn for years, and looked terrific, without going hungry. It may not just have been because I was having lots of raw plants. It could also have been because during that time I had zero grains, butter and animal protein, any one of which I could have been allergic to at that time. A key to discovering what you are allergic to is that you eat it nearly every day, and you *just love* it. In my case, I believe it was grains, and also butter.

The important rule is that you must **never heat anything over a temperature of 110°F**. When you first think about eating only raw food, that may not sound too tempting at first. But there are many fantastic 'uncook' books out there which have wonderful, easy recipes. Think Banana & Berry Ice cream with Maple Syrup and seed mix for Breakfast! And carrot cake for dinner. In fact, you could have ice cream and carrot cake for every meal, while you watch yourself get thin. Raw ice cream is made by mincing frozen fruit with your juicer.

When you eat raw, you can eat fruit, although it's best to also have plenty of green veges, seeds and nuts as well. Whenever you are extra serious about getting thin, avoid sugary fruit as much as possible, such as bananas, melons and grapes. This is because it can raise your blood sugar too much, and this makes you hungry. Also, your pancreas probably needs a rest so that it can heal itself and get back to correct insulin production. You can sweeten your meals with a tiny bit of raw honey or maple syrup, and get thin doing this, but again, it depends on your current condition and how much sugar you have eaten in the past.

Don't think that this has to be expensive. Eventually you may find that you are actually saving money on this plan, because you end up eating so much less, because you are no longer hungry. Also, you no longer buy processed foods which are much more expensive, for the amount of real nutrition you get.

Why don't you hear more about enzymes, polyphenols and other advantages of raw plant food? Could it have something to do with the fact that the 'health' industry's trillions of dollars in income depends on you not knowing about this? I believe that it is. Come to think of it, let's be honest and call the 'health' industry the disease industry, because that is the product they are selling. Here's a clue: the three doctors who wrote *Enzymes, the Fountain of Life* made this comment[4]:

"We were taught in medical school that oral enzymes were indicated only for digestive problems and that they were not indicated for any other medical conditions 'because they were not absorbed'. Unfortunately, in the United States and other countries, this was generally accepted as 'medical dogma'."

JUICING IS THE EASIEST WAY TO GET ENZYMES

You get enzymes from raw plants. That is, raw vegetables, fruit, seeds and nuts. When you first get started eating raw food, the best and easiest way to concentrate your intake of enzymes and all kinds of other nutrients is by fresh juicing. It must be *fresh-squeezed* juice. Store-bought juices have their enzymes destroyed by processing. The difference between fresh-squeezed and store-bought juices is as great as black and white. Fresh-squeezed is power-packed with nutrition the way nature intended, including enzymes, life energy and polyphenols. Store-bought juice is a dead, fattening, toxic sugar drink.

In addition, the juice of the plant, like the blood of the body, contains all the essential elements that build and nourish. This makes it super easy for your body to digest, which is important, because years of toxic food have harmed the digestive system of a lot of us.

Remember that our bodies do not get energy by burning fuel like a car does, but from complicated chemical reactions that require a good supply of nutrients[5]. In the past, if you did not have enough nutrients, your body was not able to use all of the chemical energy you ate, and so stored it in fat cells. With fresh juicing, you give the body a high concentration of nutrients, and so it will finally be able to convert the stored energy in the fat cells into energy.

So, this is what I am asking you to do for the next month, and as much as possible for the rest of your life. No matter what else you eat, no matter what else you do, make yourself drink at least one full glass of fresh squeezed juice, made from mostly vegetables, once a day. Add as many leafy green vegetables as you can get hold of (not lettuce). This is because green means chlorophyll, and chlorophyll has oxygen, which we are all short of, plus light energy, magnesium and other essential things that do wonders for the body.

Chlorophyll is almost identical to hemoglobin. The main difference between hemoglobin and chlorophyll is that hemoglobin is built around one atom of iron, while chlorophyll is built around one atom of magnesium[6]. Hemoglobin is a protein in red blood cells that transports oxygen from the lungs to all the body cells, and carries carbon dioxide away from them. It is hemoglobin that makes blood red, when it is carrying oxygen. Arteries which have lots of oxygen after leaving the heart are bright red, while veins that are depleted of oxygen are dark purple[7].

Especially add parsley, ordinary or Italian. A family member of mine met a man who looked radiantly healthy, with the bluest eyes he had ever seen. The man looked 50 years old, but he said he was 83. When asked what his secret was, he said it was parsley. He drank a lot of parsley tea in his water.

Add cilantro/coriander as well to help with metal detoxifying. It is good to also do one raw smoothie (recipes are later in the book) and one totally raw meal. If you want to really see the weight drop off, have only fresh juice and raw plant food for dinner, as much as you want. But only do this if it feels fine to do it. This is not a diet. This is a way of looking after your body for the rest of your life.

REDUCE 80 POUNDS IN 60 DAYS

Some people who are in a hurry to get weight off fast, drink only

100% fresh juice made from mostly vegetables, with a lot of greens, for a number of days. This is not a 'fast' as some people believe, because fresh juice is *food* which is super nutritious. The nutrients in the juice enable the body to do the chemical reactions that turn your fat into energy[8].

If you watch the inspiring documentary *Fat, Sick and Nearly Dead*[11] (which uses the same format of *Super Size Me*, only in reverse) you will see two very overweight men who ingested only fresh-squeezed juice and water for two months, with great results. Currently the DVD has over 600, five star reviews on the Amazon website, which is amazing. The men felt great, and had lots of energy while doing this, after they got over the first horrible four days of detoxing. Joe Cross, the producer, originally weighed 300 pounds with a very big belly, and in *60 days reduced by 80 pounds*. He encouraged another man, Phil, a truck driver, who weighed 400 pounds to ingest only fresh juice and water for two months. Phil reduced by *95 pounds after 61 days* of juicing. He then went on to lose another 100 pounds in the following 9 months.

This was the recipe they used. It's a very good one, because it's low in sugar. You could leave out the ginger if you don't care for it. I suggest you use this recipe as often as possible, because this recipe is particularly good at making you UN-hungry, because it's low in sugar, and most overweight people need to keep off sugar as much as possible, even if it is natural.

THE "FAT, SICK AND NEARLY DEAD" JUICE RECIPE

- 6 Kale Leaves.
- 1 Cucumber.
- 4 Celery Stalks.
- 2 Green Apples.
- 1/2 Lemon.
- 1 piece of ginger.

There is a great benefit to living off just fresh-squeezed juice for a while. For one thing, it makes preparing meals really easy, even if you are travelling. Just take your juicer with you. You can start on it right away, even if you haven't learned anything yet about healthy food preparation. Another benefit is that if your digestive system is blocked up with meat, or destroyed by gluten, it's a lot easier for the body to absorb nutrition from juice than from normal raw plant food.

Juice should be consumed within 20 minutes of making it, before the enzymes break down.

However, there is one major problem with having only juice - you do not have any fiber, and this can cause constipation. I suggest that before you drink your juice, you eat 1-2 tablespoons of raw seeds or nuts just before you juice. You could eat my Seed & Nut Mix – see recipes for instructions. Another good idea is to stir in some ground flax seeds or chia seeds. After all, juicing is unnatural. It is better to eat *whole* the things you juice. Seeds and nuts give you good oils, plus you get fiber which will help to keep your bowels working properly. Smoothies also have fiber.

Plus, part of the process of digestion is *chewing*. Without chewing first, it's harder for your body to understand that you just ate. It may not properly prepare the digestive system to receive food. Chewing is also important for mixing saliva with the food. Your body produces over two pints of saliva a day for a reason. One reason is that it contains enzymes for digesting carbohydrates[9].

Fiber is the parts of plants that we cannot digest. While we can't digest it, fiber is still very important for health and keeping thin[10]. And the fiber that is lost from juicing can help your digestive tract absorb excess estrogen, and fill you up. Also, raw seeds are super good for weight loss because they have lots of good fats and magnesium, the essential mineral that most of us are short of and is essential for fat loss. If you eat some seeds before juicing, it will reduce your hunger much more than if you only drink juice.

Remember to keep having plenty of water as well, especially before breakfast. While juicing is a fantastic thing to do, in the long run, you will have to develop the right habits to maintain your slim body size, and eat whole plant foods as well. There are benefits to whole plants. For example, it was recently discovered that the skin from apples has ursolic acid, which reduces obesity[12]. And fiber helps you to feel full, absorbs estrogen and helps your digestion. Unless you are super overweight, what is more important than fast weight reduction is to reduce fat steadily while you get in the right *habits*. If you do that, the fat will go, and stay off permanently.

Eventually, to develop new food habits that will allow you to keep the body you deserve for the rest of your life, start having totally raw meals as well. These never have meat, fish or dairy in them. They are made from fruit, vegetables, nuts, seeds and soaked lentils. If you get sick of cold food, you can add hot water to warm them up before serving, or sometimes cheat and add a little of something cooked, say some mushrooms lightly sauted in organic salted butter.

You will find that when you eat a totally raw meal, you eat a much smaller amount. Your body won't give off those "more, more" signals that eating a cooked meal does. You can even have raw fruit for taste and variety, to give your body all of those different molecules that it needs for the thousands of different chemical reactions that it has to do, but do it in moderation.

Right now, even if you don't have any special kitchen appliances, here are a few suggestions:

- Frozen blueberries and pumpkin seeds for breakfast. Plus a raw fruit & seed smoothie if you need more.

- Super salad for lunch. See recipe section. Not just lettuce, it also has other greens, fresh basil, fennel, celery, cucumber, olives, avocado, carrots, green onions, apples, pears, pumpkin seeds, sesame seeds and walnuts. Sweeten with ¼ tsp. 100% maple syrup, and tart it up with lemon juice.

- Fruit salad plus seeds, 1/4 tsp. raw honey & lemon juice. As much as you want.

- Sliced apples with home made nut butter (see recipe).

Once you have a blender, here are more easy ideas to get you started:

- Carrot cake. (See recipe chapter)

- Warm, raw soup for lunch or dinner. You just blend vegetables (like tomatoes, cucumber, avocado and fennel), a tiny bit of fruit (like grapes) and nuts or seeds. Then add hot water and Celtic sea salt. Try my warm Gourmet Fennel & Grape Soup inspired by Iron Chef Geoffrey Zakarian as soon as you can. It's delicious!

- Olive tapenade. Blend black olives with basil, lemon juice and salt. Eat by itself or with celery or on green leaves.

It's important to add salt to your raw meals, but it must *never* be toxic table salt. It must be Celtic sea salt. I will talk more about this in the chapter on salt.

Surprisingly, even though fruit contains natural sugars, there are nutrients in fruit which help with weight loss, in addition to alkalizing your body. Fruit is also good for us because it's one of the few plants that have few toxins. Plants make toxins to stop animals eating them, so most plants have small amounts of toxins. Fruit *wants* to be eaten, so that you spread the seed, so that's why it has less toxins. That's why pregnant women will have less pregnancy sickness if they have more fruit and water, and less vegetables.

TOO MUCH RAW FRUIT HAS TOO MUCH SUGAR

On the other hand, fruit has natural sugar. This problem is worse these days than in the past, because plants have been bred to be unnaturally super-sweet. While the sugar in fruit is a lot more nutritious and vastly less toxic than processed sugar, too much can still cause problems, especially if you are overweight. This has little to do with calories. It is because:

1. Sugar feeds microorganisms inside you, including *Candida*, which breed in bigger numbers, and release their own kind of excrement, which is toxic[13].

2. These microorganisms produce gas, which can bloat and swell your belly.

3. The more sugar in your blood, the more work your pancreas has to do making insulin, and most people need to give their pancreas a rest.

4. The more sugar in your blood, the hungrier you will get soon after eating.

Yes, some people get totally thin eating nothing but tons of raw fruit. There are pictures on the internet that attest to that. And it's better to have nothing but raw fruit than to continue to eat cooked food. But if you look at the blood of these people, you may find, as Dr. Cousens has done[11] by looking at blood under a microscope, that these people have health problems, from overgrowths of microorganisms and the yeast *Candida*. The key is to have balance. Go easy on the super sugary fruits, or avoid them altogether in the early stage, although you should be able to have them later, once you are on a maintenance plan. These include:

- Bananas.
- Dates.
- Grapes & Raisins.
- Melons.
- Mango.
- Nectarines.
- Oranges, pineapple.

In addition, when you are juicing, you concentrate the sugar. So if you are working on avoiding sugar, you will want to keep sugary fruit such as pineapple out of your juice as much as possible.

COOKED FOOD INCREASES WHITE BLOOD CELL COUNTS

We know that cooked food is toxic, because it increases the number of white blood cells[14]. This means that the body considers cooked food as a foreign body. No wonder people lose so much fat and gain muscle when they go on a 100% raw diet!

RAW FOOD HAS "BIOELECTRICITY"

According to Dr. Cousens M.D., another reason why raw food is so much better than cooked food is because it has more 'bioelectricity'. This gives you real energy, not the fake energy that is really chemical stimulation that comes from caffeine or from high blood sugar from foods such as processed sugars or grains. Experiments with mice showed that mice fed raw food had a massive *three times* more energy and endurance than when fed cooked food[15]!

A raw food program is not just another calorie restriction diet. Eat as much raw food, and drink as much fresh-squeezed vegetable juice as you want. Do this only three times a day, in order to get your leptin working properly. At the beginning, eating raw food may make you ravenously hungry. Don't be alarmed. Your body is just deliriously happy to finally get hold of some real nutrition. Keep juicing and having as many 100% raw meals as possible. Before long, you will see your body slimming down, no matter what size meals you are eating. You will quite likely find that eventually the size of your meals drop considerably. The more totally raw meals you have, the faster you will get slim.

Anytime you think that you are eating too much food, or get any bloating, just add more raw seeds or nuts to your diet, and reduce the amount of high sugar fruits. The more variety you have, the less chance you will get any toxins from overloading on one thing, and the more likely you will give your body the particular nutrients it wants. You could try my power ball mix (see recipes).

If you are really keen to get thin, consider going fully raw until you get to your ideal size, and then going on a maintenance plan where you have some totally raw meals, but gradually have more cooked plants, so long as you never have toxic food including GMOs, soy, wheat and you also greatly limit other grains.

I am not telling you, as many raw foodists will, to give up eating cooked food forever, because I want you to eat lots of raw food for the rest of your life, and to regularly have 100% raw meals. I don't want you to 'throw the baby out with the bathwater' by doing what I did originally, and find out that "it's too hard" and go back to your old ways. By permitting yourself to have cooked food at one or two meals each day, you won't feel deprived. Also, if you really must have something cooked, try adding a little cooked food (such as steamed asparagus or sauted mushrooms) to an otherwise raw meal.

I have seen some people go raw for a while, then go back to cooked food, several times in a cycle. I have done this myself. I believe it's a bit like when people give up cigarettes. I have read that most people give them up three times before being successful. Likewise, most of us are addicted to the toxins that are produced by cooked food, and so it can take a while before our taste buds become sufficiently used to us eating raw food, that it becomes something that we want to do, permanently.

HOW WILL I GET ENOUGH PROTEIN?

This question was addressed in the chapter on meat. I will add a little to this now. Common vegetables have much more protein than you need, and contrary to popular myth, they're complete proteins as well[16]. We need only 2.5 to 11% of our calories from protein, according to peer-reviewed research and the official recommendations.[17],[18],[19], and that amount is easily supplied by common vegetables[20]. (See the graph in the meat chapter).

All of our proteins are made from 22 amino acids. The body cannot use protein in its original state. The protein you eat must first be broken down into amino acids before it can be used. The body must then rebuild whatever new proteins it needs from the amino acids. It is the amino acids in a protein that are important, not the protein itself. Breaking proteins down is a big job. While some proteins are made of only 5-10 amino acids, other proteins are enormous and highly complex, containing *thousands* of amino acids. There are two main sources of amino acids[21]:

1. From food. If the food is a protein, your body has to break it down into amino acids before it can use it to build protein. If it's raw juice or raw plant food, it can use the amino acids immediately to build protein.

2. From processes within the body. This kind of protein is called

endogenous protein. Endogenous protein comes from amino acids from cell wastes, within the body. These proteins are continually circulating and form what is known as the *amino acid pool*[22]. The fact that the body can make protein from its own cell wastes is not widely known. This protein from within the body is an important source of amino acids that is often overlooked by conventional nutrition writers.

Many times, up to *two-thirds* of the body's total protein needs are supplied from endogenous protein and not from external dietary sources. The amino acid pool is like a bank that is open twenty-four hours. The liver and the cells are continually making deposits and withdrawals of amino acids, depending upon the concentration of amino acids in the blood.

COOKING DESTROYS 50% OF PROTEIN!

According to the Max Planck Institute, cooking foods usually results in destroying 50% of the protein. Cooking also destroys 60-70% of vitamins and minerals that can be used and up to 96% of the B vitamins.

COOKING DESTROYS 10,000 BENEFICIAL PHYTONUTRIENTS!

Cooking also destroys 100% of enzymes and phytonutrients[23]. Phytonutrients are compounds in plants, apart from vitamins, minerals, and macronutrients, that have a beneficial effect on the body[24]. There are over 10,000 of them!

They are antioxidant, anti-inflammatory, antiviral, antibacterial, and boost the immune system and *cellular repair*. All of those activities will help you directly or indirectly to get thin. Highly colored vegetables and fruits tend to be highest in these chemicals.

Antioxidants are particularly important because they fight free radicals. The body produces free radicals as part of its normal chemical reactions, but free radicals are like red hot particles that damage anything they touch. They *must* be neutralized by antioxidants. There are many different kinds of antioxidants, and raw food has them, including vitamins A, C and E, and minerals such as magnesium.

That's another reason why the more variety you have in your raw juice & food, the better. It's crazy to think that so-called 'authorities' tell us that pretty much all we need is some protein, calcium and a few extra vitamins. The trouble is that most scientists, and the drug companies that pay their wages, only see in terms of a specialized few items at any one time. They don't think in terms of the *massive complexity* that is nature.

This is why you don't need most of the supplements available. Although, there are a few exceptions - please see the chapter on supplements. You can swap most of your supplements for *whole* raw meals and juices, as well as superfood mixtures, available either online or from a health food store.

The Food Mafia have pushed the "complete protein" idea as a marketing gimmick. But the "complete protein" idea falls apart if we realize that the amino acids in many of the so-called complete protein foods cannot even be fully used by the body. Meat, for example, is usually only the muscle meat of the animal, which is particularly low in some of the essential amino acids.

As you saw in the graph in the chapter on meat, a varied diet of fruits, vegetables, nuts, seeds and sprouted lentils can furnish us with all the essential and non-essential amino acids, along with all the other nutrients we need, in a form that is easily and efficiently used.

You will find that when you eat totally raw meals, you end up consuming a *lot* less calories. This is because you get complete nutrition eating 50-80% less food. In addition, your body doesn't need extra nutrition for ridding it of all the toxins in normal food. This is why people on a raw diet naturally reach an optimum diet and weight, without having to think about quantities at all.

Do you think that if you were healthier and happier, it would be easier for you to keep away from the more fattening foods? Then you might be interested in an experiment that Dr. Francis Pottenger performed on 900 cats for ten years[25]. Some cats were fed only pasteurized milk (that is, cooked milk) and cooked meat. Other cats were fed what is a normal, healthy diet for cats – raw meat. The cats fed cooked food became ill, antisocial, aggressive and exhibited deviant sexual behavior. Please note that humans should never eat raw meat because of parasites, but this experiment does give us clues that cooking does more than we have been lead to believe it does.

Amazingly, it took *three generations* of raw food for the cats to return to normal. This study also showed something that scientists are only just starting to figure out. Physical degeneration caused by a poor diet and cooked food in the mother is inherited by her children and passed on to the third generation.

The reverse is also true. When a mother's diet is nutritious and has few toxins and more raw food, not only does she benefit with good health, so, too, do her offspring. Pottenger saw that with each successive generation of kittens they produced, each kitten was healthier than the prior one[26].

COOKED FOOD MEANS AGEs.
AGEs AGE YOU

Yet another study also shows how raw is better: AGEs are "Advanced Glycation End Products", and we are only now just learning about them. AGEs, by coincidence, age you. They also cause a host of health problems including joint problems, stiff blood vessels, cataracts, dementia, arthritis and serious complications from diabetes such as blindness. *Animal products have the most AGEs.* Plus, the more you cook food and the higher the temperature, the more AGEs you get. Broiling and frying increase AGEs by 1,000 times. That is why you should steam rather than fry[27]. If you eat raw plant food, you eat a massive amount less AGEs.

Modern science will probably not grasp the fantastic benefits of a raw, or mostly raw plant-based diet based on fruit, vegetables, nuts, seeds and legumes, for many decades, if ever, because:

1. Science fragments things into tiny little subjects. Our bodies are infinitely complicated.

2. There's no money in it. They want to focus on the pathetic few nutrients that are in the food that the Food Mafia and many people

in the government want you to waste your money on, so that you can enrich them and save them paying Social Security.

3. On the flip-side, the $2.2 trillion income to the Medical Mafia depends on people being unhealthy.

There are numerous people and books now that teach people how to prepare delicious whole raw meals and deserts, not just juice. A 100% raw food eating plan reduces weight, hunger and health problems greatly. You can eat whatever you like so long as it's raw. This means raw fruit, vegetables, nuts, seeds, good oils such as coconut oil and honey. One does not have any dairy, meat or fish. You can make many fabulous meals with this program, some of which taste almost as good as the cooked original. My raw carrot cake in the recipes section is an example of this. On a raw food plan, you can have desert for the main meal all the time if you want.

You might think that you would get hungry going on a 100% raw, plant-based food plan. Actually, the reverse is true. Most people, including me, experience a great reduction in appetite. I once did the 100% raw food diet for 3 weeks. During this time I got comfortably into some jeans I had not worn for years. I also looked about 5-10 years younger. I had a real glow on my face. I was videoed at this time. When I compared the videos with other videos taken a few months later, when I was back on mostly cooked food, the difference was astounding. I looked so much younger on the raw food diet.

Incidentally, I was quite amazed to discover how my need for water reduced greatly on the 100% raw food plan as well. I had often wondered how wild animals get by with so little water. After all, if we need to drink 8 glasses of water throughout the day, why don't they? I believe now that the reason why we need to drink so much water is because cooked food has more toxins and so the body needs more water to flush them out.

CHOOSING A JUICER[28]

The easiest way to increase your intake of raw food is to get juicing.

To start off with, if you don't have spare cash, it's better to have a cheap juicer than none at all. But if you are serious about getting thin, it is worth putting all the money you used to spend on toxic substances towards a good juicer, partly because it will squeeze more juice out and save you on food costs in the long run. You might even be able to stop taking a lot of your supplements, because fresh-squeezed juice will do more for you than your supplements ever did. There is a list of qualities to consider, when buying a juicer, in the shopping list chapter.

Juices should be consumed within 20 minutes of being made, since it has been demonstrated that enzyme activity in juice 30 minutes old is one-half that of freshly made juice. When apple or carrot juice turns brown, it has oxidized.

CASE STUDIES OF PEOPLE WHO GOT THIN ON RAW FOOD

Here are just a few cases of people reported by *First for Women* who lost weight going on a raw plant diet:

- Carlie Nething, 5' tall, reduced by 29 pounds, going from 134 pounds to 105 pounds, while getting a more radiant skin. Her allergies and fatigue are gone and her hair is thicker.

- Matt Frazer, 6'2" tall, reduced by 100 pounds, going from 340 to 240 pounds.

- Laura Frazer, 5'5" tall, reduced by 49 pounds, going from 184 to 135 pounds. Her constipation and bloat are gone.

Alissa Cohen's great raw cookbook *Living on Live food"* reported:

- Judeen, age 60, reduced by 105 pounds after 20 months on raw plant food, and has more energy than when she was 35 years old.

- Lynn, age 35, reduced by 30 pounds in three months. Her acne and hot flashes are gone and she looks and feels better than in years.

- Christine, age 37, reduced by 100 pounds and feels fantastic.

CAUTION: NOT ALL RAW FOOD IS GOOD FOR YOU

Many raw foodists think that if it's a raw plant, it's good for you. Of course, this is not so. Wild animals are quite picky about what they eat. This may be one reason why not all raw foodists look as healthy as they could. There are a number of raw foods which you should avoid, including:

- Anything that muscle tests as negative for you.

- Arugula lettuce. Maybe this is okay for you, but for me, this always muscle tests as negative and gives me headaches. I suspect that others should omit this as well.

- Bananas that are not organic. Non-organic bananas get gassed with toxins. It could still be more slimming to have normal raw bananas than cooked food. But, also, remember that many people are allergic to bananas.

- Garlic. Anything that makes you stink as much as garlic does, is very toxic. The late, brilliant Dr. Robert Beck found that garlic is a poison for higher-life forms and brain cells. Garlic desynchronizes brain waves[29]. Some people use garlic as a natural healthy remedy when they are sick, because it kills bacteria. While it may be good to have some if you are very sick, for this reason, it is not good to have as part of your regular diet. Gardeners use it as a pesticide, because it kills insects. Anything that kills bacteria & insects directly, is toxic for you as well. If you have sleeping difficulties, including nightmares or problem getting to sleep, see what difference zero garlic for five days makes.

- Spices. Some raw food recipes use a lot of spices. Basically, the spicier something is, the more toxic it is. Plants produce these toxins to stop animals from eating them. We are the only animal that has lost the ability to heed the "stay away" warnings of plants. Most herbs are okay and often good. I believe that the only time you should consume a lot of spices is when they are cooked lightly in oil, because then they get broken down. Wild animals don't eat many spices.

- Raw cacao. Cacao contains caffeine, to protect the plant from animals that want to eat it. Caffeine is caffeine, no matter what form it is in. It is an aging drug which puts your body and adrenals under stress. Caffeine raises cortisol levels and causes leptin resistance, both of which make you fat. Caffeine is a drug, and drugs are fattening. Please see my chapters on drugs and caffeine.

- Mushrooms. Mushrooms grow in manure. Manure contains parasites. Mushrooms *must* be cooked to kill the parasites. The only exception to this is tree mushrooms.

FRESH-SQUEEZED JUICE AND YOUR BUDGET

You might think that it's expensive, but it doesn't have to be. My local supermarket sells a 25 pound bag of sweet, organic carrots by Bunny-Luv, for only $15. Raw sunflower seeds, for smoothies, sell for only around $2/lb. Green lentils which you soak for 8 hours are also super cheap.

Please try this right now: get some lentils. Any sort will do, but you could start with green lentils. Soak them in reverse osmosis water for 8 hours. This 'sprouts' them, which means that, even if you can't see a sprout, life force inside them is now activated. The complex compounds inside them are being broken down, which makes it easier for you to absorb them. Drain and store them in the fridge. Rinse them once a day, as they will keep growing in the fridge, and will produce waste which you should clean off. Nibble on these before meals, and add them to anything savory. Make a meal of just lentils, carrots, apples and lemon juice. You may be surprised how filling they are! (Congratulations! Once you do that, you are a trainee raw foodist).

Lentils are healthier than beans. Soaked lentils are super good at helping you lose weight because they have[30]:

- Soluble fiber which is very filling.

- Soluble fiber which binds with carbohydrates, which lowers blood sugar levels.

- Very good source of iron and magnesium.

DON'T COOK FOOD JUST BECAUSE OUR ANCESTORS HAD TO

There are some people who want to convince us that cooked food is better for us than raw food. One of their main arguments is that "our ancestors did it". I would like to suggest that we, as a people, are meant to evolve, mentally, morally, spiritually, technologically, financially and health-wise. Our ancestors died a lot earlier than us, in their 40s. They were in survival mode most of the time. Just getting enough food to eat of any kind to stay alive was their main goal. And they did not have refrigeration. If all I had to eat was some moldy potatoes to last me through the winter, I am going to cook them. And they did not have our methods of juicing, or mass production, or all the different species of fruits, vegetables, nuts and seeds that we have today. Neither could they fly in fresh fruit from Peru when they needed it. So, there is no comparison between our ancestors and what we should be doing today.

Anytime you need a recipe, go to the internet, and search on "raw recipe" plus whatever food you have available. For example, search on "raw recipe avocado", or search for a recipe that you want a replacement for, such as "raw recipe key lime pie" or "raw recipe apple crumble". Just remember to think for yourself. If the recipe has ingredients which you have learned are toxic, replace them with something healthy. For example, if the recipe says agave nectar (which is toxic), replace it with raw honey or maple syrup.

I recommend having at least one fresh-squeezed juice every day. Plus one raw smoothie, with some chia seeds in it for omega 3's, plus at least one meal that is totally raw. It's a good idea to have a salad with leafy greens in it at lunch. Then have what other foods, that are not too toxic, that you feel like, cooked or otherwise.

Remember, when you eat raw, you can have as much as you want. If you want to really get slim, and your skin to start glowing and your energy levels to skyrocket, you will want to go totally raw, at least for a few days every now and again. Note that you may feel a little tired the first few days as your body detoxes the toxins from cooked food.

The raw foodists would tell you to have only raw food all the time. Yes, this works, absolutely, while you do it. And maybe that is what you want to do. But I found that I did not keep this up for life. I missed having an occasional meal of stir-fry, or lentil soup, or brown millet toast with nut butter. Only a plan that you maintain for life is going to work. If you go back to your old patterns of eating, you will get back to where you were, plus some extra.

I suggest that have a lot of raw food, including a fresh juice most days, and once or twice a day have a meal that is 100% raw, but also have some lightly cooked plant-based foods with some meals. As much as possible, have something raw with every meal, to provide digestive enzymes so that you can absorb nutrients. The only food that you have to watch how much you are eating is the cooked food, because it has toxins in it and is depleted of nutrients, and sugary fruit, especially when you are juicing. Generally, if it's raw, have as much as you want. But if you find you get hungry afterwards, or get bloated, cut down on the amount of sugary fruit next time.

It's important to have as much variety as possible, and every now and again go a week without a particular food, to prevent you becoming temporarily allergic to that food, as I discussed in the chapter on allergies. For example, after we had been doing a lot of juicing, my husband complained of feeling tired. Muscle testing indicated that he had become negative to spinach, which we had been juicing a lot of, but not to kale, which we had not juiced for weeks.

Cooking creates unnatural toxins. As Dr. Mark Hyman M.D. says, "Our immune response makes us crave foods we're allergic to."[31]

If you are serious about getting thin, please make at least one meal every day totally raw, with fruit, vegetables, nuts, seeds, sprouted legumes and / or juice. And, once or more a week, have a whole day that is 100% raw. The more you do this, the more you may want to do this, as you feel less hungry and feel the fat melting off your hips, and eventually, if not immediately, see the weight dropping off on the scales, to levels that you never thought were possible.

This food plan begins, not with a recipe, but with buying the right food. Please see my "shopping list" chapter. Once you have the food, if you can't think of a way to eat it, you can always find a recipe on the internet. In addition, there are lots of raw food uncook books to help you. Many people have not only lost weight, but also lost pain and health problems by going on a raw food diet. If you want to learn more about a raw food diet, a good place to start is with is the cookbook, *Living on Live Food*, by Alissa Cohen or *Rawsome* by Brigitte Mars.

REFERENCES

1. *First for Women* magazine, 5/7/12
2. *The Magnesium Factor*, Mildred Seelig M.D., page 11
3. *Enzymes, the Fountain of Life*, 1994, D. Lopez M.D., R.Williams M.D. Ph.D., K, Miehlke M.D.
4. *Enzymes, the Fountain of Life*, 1994, D. Lopez M.D., R.Williams M.D. Ph.D., K, Miehlke M.D., page 4
5. *Excitotoxins* by Dr. Russell Blaylock M.D., 1997, page 23
6. science2be.wordpress.com/2012/09/03/the-amazing-similarity-between-blood-and-chlorophyll/
7. en.wikipedia.org/wiki/Hemoglobin
8. *Excitotoxins* by Dr. Russell Blaylock M.D., 1997, page 23
9. www.macrobiotics.co.uk/chewwell.htm
10. www.webmd.com/food-recipes/features/get-the-facts-on-fiber
11. www.jointhereboot.com/
12. www.sciencedaily.com/releases/2012/06/120620212855.htm
13. *Rainbow Green Live-Food Cuisine*, 2003, by Dr Gabriel Cousens, M.D.
14. *Rainbow Green Live-Food Cuisine*, Gabriel Cousens M.D., 2003, page 117
15. *Rainbow Green Live-Food Cuisine*, Gabriel Cousens M.D., 2003, page 117
16. *The McDougall Plan*, John A. McDougall, M.D., (1983) pp. 98-100
17. *Diet for a New America*, John Robbins, 1987, p. 172, citing the American Journal of Clinical Nutrition
18. Dietary Reference Intakes for Energy, Carbohydrate, Fiber, Fat, Fatty Acids,

Cholesterol, Protein, and Amino Acids, Food and Drug Administration, Institute of Medicine of the National Academies, 2005. (Protein Estimated Average Requirement and RDA for adults is 0.66 and 0.8g per kg of ideal body weight, respectively. These are married to the daily energy requirements listed in the same report for various genders, ages, heights, weights, and activity levels, to get the range of percentage of calories from protein.)

19. Protein and Amino Acid Requirements in Human Nutrition (PDF), World Health Organization (2002). Recommendations on p. 126. Recommendations are an "average requirement" of 0.66 g of protein per kg of ideal body weight, and a "safe level" of 0.86 g/kg.

20. USDA National Nutrient Database for Standard Reference (accessed August to December 2009) FRUIT: Average of Apples, Pears, Grapes, Bananas, Plums, Oranges, Grapefruit, Watermelon, Strawberries, Peaches, Nectarines, Cantaloupe. VEGETABLES: Average of Broccoli 27.2%, Carrots 8.7%, Celery 17.3%, Corn 13.4%, Cucumber 17.3%, Green Beans 21.6%, Lettuce iceberg 25.7%, Mushrooms white 31%, Onions 12.4%, Peas 28.8%, Potato 10.8%, Spinach 49.7%, Tomato 19.6% (accessed December 2009)

21. www.rawfoodexplained.com/proteins/the-importance-of-amino-acids.html

22. www.rawfoodexplained.com/proteins/the-importance-of-amino-acids.html

23. api.ning.com/files/d9-oESjvOsA8NueA1LRdyN4QN*cqJC1CH-aBD11tn-Zo_/CookedFood.pdf

24. lowcarbdiets.about.com/od/glossary/g/glossphyto.htm

25. *Diet Wise* by Prof. Keith Scott-Mumby, 1984, page 52

26. www.wakingtimes.com/2013/01/23/common-modern-foods-which-cause-dna-damage/

27. *Wheat Belly*, William Davis M.D., 2011, pages 140-141

28. www.DiscountJuicers.com

29. www.relfe.com/health_benefits_of_garlic.html

30. health.howstuffworks.com/wellness/food-nutrition/natural-foods/natural-weight-loss-food-lentils-ga.htm

31. *Woman's World*, 7/9/12, page 18

CHAPTER 34

WEIGHT IS MISLEADING

Most of us, and most weight loss books and articles, define our level of success in being thin purely by how much we weigh. And yet, while eventually we want to reduce weight, focusing only on weight can be very misleading.

For example, did you know that some models are technically obese? Their percentage of fat to muscle is too high. This percentage is called the Body Mass Index (BMI). A lot of thin people are actually fat. Lately more people have come to realize this. Men should have body fat figures of 10%-18%. Women should be 16%-22%[1]. These figures vary somewhat from expert to expert, but one thing is certain - High body fat is unhealthy and not the way nature intended.

IT IS ONLY FAT LOSS THAT LOWERS THE CHANCE OF DEATH

In *The Magnesium Factor* the author discusses how some thin people are as dangerously unhealthy as some heavy people. One study showed that *weight loss* increased the death rate, while *fat loss* lowered it[2]. So, let's focus on giving the body what it wants, which is an absence of toxins, plus more nutrition and all the other keys of natural living, such as sunlight, positive emotions and exercise that does not stress the body.

There are four body-fat tests to choose from. I recommend you get this done every now and again. Be prepared to be shocked at what you learn the first time.

1. **Hydrostatic**. This works by how well you float. Fat people float better. It is a highly accurate test. This is done at a center that offers this as a service.

2. **Skin fold**. Done with calipers, by yourself or an expert. Only an expert will give you a reliable result.

3. **Electrical machine**. You can do this at a gym or buy one. Some people believe this is not very accurate, but it is better to do this than not at all. Do not do this if you are, or may be, pregnant, as it puts an electrical pulse through you.

4. **Infrared lights**. Not recommended, because they test only the biceps.

A lot of thin people with a high Body Mass Index work to improve it by exercise alone. However, I believe that if thin people followed the guidelines in this book, they would improve their Body Mass Index better than just through exercise alone. Muscle requires *good nutrition* to build, and that means removing toxins from the diet and adding more nutrition, particularly from fresh juicing and raw plants. (Please see the chapter on raw food for more information).

Judging your success at getting thin by weight loss alone does not work. Haven't we all met people who looked great, but were quite heavy? And, alternatively, people who seemed larger than they should, who didn't seem to weigh as much as they looked?

I once had a job looking after racehorses where I was walking about 8-10 miles a day. After a number of months, almost everyone I met complimented me on my new body. However, I ignored all their compliments and continued to feel depressed about my body because I *weighed exactly the same*. I kept feeling depressed about my weight, even though I dropped a size of jeans during this time. I realize now that while my weight was the same, my body had reduced in size considerably. In fact, it is quite possible that if I had tried, I might have even got into jeans that were two sizes smaller. I just did not think to try. I believe now that not only do exercise and raw plants give us more muscle, which weighs more than fat, volume for volume, but something else is going on. There was no other way I could account for how my body was so much smaller, without being any lighter.

When I started this program, there was a time when I lost only three pounds, and because one day I had enjoyed some ice-cream at lunch time the day before, I was feeling a bit mad with myself. Okay, I had eaten it at lunchtime, which is the best time to eat treats, and it was organic ice-cream, so at least it wasn't GMO, but sugar is sugar, a toxic substance that the body doesn't like, whether or not it's organic. But then I remembered that I should try on a pair of jeans that is one size smaller than the current size I was wearing, once a week. What a lovely surprise to discover that I fitted into them quite comfortably, with only a 3 pound difference!

On the reverse side, I can remember times in the past when I was eating more toxic food and was not doing exercise or juicing or raw food, and although I weighed almost the same, I nearly had to go *up* a size in jeans.

VOLUME FOR VOLUME, MUSCLE WEIGHS MORE THAN FAT

Muscle density is about 1.06 g/ml[3] and fat density is about 0.9 g/ml.[4] Therefore, one liter of muscle weighs about 1.06 kg and one liter of fat weighs about 0.9 kg. In other words, muscle is about 18% denser than fat. It takes up less room. That's why you can be thinner and still weigh the same.

Some people are under the impression that volume-for-volume, fat weighs three times more than muscle. However, this figure refers to what is called "energy density" and is not the same thing as the amount of volume it occupies.

In addition, exercise also increases the size and density, and therefore the weight, of your bones. For example, horses that do long distance training (100+ miles) get super-dense bones that are virtually unbreakable.

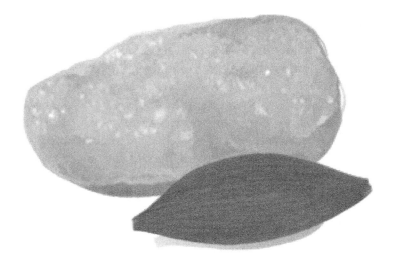

Weight for weight, muscle takes up less room than fat does

MUSCLE IS DISTRIBUTED PROPERLY. FAT ISN'T

There is yet another reason why the scales don't show the true picture. Part of the reason fat distorts your shape and makes you less beautiful is because fat is not evenly distributed over your body. For example, men typically build up more fat around their belly and women generally store more fat around their hips and thighs.

If we gained fat evenly over our whole body then fat gain would look exactly like gaining muscle! There would be less definition, but proportions would always be good. But, this isn't what happens. As we gain more and more fat, both men and women start to look more like blobs because their proportions get all messed up.

I told the information on this page to a friend who is 54 years old and 5.75" tall. She had this to say (dress sizes are U.S. dress sizes):

"I was a size six when I was in my late teens and twenties and even into my 30s. For most of my adult life I have worn a size 9-10 because it fits loose and seems most comfortable. I was even a size 12 for about a year. Last year I decided to remove meat and dairy from my diet. I also cut back on cooked food. I was not trying to lose weight, but to be healthier. I still have some organic eggs but I've managed to avoid meat.

Now here is a great side effect from going mostly raw. After a year of avoiding toxic food and eating raw meals a lot more often, I suddenly noticed I am able to fit into a *size 8* (although sometimes, depending on the clothes maker, the fit looks slightly tight). But what is even stranger is that *I weigh the same as I did before*: 145 pounds! That is more than what I weighed when I wore a size 12! I used to *weigh 142 and wear a size 12*. Now I can fit into size 8-10 and weigh 145 pounds! Today I was wondering about that when I was shopping for clothes.

Suddenly while trying things on I realized that it was weird that I could fit into a size 8, but that when I weighed myself this morning the scale says I weighed more than when I wore size 12!"

A few months later I encouraged her to go shopping and try on size 6 clothes. She was shocked to find that she fitted into everything that was *size 6*. She emailed me:

"What is so weird is to **weigh 139 pounds right now and to fit a size 6 whereas in the past, the same weight would be a size 12.**"

I believe that the changes observed in myself and my friend can be partly accounted for by various factors, including:

1. Volume for volume, muscle weighs more than fat.

2. Exercise and good nutrition increase bone density. There are studies to back this up. For example, one study found that resistance exercise, even in the elderly, increased bone density by 9%[5].

3. Muscle distributes properly over the body. Fat does not.

But, these do not explain all the observations of myself and others, whereby people can vary by *up to 3 different dress* sizes, while still weighing much the same, if they eat mostly raw plant food. I truly believe that there is something else going on, whereby people who are eating less toxic and more raw plant food get *more dense*. Their bodies take up less volume for other reasons than just those listed above. After all, we have never seen what we look like on a molecular level. For example, maybe the reason for this is that healthy cells contain more dissolved minerals, which adds to their density (weight per volume).

The more information we have, the better. I still think it's a good idea to weigh yourself first thing every morning. (What you weigh later in the day does not count). Use a scale that shows tenths of a pound. This is because it is my belief that when there is a sudden increase in weight in one day, of two or more pounds, when you ate roughly the same amount of food as you normally do, that this is not due to your body creating a whole extra two pounds of fat. It's mostly a reaction, which may be fluid retention, from something you ate that is *toxic for your body*. Muscle testing can help you to identify what that particular food is.

Weight does give us information. And we do want to get weight off because it's putting stress on the body. But, do more than just weigh yourself every morning. Also look at yourself in the mirror, feel your body and try on a size smaller pair of jeans every week. Also measure your waist.

Don't give up on this new food plan just because you don't see the changes you want on the scales after just one week or even one month. Think of what you are doing as building a new foundation, as if you are building a building. It takes a long time to build the foundation, but once the foundation is in, the building goes up quickly. Your body will be changing for the better, but it may have to make changes on the inside first, before it makes the more cosmetic changes you would like to see on the outside.

Right now, please, buy a pair of jeans or shorts the next size down. Try them on once every week. If you have been following the food and exercise and other advice in this book, and especially if you have started juicing and having fully raw meals, you may get a shock and find you actually fit into them! Once you fit into those pants, buy a size smaller again, until you are at your ideal size, rather than ideal weight.

REFERENCES

1. articles.latimes.com/1993-02-16/news/vw-40_1_body-fat-test
2. *The Magnesium Factor* by Mildred Seelig, M.D., 2003, page 109
3. *The Journals of Gerontology Series A*: Biological Sciences and Medical Sciences 56:B191-B197 (200).
4. Association of adiponectin and resistin with adipose tissue compartments, insulin resistance and dyslipidaemia. Farvidl, Ng, Chan, Barrett and Watts
5. www.naturalnews.com/010528.html

CHAPTER 35

EXERCISE #1
WALKING

We've heard it over and over again, that exercise is important for any fat reduction program. You are going to learn a number of reasons why a simple 30 minute walk, six times a week, will contribute to giving you the body you want, and it has little to do with burning calories. If you are one of those people who have tried exercise, but found that it either did not work for you, or you could not keep your program for life, then you may find some helpful knowledge here.

The magazine *Woman's World*[1] showed a woman named Diane Carbonell who failed at 500 diets, but then reduced by 305 pounds by adding a 30 minute walk to everything else she was doing right. She lost 158 pounds and now wears a size 6!

By accident she discovered a trick that can help you to burn even more off. Once you are feeling stronger, and enjoying walking, every now and again do a speed up for a short distance. Intervals of fast and slow work are called "interval training". An Australian study found that women who did interval training were *three times* more likely to lose weight than those that stuck with a consistent pace.

I know a family who also reduced a lot of weight purely from taking a 30 minute walk after dinner. A Japanese study found that taking a 30 minute walk immediately after dinner seems to trigger 100% greater weight reduction than walking on an empty stomach. But, please, if there is some reason why you can't walk after dinner, just walk whenever you can. For example, while we lived in Florida, I put off walking because of the heat. Eventually, I realized that it *has* to be done. It is as important as brushing your teeth. I got up 30 minutes earlier and started walking nearly every day.

First[2] magazine also showed success stories of women who reduced a great deal of weight by walking just 30 minutes a day.

- Cari Trapp reduced by 220 pounds. 35 years old and 5'11", Cari went from 394 to 174 pounds in five months, by walking. www.CariTrapp.com.

- Taisha Hayes reduced by 130 pounds. 30 years old and 6', Taisha went from 280 pounds to 150 pounds, dropping 12 pant sizes! She did this by exercise, starting with just a 10 minute walk each day. www.THayesFitness.com.

- Kim DiMondo reduced by 113 pounds. 39 years old and 5'4", Kim went from 260 pounds to 113 pounds, by walking. Plus she healed her excruciating hip pain. She marvels, "I couldn't believe something as easy as walking worked so well." www.Life360Coaching.com.

- Shannon Hammer lost 107 pounds. 42 years old and 5'5", Shannon went from 230 pounds to 123 pounds, by walking and a food journal. www.PositivePortions.com.

30 MINUTES OF WALKING A DAY LOWERS YOUR "SET POINT"!

Most of us have been conditioned to believe that there is a magical weight that our body wants to stay at all the time, called our "Set Point", and that there is not much we can do to lower it. It is believed by many that the set point is a reference point around which the body tries to keep a stable weight. An example of another set point is body temperature – if temperatures go above or below 98.6°F (for example, from infection or exposure to a cold environment), there are a variety of physical mechanisms that "kick in" to try to get back to, and maintain, normal body temperature[3].

But new discoveries have found that the set point is not set for life. It can be lowered by regular walking! This is because the set point is affected by the master hormone in the body, leptin. Leptin is secreted by fat cells. It affects appetite and metabolism.

Leptin helps to keep your body in its natural, optimal, thin shape. Virtually everyone who is overweight has what is called leptin resistance.[4] I believe that this is because we have moved so far away from the laws of nature, and it no longer works properly. The wonderful news is that *regular* walking lowers your "set point" by *restoring leptin sensitivity*[5].

This was discovered in a study by the University of Cincinnati, co-authored by Silvana Obicia, M.D. Vigorous exercise is not necessary, and I will be discussing later why stressful exercise is often detrimental, in the chapter on resistance exercise.

In addition, in *Your Body's Many Cries for Water*, Dr. Batmanghelidj M.D. says:

> "Proteins are more accessible and broken down more easily than fat[6]...When muscles are inactive, they are more easily attacked and their protein is broken down for conversion into sugar. However, if muscles are used, they begin to metabolize some of their stored fat as a choice source of energy."

Here's another reason why exercise is essential to losing fat. Exercise removes toxins. That is why you are not fat, you are toxic. Everyone who does not exercise is literally drowning in their own waste products. This clogs the body with toxins so that nothing works as well as it should. In addition, toxins cause symptoms such as pain, tiredness and brain fog, which in turn are more likely to cause the person to eat 'comfort' foods.

This is how it works: Every cell in the body produces waste products, in much the same way that exhaust comes out of the back of the car.

They are left-over materials from the thousands of different chemical processes that the cell has to perform to keep you alive, even if you are eating and drinking only food that is positive for your body. Now, if you are like most people and eating and drinking foods that are negative for your body, there are even more toxins to remove, because you have consumed substances that the body wants to get out of the body as soon as possible.

Nutrients are moved *to* the cells, by the heart, through the blood, by muscles in the blood vessels, and valves that prevent back flow. Waste products, which are toxins, are removed *from* the cells by the lymphatic system. However, the lymphatic system does not have muscles and valves to move the fluid along. The only way that toxins can move through the lymphatic system and out of the body, is if the muscles in the body move. This is done only by stress-free exercise or massage.

So, since so many people get almost no exercise, that is why I say that many people are literally drowning in their own waste products.

What kind of exercise is best for removing toxins? It turns out that plain old walking is the best, because this uses every single one of the more than 600 muscles in the body, without doing any damage. (Experts do not agree on exactly how many muscles there are in the body).

Toxins cause stress. They clog up your brain so you just don't feel right. 60% of participants in a YMCA survey said they were too stressed to exercise. But research shows that walking can reduce feelings of tension within just 21 minutes. Again, this is because walking moves toxins through the lymphatic system, so that they can finally be removed from the body.

THE DIFFERENCE BETWEEN "AEROBIC" AND "ANAEROBIC" EXERCISE

Living cells are not heat engines. They do not use heat energy to work. Instead, they use chemical energy from chemical reactions. When we do exercise, these chemical reactions vary, depending on the type of exercise. The chemical reactions during exercise are usually a mix of aerobic and anaerobic.

"Aerobic" means "with oxygen". Aerobic chemical reactions in the body produce safe wastes, water and carbon dioxide. Walking is aerobic. Aerobic exercise is easy on your body.

"Anaerobic" means "without oxygen". Anaerobic chemical reactions in the body produce lactic acid. It is lactic acid that causes pain, and builds up to eventually stop muscles from contracting. Anaerobic exercise, such as fast running, is hard on your body.

By the way, so-called "aerobic" exercises are mostly anaerobic, because you can't do them for more than short periods of time without causing pain.

Aerobic exercise is exercise that you can do for hours, with virtually nothing stopping you. This is walking, and slow jogging (for slightly fit people) and faster running that you can do indefinitely (for very fit people). As you do more aerobic exercise, your body builds more muscles, blood vessels and blood cells, without damage, so that when you do anaerobic exercise, your body will be able to run on aerobic chemical reactions for longer, before it has to switch to the much more inefficient anaerobic reactions.

The longer you do aerobic exercise before you switch to anaerobic exercise, the more successful you will be. This advice is from Arthur Lydiard[7]. Lydiard is one of the greatest running coaches of all time. With his training, which was revolutionary at the time, runners from New Zealand, including Peter Snell, won many gold medals during the 1960s Olympics.

Stressful, anaerobic exercise is very inefficient. It produces lots of toxins, such as free radicals[8], and also breaks down muscle, which the body has to repair. You already have enough toxins to remove from the body without making any more!

"USE IT OR LOSE IT"

This was a favorite saying of my kinesiology teacher, David Bridgman. This saying will become more important to you once you get older – say, somewhere around 45 or 50 years old.

The body is sensible. If you are not using something, then it figures it does not need it. If you don't use muscles, they atrophy. (In addition, if you don't use your brain, it atrophies. People should continue to learn throughout their lives). This is backed up by the book *Your Body's Many Cries for Water*, which says:

> "When muscles are inactive, they are more easily attacked and their protein is broken down for conversion into sugar. However, if muscles are used, they begin to metabolize some of their stored fat as a choice source of energy[9]."

You want more muscle and less fat for a number of reasons:

- It feels better.

- Weight for weight, muscle occupies less volume than fat, so you look smaller.

- Muscle burns calories. Fat does a lot less (although fat cells are very important for making leptin, so they should not be sucked out by liposuction). In fact, muscle burns up to 25 *times* more energy than fat does[10], even when you are sitting down doing nothing!

But remember that doing exercise does more than just "burn calories". It gets your leptin working properly so that your body burns fat and regulates hunger better, clears away toxins and makes your whole body work better and become younger.

MUSCLE BURNS MORE CALORIES THAN FAT

If you look at a picture of a muscle cell under an electron microscope, you will see all kinds of components, that are performing all kinds of activity, just to stay alive. That means that muscle cells are burning a lot of energy, even when you are not using them, like when you are sleeping.

Next page: Top - Rat muscle cells under an electron microscope. Bottom - Artist's rendition of fat cells under an electron microscope.

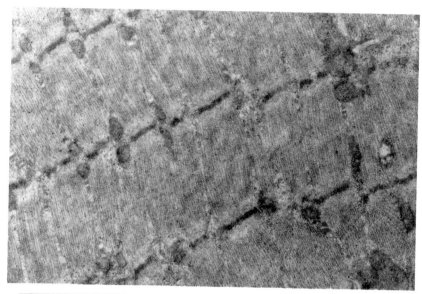

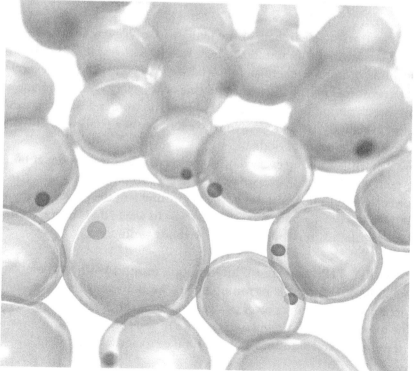

On the preceeding page you will see a picture of rat muscle fibers. I took this photo myself using a $1.5 Million electron microscope, while studying for a Master of Science degree at Sydney University.

But if you look at a fat cell under an electron microscope, you will see a lot less components. Just about the only thing you will see in a fat cell is one huge lump of fat that looks like a lump of butter. While we now know that fat cells are vital, because they produce leptin, the most important hormone in the body, obviously, they require a lot less energy to maintain.

One final reason why you should walk: Excess estrogen causes an increase in fat tissue. Making matters worse, the more fat you have, the more estrogen you make, which then makes you fatter[11]. Just like with other toxins, stress-free exercise is very good at lowering estrogen levels[12].

FAST AND SLOW INTERVALS ARE MUCH BETTER THAN CONSTANT SPEED

Australian researchers of the University of New South Wales and the Garvan Institute found the best weight loss results came from 8 seconds of intense exercise followed by 12 seconds of light exercise for 20-minute periods. They tested this on 45 overweight women over a 15-week period using a stationary bike. The women lost three times more weight than other women who exercised at a continuous regular rate for 40-minute periods.[13]

So, while walking every day is best because it lowers your set point, even if you can't walk every day, find at least 20 minutes about 3 times a week. Spend a few minutes at the beginning and the end to warm up and to cool down or stretch. The best way to warm up is to start doing your regular exercise moderately for about 5 minutes.

EASY TIP: Getting up and moving around your workplace or home for just a couple of minutes once an hour may have the same metabolism-boosting power as sweating for an hour at the gym! Why? The most effective fat-reducing enzymes in your body are found in your leg muscles, and standing up is all it takes to activate them[14]!

IMPORTANT: WHY RUNNING MAY NOT BE GOOD

I was guided to write this extra piece by an unfortunate event that happened yesterday at time of writing. A 49 year old man in a gated community near where I live, who looked healthy, was out jogging with his wife, when he dropped dead of a heart attack. I can't imagine how awful that was for his family.

This is not the only time that someone young has died of a heart attack while running. The man who got people running, Jim Fixx, author of *The Complete Book of Running*, died at age 52, also of a heart attack, after his daily run[15]. That is a bad example to follow.

You see, the problem is that while a lot of people look healthy on the outside, we cannot see how toxic and unhealthy they look like on the inside, in their organs and in their cells.

If you are eating or drinking animal protein, dairy, alcohol, caffeine, MSG, aspartame, wheat, microwaved food, restaurant and junk food, then running could very well be the most dangerous thing you ever did. On the other hand, walking could be one of the best things you ever did, because that does not stress the body.

If you still insist on running, please do your best to not run on hard surfaces. I knew a chiropractor who said that many runners she saw had damaged knees. Our bodies were designed to run on grass, which is much softer. Some extra points to consider:

1) Please walk outside rather than inside as often as you can, because your body needs sunlight (real Vitamin D) for fat loss, as well as avoiding the flu and growing strong bones. You can bet that Vitamin D supplements don't have all you need. Wear a sleeveless shirt at least. If you can do so safely and modestly, bare as much skin as possible.

2) Carry a metal stick (called a "whappy stick" in Australia) or baseball bat, for protection against wild dogs and wild people.

3) So long as you can find a safe place to exercise, it's very important to exercise away from traffic. If you walk or run near traffic, you

are sucking in a whole lot of carbon monoxide, as well as poisonous lead[16] and other harmful chemicals that your body will have to detox, rather than detox the toxins in your fat cells. There is an exponential decline in concentrations of many air pollutants, with increasing distance from busy roads. If you can't avoid the roads completely, then at least avoid rush hour.

4. Do not use a treadmill. Walk on the ground. You can even walk in one spot. I was told by a naturopath that it was discovered that a person with type II diabetes normally would see a good drop in excess blood glucose level after exercise (walking, jogging, etc.). This would be around 10-15%, which is good. However, accidentally, some researchers discovered that when a diabetic got on an electric powered treadmill, their blood sugar actually *went up*!

They repeated this with different patients. They came to believe it was because of the large electromagnetic fields coming off the machine, because they had the same people walk around outside at a comparable speed and their blood sugar fell. While not all people have this sensitivity, it still shows that a treadmill is interfering with the body's electromagnetic field.

Another reason why I suggest not using a treadmill is that I have noticed that although I felt fit after using a treadmill a lot, when I tried to walk the same distance on normal ground, I did not feel as fit as when I 'walked' the same 'distance' on the treadmill. This may be because on a treadmill I am just picking my feet up and down, which is easier work than actually carrying my body along the surface.

5. What is the best time to walk? While some say the best time is after dinner, others say that it doesn't really matter when you walk[17]. Just don't do it very late if you can manage it, because it can interfere with your ability to get to sleep. What does matter is that you find the best time that fits in with your timetable so that it becomes a *habit* for life.

Lower your set point. Clean out your toxins. Do *whatever it takes* to walk for 30 minutes in one block of activity, at least 5 times a week. Everyone can walk! Turn off the TV. Turn off the internet and get going. It's more important than brushing your teeth.

REFERENCES

1. *Woman's World* magazine 10/10/11
2. *First* magazine 10/10/11
3. www.nedic.ca/knowthefacts/documents/setpointwhatyourbodyistrying-totellyou.pdf
4. *Hormonal Balance: Understanding Hormones, Weight and Your Metabolism*, by Scott Isaacs, M.D.
5. *First* magazine 10/10/11
6. *Your Body's Many Cries for Water*, by Dr. Batmanghelidj M.D., page 102
7. *Running to the Top*, by Arthur Lydiard, 1995
8. *Excitotoxins*, by Dr. Russell Blaylock, 1997, page 111
9. *Your Body's Many Cries for Water*, by Dr. Batmanghelidj M.D., page 102
10. *Outside* Magazine, Jan 2002
11. *The Anti-estrogenic diet*, by Ori Hofmekler, 2007, page 6
12. *The Anti-estrogenic diet*, by Ori Hofmekler, 2007, page 30
13. www.articlesnatch.com/Article/Lose-Stomach-Fat---Best-Stomach-Fat-Exercise-In-Your-50s/2551196
14. *Woman's World*, 11/26/12
15. en.wikipedia.org/wiki/Jim_Fixx
16. www.cprm.gov.br/pgagem/Manuscripts/legretm.htm
17. www.webmd.com/fitness-exercise/features/whats-the-best-time-to-exercise

CHAPTER 36

EXERCISE #2
RESISTANCE EXERCISE

Resistance exercise is important, in addition to walking. But most weight builders and athletes have it totally wrong. "No pain, no gain" is false. The real motto should be *"No pain, real gain"*.

I learned this from John Douillard[1], the author of the brilliant book *Body, Mind & Sport*, which I highly recommend to you. This book will convince you why you must do less, to accomplish more. Why is this important to you? Because if you look at nearly all of the people who successfully got slim, and *stayed* slim, you will see that exercise was involved. There are two kinds of exercise that are needed to get you really looking your best:

1. Aerobic ('with oxygen'). This is covered in the chapter on walking.

2. Resistance exercise, where you focus on building muscle.

EXERCISE MUST BE PAIN FREE

Exercise that is strenuous and causes pain harms your ability to get thin for a number of reasons including:

- You won't continue with it.

- Strenuous exercise breaks muscles down. Muscles help you get thin.

- Your body must spend valuable resources and time *repairing* damaged muscles, when what it really wants to do is build brand new muscles. Therefore it doesn't have the time or resources to deal with reducing fat.

- Magnesium is critical to getting thin, and most of us don't have enough. The more intense the exercise, the more magnesium you burn. In fact, if magnesium levels are very low, an intense amount of physical exercise can even be life threatening, regardless of how fit or strong a person is[2].

- Any stress, including stressful exercise, causes the release of cortisol. High cortisol levels make you fat, especially in the belly[3].

- When exercise is too intense, the body holds onto extra water to cool the muscles down. This results in fluid retention[4].

To be successful, exercise must be part of your life, not just something you do for a few weeks. It needs to be part of your daily program. It must be as important as brushing your teeth. Most of us give up resistance exercise for at least one of the following reasons:

1. We don't have the time.

2. It hurts, or it makes us feel awful. I believe that there is a part of our mind that programs us unconsciously to not repeat anything that has hurt us in the past.

So, in addition to lifting a few weights, I suggest that you do just five movements called the "Five Tibetan Rites" which take care of both of these problems. They come from a book, *Ancient Secret of the*

Fountain of Youth, which sold two million copies. (Book #1 is the one to get, not #2). These exercises:

1. Take literally only minutes a day. You start with only one minute, once or twice a day. And work up to only 8-10 minutes a day.

2. Don't hurt, so long as you always apply the rule – "no pain, real gain."

3. Make you feel noticeably more *alive and energetic*. That's because they do more than just build muscle. They also get the energy centers in your body flowing. The ancient Tibetans believed this was one of the keys to *eternal youth*.

4. Can be done in your bedroom or hotel room.

5. Save you gym fees.

6. Tighten your body, and increase your metabolism.

I believe that it is harmful for a person who is older, overweight or unfit to try to follow the instructions of the people on fitness TV shows or videos. These people are already slim and fit, and usually young. Forget about them. I am going to teach you how to eventually look like them, but if you follow the advice they give before your body is the same as theirs, I believe that you will end up giving up on exercise altogether.

Douillard obtained much of his "no pain, real gain" information from studying Ayurveda. Ayurveda, is called "the knowledge for long life". It is a natural system of medicine that comes from India and dates back to at least 2000 BC. Inherent in Ayurvedic principles is the concept that you are capable of taking charge of your own life and healing.

Here is my favorite part of Douillard's book, that should convince you that it is time to stop listening to the advice of virtually everyone who thinks they know how to get fit. Listen to the real expert - your body. Standard science and fitness research doesn't know anywhere near as much as it thinks it does.

"Is the Sky the Limit⁵?

Ninety miles south of Phoenix, Arizona, live the Tarahumara Indians, a native Mexican tribe with an unfathomable skill in running. The Tarahumara run from their first steps to their last; it is their way of life. These remarkable people can run down deer and horses; they can run 50 to 100 miles in a day with ease, and up to 150 miles seemingly without effort. They have been known to run 40 to 50 miles at a time, taking only the briefest of breaks. Even more striking, they are said to improve with age, and the young look up to their grandfathers as the runners with the greatest skill.

A few years ago, a group of North American researchers visited the Tarahumara to study their feats. They staged a 26 mile run - a marathon, a run the researchers considered most grueling and demanding. The Indians laughed at the distance, regarding it as child's play!

The test took the Indians over rugged, extremely mountainous terrain in the scorching heat of the Mexican desert. The runners averaged 6 miles per hour including breaks. They took no food or water. At the end, they stood calmly near the finish line, breathing effortlessly, as the researchers examined them in disbelief. Pulse rates averaged about 130 beats per minute, and blood pressure, which had been low at the start, was even lower at the end of the run.

The scientists concluded that what they had witnessed *was not humanly possible*! Yet the Tarahumara were decidedly human, possessing no "super gene" or any other unique physical quality."

In Douillard's *Invincible Athletics* course, he teaches people to remove all strain and to *only* do what is comfortable. At first, people find it hard to think they are doing anything if they don't feel anything, because we've been brainwashed into thinking that if it doesn't hurt, it's not doing anything. In fact, the reverse is true.

Every time you do *any* exercise at all, you are telling the body to build more muscles. You are telling the brain "I am using this muscle, so make it stronger and bigger." If you do it daily, without *any* stress or pain, the body will build and build and build those muscles, as well as the extra blood vessels needed to nourish those muscles. If there is no pain, which means there is no stress or damage, the body won't waste time, energy and resources by stopping and repairing damaged muscles. It will just keep building more and more *new* muscle, and more and better blood vessels.

This is why you must not look for immediate results if they don't show up as soon as you like. Depending on your level of fitness, the early weeks of exercise are not to burn calories or tone muscle. They are simply to make your body just a *little* stronger, so the next day it gets just a *little* stronger, and so on *forever*. It's like planting a tiny seed to grow an oak tree. You have to nurture your body at the beginning by being super easy on it.

Pain is always the body's way of telling you that you are doing something wrong. You have to listen to your body, not your wants, not your ego, not your mind and not what other people think.

Here's one story from Douillard's book of a man who was overweight and stressed out, but also wanted to run a marathon. He had damaged his body because, like most of us, he was conditioned to expect and produce pain during workouts. At first, he found it hard to do workouts with zero pain at all times. But he continued with Douillard's program and kept all pain from his training, until eventually he was able to report -

> "John, I'm 38 years old. I've never been an athlete... I took your course to give my running one last try. Since then, I've lost 30 pounds and 6 inches of girth without trying or dieting. I don't get sick or anxious anymore, and I've got more vitality than I've ever known.
>
> Yesterday... I ran 17 miles. I felt absolutely fantastic the whole way. I felt as good when I stopped as I did when I started. The amazing thing was that I ran a 6 minute mile pace for the entire 17 miles.

It was unbelievable. I was in the Zone, I felt like I was running on air. It was the easiest thing I've ever done."

Even more amazingly, he was able to maintain a heart rate of 120 BPM (beats per minute) while maintaining a 6 minute mile pace! He achieved this because he let his body improve from the inside out, with the smallest amount of effort possible. He got into "the Zone" - a mental 'high', a time of top performance where there are no thoughts, no pain and there is only an inner feeling of calm. It's an inexhaustible source of power and peace. (Note: There are two kinds of 'zone'. One occurs when there is a perfect joining of mind and body. The other, which Douillard calls "The Illegitimate Zone", and which is more common in our society, is from a breakdown in communication between the mind and body, and occurs when the body produces all kinds of painkillers to help a person endure an ordeal that the body is not fit for).

Gold medalists feel the Zone, and you can too. Douillard explains in his book how all of us, not just athletes, can experience "The Zone" regularly. The key is to exercise with *no pain* or stress at *any* time. You may not have the time or desire to become an athlete, but I thought I would let you know of the possibilities. I am telling you about this to convince you why you must do a few minutes of a particular resistance exercise that I will describe to you, called the "Five Tibetan Rites", every day. But you must do it with absolutely no pain at any time, either during or after the exercises.

Ancient people believed in exercise, not to reduce weight, but to live a more full life. If you want to develop spiritually and to feel wonderful, not just look wonderful, you need a strong body. You can have that, even in old age, as long as you exercise regularly with the goal of making it as *effortless* as possible. You must give your body little frequent signals of what is required of it, plus time to adjust to the new exercise so that when the next level is started, it too is effortless.

THE FIVE TIBETAN RITES

The five movements that I suggest you do at least once every day are called the Five Tibetan Rites. It's called a "rite" because it's an ancient customary practice. It has no effect on one's religion or spirituality, other than improving the energy flows in your body.

The Five Tibetan Rites is a system of exercises reported to be more than 2,500 years old, which were first publicized by Peter Kelder in a 1939 publication entitled *The Eye of Revelation*. Kelder's booklet states that, while stationed in India, British army officer Colonel Bradford (a pseudonym) heard a story about a group of lamas who had apparently discovered a "Fountain of Youth". The "wandering natives", as he called them, told him of old men who inexplicably became healthy, strong and full of "vigor and virility" after entering a particular lamasery. After retiring, Kelder's Colonel Bradford went on to discover the lamasery and lived with the monks where they taught him five exercises, which they called "rites".

Later they were described in the book *Ancient Secret of the Fountain of Youth (Book 1)*, by Peter Kelder, which sold two million copies. The following is among the editorial reviews at amazon.com for Book 2:

"I have done the Five Rites and passed *Ancient Secret of the Fountain of Youth* on to many friends over the years. I recommend them without reservation." -Martin Sheen

The lamas described 7 spinning vortices of energy (chakras), that start in the body and flow into and out of the aura. As we grow older, the spin rate of the chakras diminishes, resulting in ill-health. The spin rate can be restored, which results in improved health, by performing the Five Rites on a daily basis.

While most people can't see the chakras, that does not mean that they don't exist. After all, our bodies move around because of the life-force within them, and we can't see that either. There are people who can actually see the chakras, especially people who meditate a lot. The ancient people in India and China all knew about them. Muscle testing confirms that the chakras exist. Notice from the picture on the next page, that the chakras go out past the body, both in front *and* in the back. This is the reason why you can tell when someone comes up behind you, even when you can't hear them - because they stepped into your chakra.

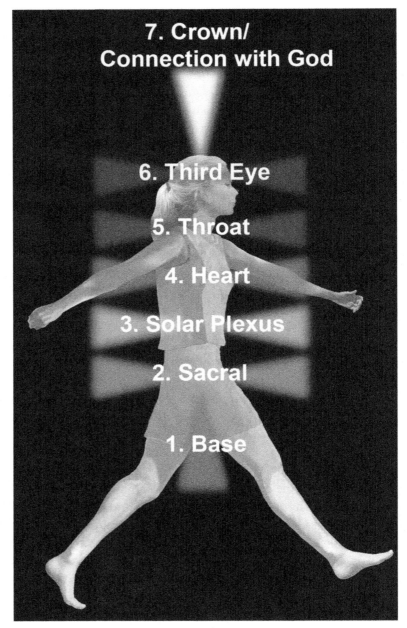

Seven chakras, front and back.

BODYWEIGHT EXERCISES

The Five Tibetan Rites are bodyweight exercises. That is, they use your own bodyweight to provide resistance, without the need for any weights or machines. Walking up stairs and pushups are also good bodyweight exercises.

Bodyweight exercises *look* simple and easy, but they supply an amazing amount of resistance for your body to work with. I believe that they are the best exercise for getting fit, with one major proviso: As with any resistance exercise, be super careful when doing them. Start off with just a *tiny* amount. Increase very gradually in the coming weeks.

When I first learned about bodyweight exercises, I started doing them with gusto. I got a DVD from an 'expert' who taught bodyweight exercises that are different from those I am going to teach you. Shortly after following the 'expert's' instructions, I developed a swelling on my leg which did not heal for years. The expert never explained how stressful the exercises were to the body, or to build up to them very slowly.

Please, I know what it's like to be old, overweight and unfit. Do not follow the fitness advice of people who are strong and thin and super fit already. You must listen to your own body and give it oodles of time to respond to the challenges you give it.

Plus, keep having fresh-squeezed vegetable juices with leafy greens, raw plant food and raw seeds to keep up your magnesium levels.

HOW TO DO THE FIVE TIBETAN RITES EXERCISES

First of all, walk on the same spot, swinging your arms, to clear out toxins that were produced overnight.

On the first day, do each Tibetan Rite exercise only once, in the morning. That's all. Unless you are very young and fit, do not add another repetition for at least a week or more. Even if you are young and fit, I suggest you don't increase the number of repetitions less than once every three days. Also, the exercises can put pressure on your joints. Work up to doing each exercise 21 times, at least once a day.

If you think you can't do these exercises at all, do the best you can, no matter how little it is. Each time you do what you can, your body will start to work on giving you the muscles needed so that you can do them better next time. Patience and perseverance is the key.

WARNING! These exercises are a lot harder than they appear. You will probably be using muscles you have never used before, even if you are fit. If you get any pain at all after doing them, start again with only one or two repetitions. The key is to doing resistance exercise with zero pain, at any time.

I had a friend of mine who was in her fifties and after she did each exercise just once, she was in pain for a week afterwards. If this happens to you, do not do them again until all of the pain is gone, plus an extra day for good measure. If you have to wait a week or more before starting them again, do so. If you are very unfit, and can work out how to do *half* an exercise to start off with, then please, do that! I cannot overstress that it's important to do these with no pain, during and afterwards. It doesn't matter if it takes months to be able to do just four repetitions. The goal is to do these for life, and you will only do that if you don't experience pain from doing them.

So long as you are not in pain from doing these exercises, it is very important that you *do not miss a day.* Make sure you do them at least once a day, preferably in the morning, so that you have all day to do them if you forget. If you miss a day, start over again at one repetition, because if you miss a day, and go back to where you were last up to, you may hurt yourself, and have to wait many days for the pain to go and to start again. Plus, once there is pain, there could be an unconscious thought to not continue with them. Even if it takes you several months to get past three or four repetitions, just keep doing them every day, without pain.

You are building a foundation for the rest of your life. Just as when you make a building, it's building the foundation that takes the long time. Once the foundation is built, the building goes up very quickly.

Do the Tibetan Rites every day, no matter what. It only takes a few minutes! After several months, when you are totally in the **habit** of doing them every day, and there is no way that you would ever miss out on them, if you still don't have the body you want, and want to accelerate your results, do some of them in the evening, in addition to your morning exercises, to tell your body what you want it to work on overnight. You may be amazed at the difference this makes.

ALEXANDER TECHNIQUE

Before I tell you how to do the Tibetan Rites, I want to give some tips on how to get up easily off the floor after the exercises, which can be tough, especially if you are older and heavy. This comes from what is called the "Alexander Technique". It is based on the fact that your skull is like a massive, super-heavy boulder. Try this now with a friend: Get them to lie on the floor. Then cradle their head in your hands. Have them totally let go and relax. You lift and hold their head in your hands, so that you truly experience the massive weight of a skull. It's amazing that our necks carry it around so easily!

Most people who go to get up off the floor lift their head up first. Do not do this. The head should always come up *last*. So, instead, keep your hands and feet on the floor, and lift your backside as high as possible. Then, tuck in your chin and roll your head up the front of your body, as though you were lifting a dead weight on a chain, which you are. Do the same thing if you want to get out of a chair. Now that you know how to get up from the floor easily, here are the exercises.

THE TIBETAN RITES EXERCISES

1. Clockwise Whirling

2. Head and Leg Raises

3. The Camel

4. The Tabletop

5. The Up and Down

These five exercises are described in detail on the following pages.

1. Clockwise Whirling

- Stand erect with arms outstretched horizontal to the floor.
- Palms face down.
- Your arms should be in line with your shoulders.
- Spin around clockwise, slowly, until you become slightly dizzy.
- Gradually increase number of spins from 1 spin to 21 spins.

Breathing: Inhale and exhale deeply as you do the spins.

Do this very slowly at first. You can increase speed later. You may think that you can increase this more than one repetition every week, but it can put quite a strain on your ankles and hips. Please be patient.

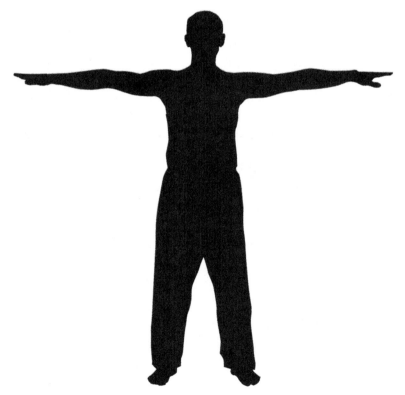

Clockwise Whirling

2. Head and Leg Raises

- Lie flat on the floor, face up.
- Fully extend your arms along your sides.
- Place the palms of your hands against the floor, keeping fingers close together. Raise your head off the floor tucking your chin into your chest.
- As you raise your head, lift your legs, knees straight, into a vertical position, or as much as you can. When you start, you may only get your legs up an inch or two. If possible, extend the legs over the body towards your head. Do not let the knees bend.
- Slowly lower the legs and head to the floor, always keeping the knees straight. Allow the muscles to relax, and repeat.

Breathing: Breathe <u>in</u> deeply as you <u>lift</u> your head and legs and exhale as you lower your head and legs.

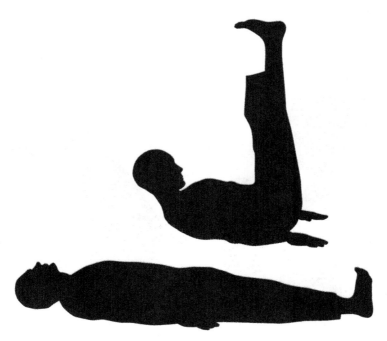

Head and Leg Raises

3. The Camel

- Kneel on the floor with the body erect.
- The hands should be placed on the backs of your thigh muscles.
- Tuck you toes under, if you can.
- Move the head and neck backward gently, arching the spine. As you arch, you will brace your arms and hands against the thighs for support.
- It should not be as far as possible, as that puts too much stress on your body. Tune in to your body.
- Return to erect position.
- Then, tuck your chin as far down as possible, against your chest.
- Lean forward as far as you can.
- There is conflicting information as to whether or not you should bend at the waist (as in the picture)[6]. It is up to you. I personally prefer to keep my back straight while leaning forward.
- Return to erect position. Then do the backward movement again.

Breathing: <u>Inhale</u> as you <u>arch</u> the spine and exhale as you do the forwards movement.

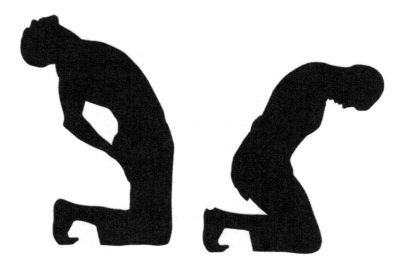

The Camel

4. The Tabletop

- Sit down on the floor with your legs straight out in front of you.
- Your feet are about 12" apart.
- With the trunk of the body erect, place the palms of your hands on the floor alongside your buttocks.
- Tuck the chin forward against the chest.
- Then drop the head backward as far as it will go (be careful).
- At the same time that you drop the head backwards, raise your body so that the knees bend while the arms remain straight.
- Tense every muscle in your body and hold for a second.
- Let the muscles relax as you return to your original sitting position.
- Rest before repeating this exercise.

Breathing: Breathe <u>in</u> as you <u>raise up</u>, hold your breath as you tense the muscles, and breathe out fully as you come down.

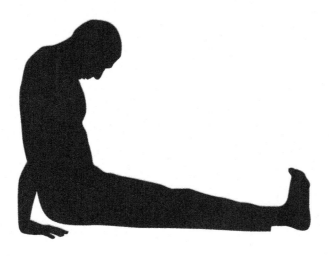

The Tabletop - breathe out

4. The Tabletop (continued)

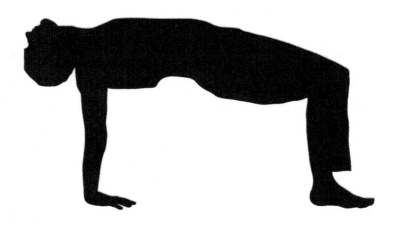

The Tabletop - breathe in

5. The Up and Down

- Lie down with your face down to the floor.
- You will be supported by the hands palms down against the floor and the toes in the flexed position.
- Throughout this exercise, the hands and feet should be kept straight.
- Start with your arms perpendicular to the floor, and the spine arched, so that the body is in a sagging position.
- Now move the head back as far as possible.
- Then, bending at the hips, bring the body up into an inverted "V".
- At the same time, bring the chin forward, tucking it against the chest.

Breathing: Breathe <u>in</u> deeply as you <u>raise the body</u>, and exhale fully as you lower the body.

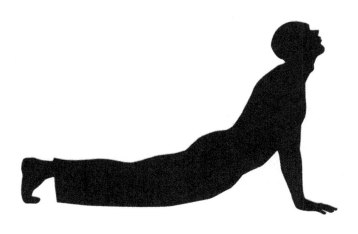

The Up and Down - Breathe out

5. The Up and Down (continued)

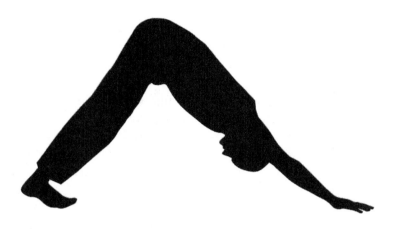

The Up and Down - Breathe in

WORKING OUT AT HOME WORKS BETTER THAN THE GYM

Here is yet another reason why doing the Five Tibetan Rites on a daily basis will help you get the body you deserve:

Woman's World magazine reported; "A study has shown that women who work out at home lose more weight than those who exercise at the gym. Forty-nine women followed the same diet and exercise route for a year. Those who exercised at home lost an average of 25 pounds; the gym goers shed 15 pounds." They suggested the reason was that it was easier to stick with the program, because it's so much more convenient.

JUST 3 MINUTES A WEEK CAN MAKE YOU FIT

An article by the BBC[7] gave more evidence as to how you can benefit enormously from an exercise that is done in only a little time:

"A few relatively short bursts of intense exercise, amounting to only a few minutes a week, can deliver many of the health and fitness benefits of hours of conventional exercise, according to new research, says Dr. Michael Mosley". (Try running or dancing on the spot).

I found it particularly interesting that this article reported that in one study,[8] where 1,000 people exercised and then had their aerobic fitness measured, while most of the people gained in fitness, 20% of the people showed no real improvement at all. The article puts this down to genetic differences, but my experience with kinesiology tells me that all of these people were greatly out of balance. The brain of these people was not sending the right signals to their muscles. I believe that some good kinesiology balances would have made a world of difference to these people. For example, I have seen kinesiology make people stronger and more co-ordinated, and improve jogging times, after just one session of kinesiology.

BREATHE THROUGH THE NOSE

Wild animals breathe through their nose, even when running fast. We should do the same, but we have forgotten how. Mouth breathing is meant to be used only for emergencies. As you learn to breathe through the nose when exercising, instead of the mouth, you will learn to take longer, deeper breaths, which are from deep in the diaphragm, not high in the chest. This will make you calmer and fitter. John Douillard suggests making a "Darth Vader"-type noise when breathing out, to fully squeeze every last bit of air from your diaphragm, so that your body can then absorb even more oxygen in the next intake.

Breathing through the nose activates the parasympathetic nervous system, which lowers heart rate and makes you calmer. Breathing through the mouth, on the other hand, increases the sympathetic nervous system, which causes increased heart rate and stress-fighting hormones, which can lead to more fat retention.

Try doing Darth Vader breathing. It may take a while to get used to it, but the more you do it, the better results you will see. At first, at times you may need to breathe through the nose only on the 'in' phase, and out through the mouth. But keep on working on it until you breathe both in and out deeply through the nose, just like a running horse.

WEIGHT TRAINING - KEEP THE 50-50 RULE

Lifting weights is also excellent, and good for adults, with one proviso. It is critical that you follow Douillard's advice and keep to the 50-50 rule. While the current thinking of most people is that one should lift 60-80% of the maximum that you can lift, Douillard says that Ayurveda teaches that you should lift no more than 50% of your maximum during training, after proper warm-ups.

This is because of what I said before: you want to tell your body what is required of it, but do it in such a way that it does not hurt the body, so that it doesn't have to waste time or resources doing any repairs. The body can then devote itself totally to building new muscles and blood vessels.

Children should not lift weights as it is too easy for them to damage themselves.

Therefore, in addition to the Five Tibetan Rites, obtain a weight bar with some adjustable weights. Start off with the lightest ones you can get. Always unlock your knees. Suggestions are to lower the bar to the knees, then stand erect, or lower the bar to the knees and then pull the bar into the chest as if you are rowing.

Do the Tibetan Rites every day, and lift some light weights, no matter what. It only takes a few minutes! Make them as much a habit as eating is, so that you can be thin and healthy for the rest of your life.

REFERENCES

1. www.LifeSpa.com
2. *The Magnesium Factor*, by Mildred Seelig, M.D., 2003, page 94
3. chriskresser.com/10-ways-stress-makes-you-fat-and-diabetic
4. *Mastering Leptin*, by Byron Richards CCN, 2002, 3rd edition 2009, pg. 88
5. *Body, Mind and Sport*, by John Douillard, 1994, page 10
6. www.t5t.com/article_info.php?articles_id=40
7. www.bbc.co.uk/news/health-17177251
8. www.pbrc.edu/heritage/index.html

CHAPTER 37

YOU NEED THE RIGHT KIND
OF SALT TO BE THIN

The media and medical system have told you a lie, that avoiding salt will help you live longer. The prevailing viewpoint is that salt is a general poison, like alcohol and tobacco. Salt has been vilified as the great devil at the dinner table. Even the health food industry has gone along with this one.

This makes no sense, because our cells all contain salt! We sweat salt. Our tears contain salt. Our blood is salty. Our cells depend upon correct levels of salt and water to produce and move nutrients where they are needed. Therefore you need correct amounts of salt to be thin.

The question should not be "Do we need salt?" We absolutely do. We cannot live without it. The question should be, "What kind of salts are good and bad for us?"

There are basically three kinds of salt:

1) Sodium Chloride. Normal table salt. This is toxic and bad for your weight and health, as you have been told.

2) So called "sea salt". This should be good for you but unfortunately

it has been processed and many of the valuable minerals removed. It's also toxic.

3) "Celtic sea salt" or "macrobiotic, hand-harvested, sun-dried sea salt". This is *very good for you*! And delicious!

The following information is mostly from Dr. Jacques de Langre, a California biochemist who has studied the health benefits of salt for over 35 years. He has a Ph.D. in biochemistry from the University of Brussels. He wrote two books on this topic, *Sea Salt's Hidden Powers* and *Sea Salt, the Vital Spark for Life*.

Dr. de Langre openly agrees that refined table salt, which is pure sodium chloride, is toxic to the body. Yet he believes Celtic sea salt is extremely healthy, and has the exact opposite effect of refined salt. Celtic sea salt is so named because it was first produced in France. The entire health field is very sloppy with its terminology on salt. They think all salt is the same. This is far from true. Most refined salts are a poison. But some natural salts are a very important supplement.

In America, doctors condemn salt. 99% of the world's research on salt is done on commercial table salt. This is the only salt they know of. They think all salt is the same, but they're wrong. The medical doctors have a dilemma. Refined salt can cause a lot of problems. They are correct on that point. Yet, a salt-free diet also has problems. Neither approach, taking refined salt, or avoiding it, is the answer. People desperately need salt for good health, and medicine doesn't have any solution.

In parts of France, however, when a person comes in with heart problems, high blood pressure, or other problems which are hard to diagnose, the first question the physician may ask is, "What kind of salt are you using?" There is no such opportunity here, because the only recognized salt is refined, white table salt. Some of the best scientific research on the health properties of good salt are written in French, German and Portuguese. Few American doctors have read them. This country was raised on refined salt, which we inherited from the English. So, we have not been exposed to healthy salt. There is much we can learn about food quality from the French.

You can't function without salt. You can't digest food without salt.

Your heart, adrenal glands, liver and kidneys can't function without salt. And therefore it's hard to get rid of fat without salt.

The most convincing fact that salt is critical to life is that everyone was born in a salty solution, which was our mother's amniotic fluid. Amniotic fluid is the fluid surrounding the embryo. This is probably the best biological proof we have that cellular structure is enhanced by salt. The amniotic fluid is a salty, 'mini-ocean' for the fetus. This is a prime example of why we need all of the ocean's minerals as part of our make-up. How terrible then that salt has been removed from virtually all baby foods. Where will the salt come from for these babies to produce properly functioning bodies? If you make your own baby food, you can add a tiny bit of Celtic sea salt.

Your blood needs salt to function. There was an article in the Scientific American on this topic in the July, 1963 issue, "'The Social Influence of Salt." It said, "'The chemical requirements of the human body demand that the salt concentration in the blood be kept constant." They discussed how you can *die* on a completely salt-less diet.

Without salt, there is no longer any exchange between the sodium on the outside of the cell, and the potassium on the inside. Talk about aging, this is probably the one, single, most important biological fact that must be considered when you discuss salt. A salt-free diet speeds up aging. Your cells must be bathed in a sodium-based, extracellular fluid. When the cells are not in this fluid, they will *explode*.

On the other hand, taking refined salt is not the answer. This will promote a calcification and a breakdown of cellular tissue. Both are serious health problems.

De Langre says that in most cases, high blood pressure is not measurably lowered by restricting salt intake. Even a drastically reduced sodium diet, down to less than 1/2 gram/day, often fails to show any improvements in cardiovascular problems.[1] De Langre believes that a low-salt diet can actually cause high blood pressure in some people. A salt-free diet can tire and damage the valves of the heart. The heart cannot contract normally. This will certainly make exercise difficult.

Without salt, the cells starve. Salt is an *energizer*. The more energy you have, the easier it is for the body to remove the toxins stored in the fat cells, and then get rid of the fat. If salt was so bad, why do they feed intravenous saline solutions to hospital patients? They do that be-cause the body runs on salt. Without salt, we run out of electrolytes. Without electrolytes, our human batteries die out.

A lot of vegetarians eat a salt-less diet. This is bad because there is a lot of potassium in green leafy vegetables, which needs to be neu-tralized by sodium. If potassium is in excess in relation to sodium, the body loses its ability to produce hydrochloric acid, which causes digestive problems.

God put 84 elements in salt as a buffer, to protect you from pure sodium chloride. In the USA people have been taught that salt is pure sodium chloride. When people talk about salt, they overlook completely that there are 84 buffering elements in salt to protect people from the harshness of sodium chloride in its pure state. God put these comple-mentary elements in salt so that it can be used, and also so that it can be eliminated easily in urine.

An analysis of salt goes way beyond the minerals and the chemical elements. An article in *Ocean Magazine*[2] made a fantastic defense of salt, saying sea salt is not just chemicals. It is a lot more. There is also:

- 84 of the 103 known elements.
- Magnetism.
- Bio-electric energy.
- Vital and inert gases, such as helium, neon, and argon.
- Micro organisms that are critical for the life of salt.

Sea water is a complex chemical soup, containing 84 of the 103 known elements. Our blood is like the ocean. In the ocean, sodium is buffered. In our blood, the sodium is buffered. And in our diet, the sodium should be buffered as well.

If you tried to inject pure sodium chloride intravenously, you would kill the patient. He goes into salt shock. This is well-known in medical circles. In the 1900's, a medical doctor named Jacques Loeb, from the University of California, performed an epic experiment. He put fish in a tank of water mixed with refined salt, the same concentration of salt that exists in sea water. All the fish died. If fish can't live on pure sodium chloride in dilute concentrations, how can we?

The Celtic process of drying the salt by the sun and the wind first started well over 900 years ago. Today, this same pristine process of salt-making continues. Celtic salt contains every element that is in seawater, minus the mud. There are actually more than 84 elements in the ocean, but they haven't all been detected yet. No heat is used. What remains is biologically active, pure, moist, Celtic salt. No chemicals, preservatives, or anything else has been added. This is the kind of salt that you should add to your life.

De Langre has said that he has had reports of people going to the doctor and their doctor saying, "Well, you must be taking less salt, because your blood pressure is lower." But the truth was, they didn't cut down their salt intake at all. They were taking the Celtic salt. Here's a letter from a man in Los Angeles to De Langre:

"Two weeks ago I donated blood at a Red Cross station. At that time my blood pressure was 160 over 90. Yesterday, after hardly one week of using the Celtic salt, the only new addition to my diet, I recorded a blood pressure reading of 105 over 82". (Normal blood pressure is 120 over 80).

De Langre reported that over several decades, a few thousand people have reported similar stories. Suddenly their blood pressure became normal when they switched from no salt or table salt to Celtic sea salt. Of course, results will vary from individual to individual, there are always exceptions, and other improvements to diet and life style may be needed in addition.

In regular salt, the refined sodium chloride often stays in the body long after it has done its job. Celtic salt helps to remove this excess sodium, as soon as it is no longer needed. This is because the Celtic salt has magnesium in it (and magnesium is necessary for fat loss).

It's one of the great nutritional paradoxes, that you have to give salt, in order to lower the level of salt in the tissues. The Celtic salt literally "scrounges" around the body looking for excess salt deposits in the interstitial tissue and it drains this sodium through the kidneys.

De Langre claims that if a person has low blood pressure, taking the Celtic salt will not make their pressure go even lower. The Celtic salt seems to have the ability to balance whatever function is unbalanced in the body. The more balanced your body, the easier it is to get thin.

Unfortunately, De Langre says that most sea salt that is sold in health food stores can be just as bad for your health as regular salt, because it is so highly refined. You can tell sea salt is refined if it does not have any sign of moisture at all. Refined salt is very dry salt. This tells you the magnesium has been taken out, because magnesium is a water-hugging molecule.

When salt is refined, even sea salt, the manufacturers basically extract all the precious elements out of salt so they can sell the important minerals to chemical companies for a good profit. What's left is a by-product, pure sodium chloride. To this they add anti-caking agents, anti-yellowing bleaches, and glucose.

There is a huge difference in taste between refined salt and Celtic sea salt. Celtic sea salt is delicious! Your taste buds will be gently awakened. But if you put regular salt on your tongue, your tongue will be out of commission for at least 30 minutes. You cannot taste anything else, because your taste buds are stunned and weakened. This is why you see people in restaurants piling the salt on in order to get some taste out of the food. The salt irritates the taste buds and inhibits them.

On the other hand, if you eat Celtic sea salt you don't need to eat as much food, because you are getting more nutrition from the food you eat. You will find you are satisfied quicker, so you eat less, and get thinner.

Ideally, you want to cook the salt as little as possible. It is best to add the Celtic salt to your food directly. When you cook with the salt, add the salt towards the very end of the cooking. This is when you have almost no boiling going on, just a low simmer.

Can you have too much Celtic sea salt? Of course. You can overdose on anything, even water. You have to use common sense. In healthy people, there is a built-in mechanism that tells them when the body has had enough salt. You are not as prone to start pouring the salt from the shaker as many do with refined salt.

Vegetables cannot be fully digested without being salted. De Langre believes that when you use Celtic salt, you can get up to *seven times* the nutrition out of vegetables. The more nutrition, the easier it is to get slim.

While some people like to eat salt from ancient sea beds (like Himalayan salt), de Langre also believes this is not fit for humans, because after thousands of years of rainfall through the geological layers, many of the vital minerals are depleted. The natural balance of the salt is gone. Remember that salt should be *moist.*

You can tell that good salt is good for animals as well as for us, by watching how much trouble animals go to collect salt. For example, in parts of Africa, elephants dig huge holes with their tusks to get salt, or even go down deep, dark caves to grind rocks off the walls and suck salt out of them.

Occasionally some people initially have adverse reactions from using Celtic sea salt. Some people get rashes. The salt acts as a scavenger and purges the body of many toxins from some hidden areas. It is likely a cleansing reaction by the kidneys. This is a normal reaction for people who are very toxic. If you are not toxic, it should not happen. A similar reaction is that rashes may break out under the arm pits for a while.

Visit your health food store, or go online, and get a bag of Celtic or sun-dried sea salt that is moist. It is more expensive, but it is well worth it. If you think about it, it's only the cost of about 2 ½ Big Macs®. Make sure it's moist. Get a salt that is finely ground. Salt from the very clean North Atlantic Ocean is cleaner than salt from the Mediterranean Sea. Carry a small bag of it if you are going to eat away from home. Have delicious celtic sea salt daily. Listen to your body and do the best you can to maintain the correct balance. As with all things, too much can be as bad as too little.

REFERENCES

1. *Annals-of Internal Medicine,* May 1983 issue, Dr. John Laragh, page 740
2. *Ocean Magazine,* September 1982

CHAPTER 38

MAGNESIUM:
THE MOST ESSENTIAL MINERAL

At least 80% of us don't get enough of what is the most important mineral for our bodies – magnesium. Not calcium, but magnesium. Magnesium is critical for over 300 of the body's chemical reactions, says Carolyn Dean, M.D., N.D., medical director of the Nutritional Magnesium Association, and author of the excellent book, *The Magnesium Miracle*[1].

We have been brainwashed into thinking we need lots of calcium, partly by a dairy industry that depends upon you believing that, to maintain their high profits. The truth is that most of us are suffering from magnesium deficiency, partly because we have too much calcium[2], because the two must be balanced.

It's possible that more than 80% of us are lacking magnesium, because you can't tell how much you have from a blood test. It's how much is inside each cell that's important, and this can vary enormously from the concentration in the blood.

LACK OF MAGNESIUM IS A MAJOR CAUSE OF OBESITY

Lack of magnesium is a major cause of at least twenty-two diseases, including obesity[3]. Other diseases include blood clots and insulin resistance (which means diabetes).

Much of modern heart disease is caused at least partly by magnesium deficiency[4]. But don't expect the medical establishment to tell you this, because heart disease brings in about $450 billion a year[5].

Magnesium helps maintain healthy cortisol levels. Cortisol is a hormone related to stress. Yale University found that when cortisol levels are raised, even for just a few hours, the body stores more fat, especially around the belly. Dr. Dean explains: "Cortisol causes fat cells in the belly area to store ... fat because the body perceives almost any stress as starvation stress[6]."

HIGH CALCIUM = LOW MAGNESIUM

We have been taught that we need calcium from dairy food to protect us from osteoporosis, but in Asian and African populations where people have very low daily calcium intake, there is little osteoporosis. When magnesium levels are low, calcium moves out of the bones. And the reverse happens, when magnesium levels are high, calcium moves into the bones[7].

High levels of calcium cause low levels of magnesium. High levels of calcium also cause low levels of iron and zinc, because calcium competes with these minerals for absorption in the intestines[8]. Both iron and zinc are essential for proper health, and therefore essential to get you thin. For example, zinc is a component of insulin.

MAGNESIUM IS ESSENTIAL TO BREAK DOWN FAT

Here are some important facts about magnesium, that relate directly or indirectly to getting thin. Most of this information is from the excellent books *The Magnesium Factor* by Dr. Mildred Seelig M.D. and *Transdermal Magnesium Therapy*, by Dr. Mark Sircus, M.D.

1. Magnesium is essential to break down fat, because it's part of the enzymes that do that[9].

2. Magnesium is essential for a healthy use of carbohydrates, fats and proteins[10].

3. Refined carbohydrates such as grains use up magnesium, whereas seeds, nuts, leafy green plants and legumes (lentils & beans) provide magnesium.

4. Magnesium helps you get thin, but only if you have enough Vitamin D to absorb it. Alternatively, Vitamin D speeds fat loss and hinders fat-cell growth, if you have enough magnesium[11].

5. Magnesium deficiency increases insulin resistance, which is a cause of diabetes and obesity.

6. Magnesium is essential for proper muscle and nerve function, which indirectly affect your ability to lose weight.

7. Magnesium deficiency may cause aggression or depression, both of which may cause you to look for 'comfort foods'. If you have children who are aggressive, consider lack of magnesium as part of the problem.

8. Magnesium is paired up with calcium. The *more calcium* you take in, the *less magnesium* you absorb. When calcium is too high, but magnesium is just right, when you excrete calcium, magnesium goes too, so that you end up with low levels of magnesium[12].

9. Magnesium is essential for removing toxins[13], which you have to do to get rid of fat.

10. While the magnesium levels in our food have dropped dramatically, we need higher levels of magnesium than in the past, because there are so many more toxins in our food and our environment.

11. Even our thoughts, via brain neurons, are dependent on magnesium[14].

12. Magnesium controls the uptake of many hormones and nutrients[15]. Nutrients are essential for reducing fat.

13. Lack of magnesium causes negative moods[16]. This is partly because serotonin levels will be lower. It's also because, while calcium excites nerves, magnesium calms them down.[17] Negative moods can lead to eating co-called 'comfort' foods.

14. Low magnesium levels cause fluid retention[18].

15. Magnesium is not promoted because drug companies don't make money selling it.

16. Magnesium supplementation lowers cholesterol up to 23% and triglycerides by up to 42%[19].

17. Any emotional stress reduces magnesium levels. Intense stress causes massive reductions in magnesium levels, and this produces even more stress[20].

18. Magnesium is essential for hundreds of the enzymes in your body to work properly[21].

19. In the case of Type II diabetes, where insulin sensitivity has been lowered, magnesium supplementation can restore the ability to lower blood sugar[22].

20. Low magnesium causes low potassium levels, even if the intake level of potassium is high[23].

The following fact from Mark Sircus' excellent book *Transdermal Magnesium Therapy*, which I highly recommend, is indirectly related to getting thin, but it is so important that I thought you would like to know this: There is usually 10,000 times more calcium outside of cells than inside. Whenever you get more calcium inside the cell, you will have a deficiency of magnesium. And it seems that there is always more calcium inside the cell at the time of death. So, whenever any-one is seriously ill, part of your plan must be to restore magnesium[24]. (Note: Since dairy has high calcium and low magnesium, no wonder so many people heal their health and weight problems when they give up dairy products).

Unfortunately, our bodies have a lot less magnesium than they need for at least five reasons:

1. Processing food removes magnesium. For example, if you in-gest the oil that your body needs in a natural way, by eating whole seeds, you get plenty of magnesium. But oil from a bottle has zero magnesium[25].

2. We don't eat enough of the foods which are high in magnesium, such as vegetables, particularly leafy green vegetables, nuts and seeds, whole grains, legumes and fruit.

3. Modern farming practices deplete the soil. Most importantly, modern fertilizers and pesticides kill soil microorganisms. Plants need microorganisms to absorb minerals from the soil. Therefore, even the good foods we do eat, unless they are organic, contain a lot less magnesium than they used to. For example, the average person's daily diet in 1909 had 408 mg, but in 1985 it was down to 228 mg.[26].

4. Boiling washes away magnesium and other valuable minerals and vitamins. Only steam or stirfry, or even better, eat it raw, or at least eat part of it raw.

5. We consume toxins, and the more toxins we have, the more magnesium we need to remove those toxins. For example, alcohol, caffeine and sugar deplete the body of magnesium[27]. So do drugs such as insulin.

There is evidence that people can benefit from taking magnesium supplements[28]. Mildred Seelig recommends working slowly up to 480 milligrams a day[29]. Mark Sircus says that oral magnesium chloride is "well tolerated and gets absorbed very quickly[30]. However, Sircus mainly believes that magnesium supplements are not enough, because some are made from the wrong kinds of magnesium, the rate of release cannot be controlled and interaction with substances such as calcium interferes with absorption[31].

The best ways to increase your magnesium levels are the following.

1. Fresh juice and eat raw leafy green plants. Think of Italian parsley, parsley, kale, spinach, collard greens and beet greens (organic only so they are not GMO).

2. Eat raw seeds and nuts.

3. Eat spirulina and chlorella. Tablets are easier to eat than powder.

4. Eat lentils and beans. Soak them for 8 hours to sprout them to improve nutrition. Store in fridge, and rinse once a day until needed.

5. Fruit also contains magnesium. Eat raw.

6. Greatly limit your intake of dairy products.

7. Limit your intake of grains. If you eat any grains, make sure they are whole. Preferably soak them in water for 8 hours before using to break down the phytic acid in them. No wheat (white flour is processed wheat flour).

8. Eliminate toxins, including sugar, from your diet.

9. Greatly reduce your intake of oils, which fill you up but have all the magnesium removed from them.

10. Replace the salt you are using with sun-dried sea salt, such as Celtic Sea Salt, available from health food stores or online. Regular sea salt has a lot of the valuable minerals removed from it.

11. Have warm foot baths with one tablespoon or more of magnesium chloride* (food grade or aquarium grade). Soak for at least 20 minutes.

12. Use magnesium oil for deodorant, and rub it all over your body, so long as it does not sting you. Magnesium chloride occurs naturally in sea water. It is produced by extracting it from the sea by solar evaporation[32]. It is easily assimilated and used by the body[33].

TO MAKE MAGNESIUM OIL

Mix one part magnesium chloride (food or aquarium grade) to two parts water (or more diluted, it if it stings too much)[34].

Absorbing magnesium through the skin is especially recommended because some people are so low in magnesium, that they have lost the ability to absorb magnesium through the intestines. However, they can still absorb it through the skin[35].

Some people even recommend having higher concentrations of magnesium chloride, or even spraying diluted magnesium chloride into your water[36].

Here's a thought: Since we can absorb magnesium, and also certain drugs, through the skin, what toxins are your body absorbing through the skin from makeup, cleaning chemicals and hair products? If it isn't food, maybe it should not be on your skin at all.

HAVE A MAGNESIUM BATH

There are 3 ways to do this:

1. A footbath for 20 minutes, with one tablespoon of magnesium chloride.

2. A bath for 20 minutes, with two tablespoons of magnesium chloride.

3. Spray "magnesium oil" on your body. You can use it for a healthy

deodorant.

Interestingly, Mark Sircus makes this comment in his book[37]:

"The medical authorities, and certainly the pharmaceutical companies are in a pickle with magnesium chloride. Here is a powerful medicine that is natural, non-toxic, inexpensive, and effective in a wide variety of medical situation. So what do they do? They commission a study that is essentially designed to show the opposite".

Dr. Stephen Davies criticized the scientists who wanted to show that magnesium chloride is unsafe for "clearly selecting too large a dose of intravenous magnesium, and also for giving magnesium too late and then too quickly."

If you are one of those people who has been doing well on your diet and exercise, yet the fat has not reduced enough yet, have a magnesium foot bath every day, do the other things on the list above, take Vitamin D supplements and get as much sun on your skin as you possibly can (to absorb the magnesium), as many days in the week as you can manage. See if you don't notice changes within weeks, as well as start to feel more relaxed and happy.

REFERENCES

1. *First for women* magazine, 7/9/12
2. *First for women* magazine, 7/9/12
3. *Transdermal Magnesium Therapy*, by Mark Sircus, Ac, M.D., 2007, p. 73
4. *The Magnesium Factor*, Mildred Seelig M.D., page 2
5. www.cdc.gov/chronicdisease/resources/publications/AAG/dhdsp.htm
6. *First for women"* magazine, 7/9/12
7. *Transdermal Magnesium Therapy*, by Mark Sircus, Ac, M.D., 2007, p. 53
8. *Transdermal Magnesium Therapy*, by Mark Sircus, Ac, M.D., 2007, p. 56
9. *The Magnesium Factor*, Mildred Seelig M.D., page 11
10. *Transdermal Magnesium Therapy*, by Mark Sircus, Ac, M.D., 2007
11. *First for women* magazine, 7/9/12
12. *Transdermal Magnesium Therapy*, by Mark Sircus, Ac, M.D., 2007, p. 54

13. *Transdermal Magnesium Therapy*, by Mark Sircus, Ac, M.D., 2007, p. 96

14. *Transdermal Magnesium Therapy*, by Mark Sircus, Ac, M.D., 2007, p. 99

15. *Transdermal Magnesium Therapy*, by M. Sircus, Ac, M.D., 2007, p. 263

16. *Transdermal Magnesium Therapy*, by M. Sircus, Ac, M.D., 2007, p. 270

17. *The Magnesium Factor*, Mildred Seelig M.D., page 14

18. *Transdermal Magnesium Therapy*, by M. Sircus, Ac, M.D., 2007, p. 270

19. *The Magnesium Factor* by Mildred Seelig, M.D., 2003, page 125

20. *The Magnesium Factor*" by Mildred Seelig, M.D., 2003, p. 125, pg 155-162

21. *The Magnesium Factor*, Mildred Seelig M.D., page 11

22. *The Magnesium Factor* by Mildred Seelig, M.D., 2003, page 35

23. *The Magnesium Factor* by Mildred Seelig, M.D., 2003, page 63

24. *Transdermal Magnesium Therapy*, by Mark Sircus, Ac, M.D., 2007, p. 49

25. *The Magnesium Factor* by Mildred Seelig, M.D., 2003, page 87

26. *Transdermal Magnesium Therapy*, by Mark Sircus, Ac, M.D., 2007, p. 26

27. *Transdermal Magnesium Therapy*, by Mark Sircus, Ac, M.D., 2007, p. 27

28. *The Magnesium Factor* by Mildred Seelig, M.D., 2003

29. *The Magnesium Factor* by Mildred Seelig, M.D., 2003, page 114

30. *Transdermal Magnesium Therapy*, by Mark Sircus, Ac, M.D., 2007, p. 31

31. *Transdermal Magnesium Therapy*, by Mark Sircus, Ac, M.D., 2007

32. *Transdermal Magnesium Therapy*, by M. Sircus, Ac, M.D., 2007, p. 189

33. *Transdermal Magnesium Therapy*, by Mark Sircus, Ac, M.D., 2007,p. 209

34. *Transdermal Magnesium Therapy*, by Mark Sircus, Ac, M.D., 2007, p. 36

35. *Transdermal Magnesium Therapy*, by Mark Sircus, Ac, M.D., 2007, p. 39

36. magnesiumforlife.com/transdermal-magnesium/combining-oral-with-transdermal/

37. *Transdermal Magnesium Therapy*, by Mark Sircus, Ac, M.D., 2007

CHAPTER 39

STOP HIBERNATING
GET 'VITAMIN' D3 -
A STEROID HORMONE

Vitamin D deficiency makes you fat and hungry in a number of ways, including causing leptin resistance[1]. But it's even worse than that. The very interesting book, *Vitamin D3 Miracle* by Bowles, gives evidence to show that without enough Vitamin D, your body thinks you are hibernating. That makes sense. Vitamin D is made by the skin, from cholesterol[2], when it has sunlight on it. Without enough sun, the body thinks that winter is coming, and so you need to hibernate. That is, slow the metabolism down, eat more food and put on lots of fat.

This verifies what natural health people have known all along. To have perfect health, which includes being slim, you need a balance of the right:

- Food.
- Water.
- Exercise.
- Sleep.
- Rest.
- Air.
- *Sun.*
- Positive Emotions.
- Electromagnetics.

For thousands of years humans spent many hours each day in the sun. From dusk to dawn, they were outside working in the wild or in fields, buying or selling in open markets, walking or riding on horses or in open carriages, for work or to visit friends and family (there were no phones). Children played outside. Many people stayed indoors for siesta when the sun was overhead, but apart from that, they were outside a great deal of the time. Even wealthy people, who didn't work, walked in their gardens or to visit friends, went on picnics and rode on horse-back, or in beautiful, open carriages. Only a few old and rich people stayed in doors nearly all the time and rode in only covered-in carriages – and a lot of them were fat, although not the extremes of obesity that we have today.

I dimly perceived the truth of how we all needed a lot more time in the sun when I started muscle testing my clients to find out how much time their body wanted to be in the sun each day, and was shocked when body after body gave me answers of around seven hours! I had difficulty working out how anyone could find the time to do this. Bowles suggests a solution in Vitamin D3 Miracle. We are meant to greatly increase the amount of D3 supplements we take, way past "recommended dosages".

If you think about it, obesity and many other diseases have sky-rocketed since the 1980s, when doctors started telling people to keep out of the sun and to use sun block.

'VITAMIN' D IS NOT A VITAMIN. IT'S AN ESSENTIAL STEROID HORMONE

Vitamin D3 Miracle contains some very good information. Bowles spent two months reading 52,000 abstracts and titles of science journal articles related to Vitamin D. You can do the same. Just go to www.ncbi.nlm.nih.gov/pubmed

It turns out that 'Vitamin' D is not a vitamin. It was originally thought to be a vitamin because it was found in food. But it is, in fact, a *steroid hormone* that affects almost all the cells in the body, by instructing the genes what to do. It's absolutely essential for weight loss, as well as health and strong bones, joints and muscles.

66 DISEASES RELATED TO LOW LEVELS OF VITAMIN D

From reading through the studies at PubMed, Bowles saw that Vitamin D deficiency is involved with obesity, as well as at least 65 diseases including, but not limited to, acne, alcoholism, allergies, arthritis, asthma, autism, cancer, chronic wounds, Crohn's disease, depression, diabetes, glaucoma, gout, heart disease, learning disabilities, lupus, migraines, multiple sclerosis (MS), plantar warts, PMS, pregnancy problems, pre-term births, psoriasis, strokes, toenail fungus and tuberculosis.

Bowles tells whereby in the 1920s it was found that Vitamin D2 could be made easily by shining ultraviolet light onto organic matter (food). Dozens of foods became fortified with D2. One scientist said that the average person was taking 20 mg of Vitamin D2 a day. The hospitals started emptying, and were getting ready to go bankrupt[3]. So, the unit of measurement of Vitamin D2 was changed from milligrams (mg) to International Units (IU), which is what we use today. Suddenly 20 mg became 800,000 IU. That's nearly 1 million IU, which sounds a lot scarier[4]. Note that Vitamin D2 is one third or less the strength of D3[5].

It may turn out that it's a good idea to have a UV light turned on in your fridge. And use full-spectrum bulbs whenever you can. However, do not drink water that has been affected by UV light, as it has no organic matter in it and the UV light seems to harm the energy of the water. After all, UV light is not the same as sunlight.

TAKE AT LEAST 5,000 IU D3 A DAY (EQUAL TO 15 MINUTES IN THE SUN)

Vitamin D3 is one of the important supplements to take, as it is essential for weight loss and proper muscle and bone growth, as well as protecting you from many other things such as depression, diabetes and the flu. However, most of us are very deficient in vitamin D, and don't have the time to be in the sun that our bodies need. Plus older people find it harder to make vitamin D.

Therefore, a Vitamin D3 supplement at the right dosage, in addition to getting what sun you can, is essential. Relatively recently doctors "recommended dosage" was a pitiful 400 IU a day. Now it's around

2,000 IU a day. In fact, this should be higher. Bowles tells the story of his father, a Stanford educated medical doctor, who took 2,000 IU of D3 a day for several years. That's a lot more than most people take. He then had a blood test, which showed that he was still at the very low end with 30 ng. Bowles says it's best to be over 70ng/ml, and possibly as high as 150 ng/ml. (You can purchase Vitamin D blood tests on the internet. See www.YoureNotFatYourToxic.com).

Adults need at least 5,000 IU a day to stay healthy[6] , and possibly more. How high is probably not known yet. For example, 5,000 IU may sound like a lot, but in fact it's only the amount of Vitamin D your body would make if you lay in the sun in a bathing trunks or a bikini for just 15 minutes[7]!

That's a massive difference. When you hear of a miraculous cure from a particular substance, knowing how much was given is often as important as knowing what it was. Only recently are people starting to realize that the so-called "recommended dosages" are way too low. Don't expect the medical industry to give you the correct advice on this one. This is another way that the drug companies, helped by the FDA, keep their profits high. Healthy people don't need to buy medical products.

According to the Vitamin D Council, 1000 IUs per 25lbs are recommended each day, although using a blood test is the best way to know your ideal dose[8]. African Americans may need even more, from 6 to 30 times more, depending on who you believe[9].

Therefore, get yourself a vegan, non-GMO Vitamin D3 supplement, that is 2000 IU or 5000 IU per tablet. See www.YoureNotFatYourToxic.com.

VITAMIN D TOXICITY

While the medical establishment tell us that they are terrified of excess Vitamin D (but not concerned about aspartame or GMOs), it turns out that Vitamin D toxicity is an extremely rare occurrence, and only occurred when a normal person ingested millions of IUs a day for months! In one study, pregnant women took 100,000 IU a day for the entire 9 months of their pregnancy with no ill effects, and with healthy babies[10]. In addition, Vitamin D toxicity never occurs from too much sun exposure. Note that some people now believe that high doses of D3 are safe only when supplemented with Vitamin K2.

HIGH DOSES MAY BE BENEFICIAL

In *Vitamin D3 Miracle*, Bowles tells how he did experiments on himself using high doses of Vitamin D3 to heal a number of body problems. Vitamin D3 is a hormone that is especially involved with bone and joint remodeling. Experiments with rats showed that rats that had their bones broken grew a callus on the break, unless they were supplemented with vitamin D, in which case the break healed with no callus. When Bowles took extra high doses of 20,000 to 100,000 IU a day, his joints began to hurt where he had old sports injuries. (I was astonished to read how he then took pain killers at the same time, instead of cutting back on his dosage and being patient). He seemed to get results with 4,000-20,000 IU a day. The following healed:

- Arthritic pain (after a month of 4,000 IU a day).
- 'Snapping' hip click.
- Bone spur on elbow.
- Ganglion nerve cyst reduced noticeably in size.
- Subcutaneous cyst on face.
- Snapping, clicking hurting shoulders (after 1 month of 4,000 IU a day)
- Without changing his bad diet he felt his appetite decrease, and his weight reduced by 25 pounds, going from 204 to 179 lb, after taking 20,000 IU a day for several months.
- Pain in joints from old injuries improved a lot (after two months of 20,000 IU a day).
- He can now throw a ball three times further than he could before, due to less stiffness.
- Allergies greatly reduced after a year.
- Energy increased.

Bowles stressed that if one has super high Vitamin D levels, it is important to also supplement with Vitamin K2[11]. K2 is found naturally in eggs and butter.

YOU NEED MAGNESIUM TO BENEFIT FULLY FROM 'VITAMIN' D

"In one of the biggest health breakthroughs of the past decade, scientists identified Vitamin D as a nutrient that hinders fat-cell growth and speeds fat loss. But to get the full benefits, the body needs *magnesium*[12]".

Unfortunately, one reason why we have obesity is because most people are deficient in both Vitamin D and magnesium. Magnesium is the most important mineral for the body, and is essential for getting thin. But you won't absorb enough if you don't have enough vitamin D[13].

GET REAL SUN ON YOUR SKIN

Science is only just now starting to discover things that are vital to getting thin and healthy, like healing leptin resistance, the importance of essential fatty acids, micronutrients in raw plants and Vitamin D. Much of what science is discovering just backs up the advice that natural health people have been giving for ages.

I believe that one day science will find that direct sunlight does things for fat loss that plain old vitamin D supplements do not, no matter how well they are made. While considering this theory, I became aware of how so many women are putting on belly fat, rather than all-over body fat. Now, obviously there are other reasons for this besides lack of sunlight, including rise in cortisol when one ingests toxins, but please bear with me. I believe there may be an extra way to help you to lose fat, especially belly fat, that has nothing to do with food.

Consider that when women are slim, they love to wear two piece swimming costumes. But as soon as a woman gets overweight, she covers up with a one-piece, and even starts to stop wearing sleeveless tops. Both men and women who are grossly overweight are a lot less likely to get direct sun on their skin. This, I believe, helps them to put on more fat.

So, please, try this. When you go for a walk, at least wear sleeveless. At least once a week, lie down in sun that is fairly direct. Naturally, make sure that you don't do it for so long or that the sun is so hot that you burn. And, no matter how big you are, please get some sun on your belly. Let the sunlight produce results right next to the fat cells that you want to zap.

SUNSCREEN IS TOXIC

Do not use sun screen. Sun screen is toxic, and anything that is on your skin gets absorbed into the body[14]. Babies and children especially should never, ever use sunscreen. Instead, they should get some sun, and when they have had enough, be protected from too much sun by hats and shade. Pregnant women should expose their belly to the sun.

The truth is that there is evidence that sunscreen helps to cause cancer[15]. (Remember, each cancer victim pays about $300,000 for treatment). For example, while natural Vitamin A is safe, the synthetic vitamin A found in many sunscreen brands contains substances which react negatively in the sunlight, becoming toxic to the system. 92% of the chemicals in sunscreen contain at least one of the ingredients which are harmful to humans.

TANNING BEDS "MIGHT AS WELL BE COFFINS[16]"

The above title was the title for an article at WomensHealthMag.com. Tanning beds produce unnatural radiation, and even though the manufacturers claim the light is "full spectrum", no one has ever managed to reproduce true sunlight. The article explained how Oncologists now believe that tanning beds are to blame for the alarming spike among young women in lethal melanoma cases—the second most common cancer in adults under 30.

You're not fat. You're hibernating. So, get some vegan, non-GMO 2000 IU or 5000 IU Vitamin D3 tablets, and do all you can to get into the sun as often as possible (without burning, of course). Even in winter, keep an eye out for a sunny, not-so-cold day and see if you can get out of the wind and get some sun on your belly and legs.

REFERENCES

1. *Understanding Leptin*, by Byron Richards CCN, 2002, third edition 2009, page 183

2. en.wikipedia.org/wiki/Vitamin_D

3. Quote attributed to the late famous Vitamin D researcher Dr. Carl Reich in *The Disease Conspiracy – The FDA Suppression of Cures*, 2006, page 141.

4. *Vitamin D3 Miracle*, Jeff Bowles, page 140

5. jcem.endojournals.org/content/89/11/5387.full

6. www.vitamindcouncil.org

7. *Eat fat, lose fat*, 2005 by Dr. Mary Enig & Sally Fallon

8. www.vitamindcouncil.org/about-vitamin-d/how-to-get-your-vitamin-d/vitamin-d-supplementation/

9. *Vitamin D3 Miracle*, Jeff Bowles, page 97

10. *Vitamin D3 Miracle*, Jeff Bowles, page 21

11. *Vitamin D3 Miracle*, Jeff Bowles, pages 95-96

12. *First for women* magazine, 7/9/12

13. *Transdermal Magnesium Therapy*, by Mark Sircus, Ac, MD, 2007, page 33

14. www.naturalnews.com/001264.html

15. naturalsociety.com/sunscreen-causes-cancer-what-you-may-not-know-about-sunscreen/

16. www.womenshealthmag.com/health/tanning-beds

CHAPTER 40

MSM SULFUR IS IMPORTANT FOR FAT LOSS

Deficiencies in sulfur can result in every cell and organ in the body not working efficiently. Naturally, this can contribute to fat gain as well as a host of other health problems.

After magnesium and vitamin D, sulfur in the form of MSM (methylsulfonylmethane), is an important supplement to take. Fortunately, unlike magnesium, it is very easy to improve sulfur levels with supplementation. The importance of supplementing one's diet with MSM has been grossly underestimated. In fact, MSM has been called "The forgotten nutrient"[1].

Sulfur is the third most abundant mineral in the body, after calcium and phosphorus. Half of it is in muscles, skin and bones. Sulfur is also in collagen, so it is needed for healthy nails, hair and any flexible tissues including cartilage. It is most important for healthy joints.

Most importantly, sulfur is part of the connective tissue of the body, which keeps cells together. But it does much more than just support. It is also important in the transport of nutrients and electrolytes (salts and minerals that conduct electrical impulses) and other many other substances[2,3,4,5]. Nutrients are essential for fat loss.

Shortages of sulfur reduce production of enzymes, which are needed to keep you thin. Sulfur is also important for energy production in the cells, so that means it's harder to burn fat without it. You can see from this that we must have sulfur in order for our bodies to work properly, and therefore to get thin.

Plus, if you are not exercising at all due to stiffening of any muscles or joints, or pain, lack of sulfur could be the cause. MSM is an effective pain killer. Dr. Stanley Jacob M.D. and Dr. Ronald Lawrence M.D., Ph.D. published *The Miracle of MSM*. After 20 years of experience with fighting pain with MSM, they concluded that of 18,000 patients, a massive 70% experienced benefits from the use of MSM, finding that pain diminished or disappeared altogether.

Yet another benefit of supplementing with MSM is that it helps to make healthy mucous membranes, which are the linings of many organs, such as the intestines and lungs[6]. Once the mucous membranes are healthier:

- Allergens cannot bind to the mucous membranes (thus helping with allergies).

- Parasites cannot bind to the mucous membranes (thus helping you to get thin). Amazingly, animal studies have shown that animals that had intestinal worms were free of worms after just 17 days of MSM intake!

- Toxins are eliminated more easily (and toxins make you fat)

- MSM is great for detoxing, because it is a strong antioxidant. That is, it binds to free radicals that would otherwise damage cells, and neutralizes them. Free radicals are formed by normal chemical reactions in the cell and actually have some good uses, like killing viruses and bacteria. But when we have too many free radicals from ingesting too many toxins, free radicals do great damage[7]. Think of free radicals as red hot particles that damage anything they touch[8].

- MSM drastically increases the ability to excrete toxins. Since toxins make us fat, it should be part of your fat-loss program[9].

The following story may give you some idea of how important it is to include MSM daily in your diet:

> An older woman suffered from aluminum poisoning so much that she could not speak and was confined to bed for *six years*. Then a natural health practitioner advised 2 teaspoons a day of MSM. Just two weeks later while having a warm bath to help her eliminate the toxins she smiled and *finally spoke* – "Gee, I feel much better now." Several months later she was able to lead a normal life[10]!

Remember that MSM is still an unnatural product, which has been processed. Anytime we take an unnatural supplement, rather than get our nutrients in whole food form, you can cause problems and imbalances of other nutrients. Do not take more than recommended dosages.

REFERENCES

1. *The Forgotten Nutrient MSM: on Our Way Back to Health with Sulfur.* Ley, B.M., Health Learning Handbooks, BL Publications, California: 1998.
2. Munck-Khoe, L.K. de: Vitaminen, Hardware of Software? Deel 1. Ortho 14(5), 1996: 204-211
3. Munck-Khoe, L.K. de: Vitaminen, Hardware of Software? Deel 2. Ortho 14(6), 1996: 252-261.
4. Vos, R. de: De Magie Van Het Leven Zit in De Chemie. Folia Orthica 1998 (1): 7-10.
5. Lamers, H.J.: Ferdinand Huneke, Ontdekker en Grondlegger van de Neuraaltherapie. Tijdschr. Voor Integr. Geneesk. 1996; 12(1): 18-22.
6. Herschler, R.J.: MSM: a Nutrient for the Horse. Eq. Vet. Data, 1986.
7. www.msm-info.com
8. *Excitotoxins*, by Dr. Russell Blaylock, 1997, page 45
9. www.msm-info.com
10. Owen, B.: Ask Dr. Bob?? Why MSM?? Health Hope Publishing House, California, 1997

CHAPTER 41

ORGANIC FOOD:
YES OR NO?

Unlike some natural health people, while I like organic food, if it's reasonably priced, I am not an "organic Nazi". Unfortunately, I have met overweight people who tell me that they eat only organic food, as though that is all they need to do. They may even drink organic milk, which is fattening & unhealthy whether it's skim or not, because it's toxic because it's homogenized, and because God designed cow's milk to make a baby calf weigh 1,000 pounds within two years. These people wonder why they are getting larger despite this. Therefore, I will explain some facts about organic food.

First of all, the word "natural" on a product means absolutely nothing at all. It has zero legal meaning[1]. Besides the legal definition, consider that poisons like arsenic and mercury are also natural. Companies everywhere stick the word "natural" on virtually anything these days. They realize that people want to return to a natural way of life, and are trying to fool people that their toxic products are natural. They even say that sugar is natural! Sugar cane is natural, but the processes they put it through aren't natural. Just remember, coal tar is natural, and they use that to make what they call 'natural' vitamin supplements.

I am sure you can see that this is not quite the same as eating a raw organic piece of fruit.

Organic food, however, does have a legal definition[2]. Organic food is meant to be produced by farmers who emphasize the use of renewable resources and the conservation of soil and water to enhance environmental quality for future generations. Organic meat, poultry, eggs, and dairy products come from animals that are supposed to be given no antibiotics or growth hormones. Organic food is meant to be produced without using most conventional pesticides, synthetic fertilizers, sewage sludge, bioengineering or ionizing radiation. Before a product can be labeled 'organic,' a Government-approved certifier is meant to inspect the farm where the food is grown to make sure the farmer is following all the rules necessary to meet USDA organic standards. Companies that handle or process organic food before it gets to your local supermarket or restaurant must be certified, too. Therefore, organic is definitely better for you, the environment and the future of mankind.

Unfortunately, however, a lot of so-called 'organic' products have been bought out recently by giant corporations, who are the same ones that have been feeding you toxins and GMOs for years, and are often tied in with the medical-industrial complex, that profits enormously from ill health. The diagram on the next page is an illustration of this. Please go to www.msu.edu/~howardp/OrganicMay2013zoom.png for a clearer version of the chart. It shows, for example, that Pepsi owns Naked Juice, Coco Cola owns Odwalla, Kellogg owns Kashi, M&M owns Seeds of Change and Dannon owns Stoneyfield. This is a very serious situation and it is positive proof that you must never assume anything when buying food, even organic food. It is imperative that you constantly read every label, every time, you buy a product. Never assume that a given product is "safe" because you recently purchased it and it contained no toxic substances. You must read the label every time you purchase it, as these companies are very deceptive and they frequently change formulations to include toxic ingredients, such as canola oil.

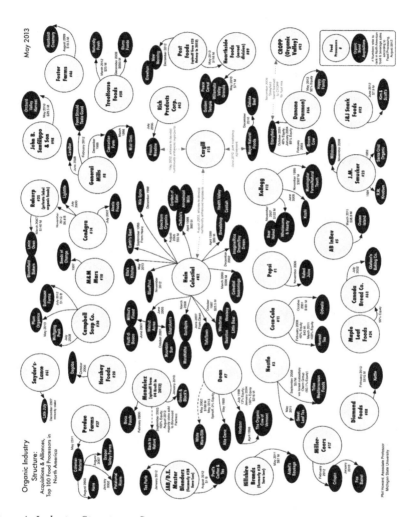

Organic Industry Structure - Source:

Michigan State University. www.msu.edu/~howardp/OrganicMay2013zoom.png

USDA SNEAKS ASPARTAME INTO ORGANICS VIA NEOTAME[3]

USDA 'Organic' food is no longer safe, if it's processed rather than just produce such as fruit and vegetables. NutraSweet, a former Monsanto asset, has developed a new and improved version of this neurotoxin called Neotame. Neotame has similar structure to aspartame, except that it appears to be even more toxic than aspartame. Like aspartame, some of the concerns include gradual damages to nerves and the immune system.

To make matters really appalling, Neotame requires *no labeling*. And it is even included in USDA Certified 'Organic' food.

No one is clear why this evil sabotage was allowed to happen. Neotame has been ruled acceptable, and without being included on the list of ingredients, for:

• USDA Certified Organic food items.
• Certified Kosher products with the official letter k inside the circle on labels.

Therefore, if you buy any *processed* food, whether USDA Certified Organic or not, that food could very well contain poisonous Neotame, because it is cost-effective, and since no one knows it is an ingredient, there is no public backlash, similar to what is happening with Aspartame. That is why you must make your own food. This is a terrible, evil situation. No wonder there is an epidemic of disease and obesity, with this kind of thing going on.

To make matters worse, consider the food chain. Many cows are being fed Neotame. A product called "Sweetos," which is composed of Neotame, is being substituted for molasses in animal feed. Most animals will not eat spoiled, rancid feed. They know that it is not good for them. So the factory farmers just cover up the unpleasant tastes and odors, and then they can feed them anything they want to. You get the neotame second hand.

That is, because of unlabeled Neotame, plus mega corporations buying out organic companies, there is now a catastrophic hidden danger about buying any 'organic' processed food that has been made by a corporation, rather than buying whole organic fruit, vegetables, nuts, seeds and lentils.

ORGANIC PRODUCE CAN BE TOXIC

Whether or not organic produce is non-toxic depends on where it is grown. For example, be very wary of 'organic' produce from China. USDA organic standards place *no limits* on levels of heavy metals contamination of certified organic foods, including mercury, lead, cadmium, arsenic and aluminum. Even further, there is no limit on contamination from PCBs, BPA and other synthetic chemicals. That is a worry even for US grown organics. That's because "organic" certifies a process of how food is grown or produced. But organic certification does nothing to address *environmental* sources of pollution.

ORGANIC IS BETTER

Generally, however, locally grown organic produce is definitely better than non-organic. I urge you to watch the excellent documentary *Food Inc.* which shows secrets of what is being done to our food these days. While the medical-industrial complex will continue to fund studies that say otherwise, a four year, $25 million study by the European Union into organic food - the largest of its kind to date – found that with regards to organic food compared to "regular" food, organic food is more nutritious than ordinary produce. For example:

- There are 40-50% more antioxidants in organic food.
- There are higher levels of beneficial minerals like zinc and iron in the organic produce.

All of this will help to get you thin. However, that being said, keep in mind:

- It's much, much better to have non-organic fruit and vegetables, than no fruit and vegetables, if you can't afford organic. Organic is about quality, but you want **quantity** of plants. The only exception to this is a few plants where a super high level of pesticides is used, such as strawberries, or bananas which are gassed with ethylene, which is used in blowtorches. In that case, if you can't afford organic, get something else.

- Something is not healthy, just because it's organic. Regarding organic meat, dairy and eggs, leading nutritionist Dr. Campbell in *Forks over Knives* says that the protein is the same, whether it's organic or not. When it comes to animal protein versus plant protein, it's not the difference in the quality of the food that is important, it's what kind of food it is in the first place.

IF IT COULD BE GMO, MAKE SURE IT'S ORGANIC

However, that being said there is one proviso. If you are eating anything that has a possibility of having been genetically modified, it is essential that you buy only organic. GMO plants are never organic. It's important to keep up-to-date on which genetically modified foods are allowed to be grown or imported into your country. In the USA, as of time of printing, they are:

- Corn.
- Soy.
- Canola (not that anyone should use rapeseed oil).
- Beets (or sugar that is not from sugar cane).
- Zucchinis.
- Papaya.
- Dairy (cows are fed GMOs, including GMO alfalfa. Plus injected with genetically modified rBGH).
- Eggs (chickens are fed GMOs).
- Meat and farm-raised seafood (animals are fed GMOs).
- Seafood (they are fed GMOs).

THE WORST FOODS WITH MOST PESTICIDES

Do all you can to buy organic of the following:

- Apple.
- Bananas (so they weren't gassed).
- Broccoli.
- Carrot.
- Celery.
- Cherries.
- Grapes.
- Kale.
- Lettuce.
- Nectarine.
- Peach Pear.
- Pepper.
- Strawberries (these have extra-high levels of pesticide).

These are lower in pesticides. It's not so important that they be organic:

- Asparagus.
- Avocado.
- Cabbage.
- Eggplant.
- Grains.
- Kiwi fruit.
- Mango.
- Nuts.
- Onion.
- Pineapple.
- Seeds.
- Sweet peas.
- Sweet potato.
- Tomato.
- Watermelon.

Please remember, while organic is best, what you eat is much more important than whether it's organic or not. Money is energy. If you have to work a second job to pay for organic produce, you are better off with the ordinary produce.

However, please keep this in mind. There is a war going on over our food, which you will see in the documentaries *Food, inc.* and *The World According to Monsanto*. Ultimately, for the future of our grandchildren, all of mankind and the earth, all our food needs to be grown organically. This will only happen when more and more people demand it with their ultimate power, what they spend their money on. Therefore, even when it's not in your budget, please do as I have done, even when I felt I could not afford it, buy at least a little more organic fresh produce than you normally do every now and again, even if it's just one apple. The more people who do this, the cheaper and more widespread organic produce will become.

Please keep in mind that unless you can afford lots of organic produce, in my experience sometimes the ordinary produce tastes better than the organic produce, and is currently more readily available. I know it shouldn't, but it seems to me that it does. And, if it tastes better, you will be more likely to stick to a whole-foods plant based diet. Quantity of fresh vegetables and fruit is more important than organic quality, and that's what you need to get thin.

REFERENCES

1. www.organicauthority.com/foodie-buzz/5-food-labels-that-mean-nothing. html

2. www.nal.usda.gov/afsic/pubs/ofp/ofp.shtml

3. Barbara H. Peterson, 2010, farmwars.info/?p=4897

CHAPTER 42

YOUR HEALTH IS LIKE
A BANK ACCOUNT

One day I was at the post office, and I heard a woman talking to another woman say how she had just put on a whole lot of weight, and didn't understand why, because "she was eating the same things that she always ate". Does this sound familiar? If you are too young for this to have happened, be warned! Everyone gets old and this could be you one day if you don't learn now. Living near the beach, I see a lot of thin teenagers in bikinis who chomp on chips and drink sodas. Yet I see very few 30 year olds with the same bodies. If only those teenagers would change their habits and addictions now, they could maintain those great bodies for life. This chapter will explain why this happens.

Our fat and weight are intricately tied up with our health. Our health is like a bank account. The following numbers are obviously totally fictitious. I am just doing the best I can to try to get you to see the health of your body from a different perspective.

When we are born, we arrive with a deposit of, say, $500,000-$2 million, depending mostly on the diet and lifestyle of both of our parents in the seven years before we were conceived, particularly the mother but also the father.

From then on, whenever we did something negative to the body, we withdrew from the account. Some things, like having a little sugar, reduced the account by only a few dollars. High fructose corn syrup used up more. Eating microwaved food and aspartame used up a whole lot more.

Unfortunately, the 'price' of some of the negative things that we spend from this account has also gone up over the years, at the same time that the credit from some of the good things has gone down. For example, an egg from 1960 may have been a $0.20. But now it costs $5.00, unless it's organic. This is because of such things as:

- The quality of our soil has gone down, due to chemical farming.

- Concentration of toxins in most animal products has increased due to factory farming and crazy breeding of animals to meet unnatural standards.

- Dangerous toxins are being added to the food chain due to Genetically Modified food.

- More products which make our lives 'better' (air fresheners / non-stick fabrics / cell phones etc)

- Nowhere near enough government oversight to see that chemical factories recycle and deal with chemicals properly, before releasing them into the environment.

- Big corporations preventing the growth of technologies which can provide cleaner, safer energy and products, but threaten their own profits. For example, search on www.Youtube.com to see Henry Ford's car that was made of plastic and hemp in 1941. It was stronger and lighter than steel! Another example is that back in 1996, my husband Michael was involved with a company that perfected a revolutionary, wonderful process that cleaned all impurities out of coal before burning the coal. It was called the "Turner-Lloyd" process and it even has a U.S. patent. This could have ended air pollution from coal factories at the same time it made the valuable impurities available for selling. But the oil companies frowned upon this technology, so that company was prevented from developing their technology, and we don't have it today.

Going back to my description of the health bank account, when we do something positive, we add to it. Unfortunately, it's a lot easier to keep the balance on the account high by not spending, than it is by adding to it. Fresh-squeezed juicing, eating lots of raw plant food and getting rid of parasites by herbs and zapping raises the account. Getting a kinesiology balance can also make a positive deposit.

Eventually, some people start to spend so much that they get down to a zero balance. When this happens, the 'bank' starts to charge *interest*. Just as with a credit card, now you have to do more than make a monthly payment. You have to *pay extra*. This is when the old ways that used to work, no longer work. This is when symptoms such as massive fat gain as well as aches and health problems really start to increase, or in extreme cases the person dies at an early age of heart attack or cancer.

Now you have to do much more than what you might have had to, had you done more earlier. Now you have to not only stop spending, but also start contributing. For example, it's no longer enough to just stop eating donuts. You might have to start paying back by eating raw plants as well. Another example may be that maybe you got by on 6 hours of sleep a night, but now a normal night of 8 hours sleep is not enough. You might need to have 9-10 hours of sleep for a while.

The following are totally wild guesses only. They are *totally inaccurate*. They are merely to give some idea of how some things cause a bigger withdrawal from, or deposit to, the account. The list does not include everything that is good and bad. It's just to give you an idea of how you accumulate health debits and credits over time. They are only an illustration to help you to understand this concept.

Debit. Subtract this amount each time for doing the following-	Credit. Add this amount each time for doing the following -
$1: Eating sugar. No exercise in a day. Super stressful exercise. Missing one hour's sleep. Eating meat, chicken. Eating dairy. Drinking one cup of coffee or tea. Drinking a soda with caffeine. Eating chocolate. Drinking bottled fruit juice.	**$1:** Having some sunlight on your skin without burning. Getting an extra hour's sleep. Eating some raw seeds. Drinking 6-8 glasses of reverse osmosis water in a day. Having spirulina or chlorella.
$2 Eating high fructose corn syrup Eating wheat. Eating something that had blue coloring added to it. Eating puffed grains (rice, wheat, corn etc). Eating garbage eaters (oysters, clams etc). Eating factory-raised pig (pork, bacon, ham, sausage). Drinking homogenized milk. Eating soy, e.g. oil, flour, beans (except fermented – e.g. tofu, soy sauce). Eating vegetable oil or margarine.	**$2** 20 minute walk. Zapping your parasites. Taking probiotics (good bacteria) occasionally. Eat raw, leafy greens (other than lettuce). Eating raw coconut oil. Eating chia or flax seeds, or brazil nuts, for omega 3s.
$3: Going a day without water. Eating aspartame. Eating MSG. Eating cottonseed oil. Eating a fast-food meal.	**$3:** Drinking fresh vegetable juice. Eating a totally raw plant meal. Having a kinesiology balance.

Debit. Subtract this amount each time for doing the following-	Credit. Add this amount each time for doing the following -
$5: Eating microwaved food or water. Kissing an animal (which gives you parasites). Eating French fries. 5 minutes talking on a cell phone. A night with a radio clock next to the head of the bed.	**$5:** Doing a parasite cleanse. Having nothing but fresh vegetable & fruit juice for a day. Meditating. Praying.
$100: Eating anything genetically modified (e.g. corn, soy, canola, cottonseed, sugar from beets, zucchinis, meat, papaya, non-organic dairy, eggs, farm-raised seafood). A night sleeping with an electric blanket.	**$100:** Forgiving others and letting go.
$200: Getting mercury dental amalgams.	**$200:** Getting mercury dental amalgams removed.
$5,000 Having one vaccination.	**$5,000** For each month you were breastfed, after the first month.
	$30,000 For the first month you were breastfed.

Keep your health account high to get thin and so that your quality of life stays high. Remember that the borrower is servant to the lender. Eating toxic foods makes you a servant to the Food Mafia and the Medical Mafia. I hope this thought makes you angry. I hope it makes you angry enough to change your life so that you free yourself from these human parasites.

CHAPTER 43

TOXIC EMOTIONS ARE FATTENING

If our bodies were just a metal machine that ate only one fuel, then we would have nothing more to worry about in order to get thin than just focusing on calories. However, living, organic bodies with a spirit inside them are totally different. For one thing, negative emotions are toxic and can cause fat gain in a number of ways. These include:

1. When we experience stressful emotions, cortisol levels go up. Cortisol tells our bodies to store more fat, especially on the belly. It also causes insulin resistance, which leads to more weight gain[1].

Yale University found that when cortisol levels are raised, even for just a few hours, the body stores more fat, especially around the belly. Dr. Dean explains: "Cortisol causes fat cells in the belly area to store ... fat because the body perceives almost any stress as starvation stress[2]." Stress can be from chemical or electromagnetic causes, and it can also be from emotional causes.

2. When we experience negative emotions, we are more likely to reach for something to eat to make us feel better for a few moments. And that food is more likely to be something that is toxic. For example, when one is feeling down, one is more likely to reach

for chocolate than brazil nuts.

3. Negative emotions cause acidity, which makes us fat. Negative emotions include:

- Anger.
- Fear.
- Jealousy.
- Overwork.
- Stress.

On the other hand, positive emotions cause alkalinity, which makes us thin. These include:

- Focusing on gratitude.
- Kindness.
- Love.
- Meditation.
- Peace.
- Prayer.
- Reading Godly books.
- Service to others.

Negative emotions cause our body to go out of balance. That means that the body does not work as efficiently, and weight gain as well as health problems occur. In particular, a person who previously kept their body in good shape, who suffers traumatic stress, may find that what used to work to keep them thin, does not work any longer. This is probably one reason why some of my kinesiology clients have lost many pounds in the weeks after a kinesiology session, because I rebalanced their body energetically back to how it was before the stress, as well as removed the emotional stress stored in the body.

WAYS TO REDUCE FAT GAIN FROM NEGATIVE EMOTIONS

1. What ever happens, say to yourself, *"This, too, will pass"*. Paste

it on the fridge.

2. No matter how bad things are, do your best to detach from them. Remember that one day you will leave your body behind and go to the Heaven of your choice, and whatever is upsetting you, will all have seemed like a bad dream.

3. Every day talk to God, and do your best to do what He wants you to do. Spending 10 minutes a day studying the Bible can help you to grow. Emily James lost 46 pounds by starting her day with a chapter from Heather Kopp's *The Dieter's Prayer Book*.

4. Meditate. This is not "emptying" your mind, as some people believe. That is impossible. It is stilling all the thoughts that go round and round in a person's head like a broken recording. Prayer is talking to God, while meditation is listening to God. Sit for five minutes and "Just *be*". Go inside, to the place that Yeshua (Jesus Christ) talked of when he said "the kingdom of God is within you". (Luke 17:21)

5. Take deep, super slow breaths. Let as much air out as possible, as deep in your body as possible. Most of us do not get as much oxygen into our lungs as we should. Do not "chest breath". Breathe deep in the lower abdomen. The lower abdomen is where your 'hara' is located – near your navel. This is the power center that correct martial arts are based on. Correct martial arts are based on chi, or life force, and the hara is the main center of chi.

6. Fill your heart with as much love as possible. If this is difficult, first think of something that you love unconditionally. You could also breathe in while you do this, and then breathe the love out and think "Yahweh" (the name of God) as you do so.

7. Get a kinesiology balance. This can greatly improve emotions. It is amazing how often people feel more happy and peaceful once this is done. I teach how to do this in my DVD training system

Perfect Health with Kinesiology & Muscle Testing.

8. Volunteer to help others who don't have what you do. Research has found that volunteering improves the health, happiness, and in some cases, the longevity of volunteers[3]. Plus it gives you something else to think about besides eating. Even unwilling children who are forced to volunteer, fare better than children who don't volunteer. You could consider doing work to help the 27 million slaves in the world today (some even in the USA) - see www.FreeTheSlaves.net. Or do work to help the 800 million people who have only filthy water, and often have to walk 6 miles to collect it. See www.WaterAid.org / www.WaterAidAmerica.org.

9. Do "Emotional Stress Release". This comes from kinesiology and is taught in my DVD training system, *Perfect Health with Kinesiology & Muscle Testing*. When we think of something that is emotionally stressful to us, any muscle in the arms or legs which previously tested strong will test weak. This is a remarkable thing to see and experience. It doesn't even have to be a particularly stressful memory. The weakness happens because the stress stored in our body causes the brain to stop sending correct signals to the muscles. The correction is very simple:

Cover the forehead lightly with one or both hands, while you think of the stressful thing. You can do this to yourself, or do it for someone else by touching their forehead with your hands. The two areas that need to be touched are the two bumpy areas that stick out, above each eyebrow and in the middle of the forehead, as shown in the picture on the following page. Emotional Stress Release works because when we are stressed, blood goes to the back of the brain. The past is stored in the back of the brain. So not only is the current situation bad, but it gets associated with painful memories from the past, which greatly magnify the stress.

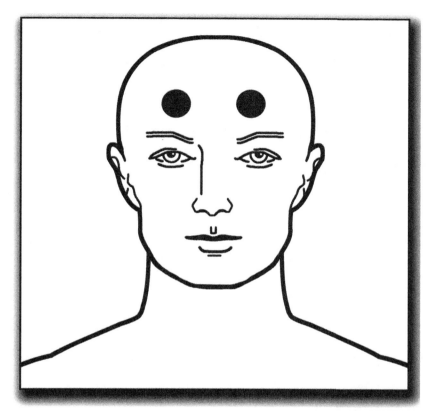

Emotional Stress Release points. Cover lightly with your hand or fingers from "Perfect Health with Kinesiology & Muscle Testing"

Touching the forehead brings the blood to the front of the brain, which erases stress from the memory. This brings you into present time and gives you new choices[4]. It has been estimated that most people use the front of their brain only 5% of the time!

You can verify that stress has been removed because when the person next thinks of the stressful memory, their muscles no longer go weak when tested. Do Emotional Stress Release anytime you are stressed, or can't think clearly. Do it for your children or even adults when they hurt themselves.

As soon as you can be quiet and private, I suggest you do this for 10-30 minutes while you review a video in your mind, of your whole life, and anything negative that happened to you or anyone close to you. If you start to cry, just keep doing it. When you do this, you will likely see 'pictures' in your mind. Keep going until the pictures go away. You might also give a big breath and feel like smiling at the end. Later on, do the same thing for your children, although they may only need a few minutes. If your spouse will let you and won't do it for themselves, do it for them as well.

Get in the habit of doing this for a minute every night, while you think about anything that might have upset you that day, before you go to sleep.

REFERENCES

1. *First for women* magazine, 2/12/12 – from "Cracking the Metabolic Code" by James LaValle NC.

2. *First for women* magazine, 7/9/12

3. money.usnews.com/money/personal-finance/articles/2012/04/04/ why-helping-others-makes-us-happy

4. *One Brain*, Dyslexic Learning Correction & Brain Integration, Gordon Stokes & Daniel Whiteside, 1992

CHAPTER 44

WERNICKE'S COMMANDS:
THE ENEMY IS SELF SABOTAGE

Have you ever tried to do so something, and given up before you completed the goal? If so, it's possible that you gave up because of what is called a "Wernicke's command".

Negative emotions can make us eat fattening and unhealthy food. But so too can negative *thoughts*. Many of these thoughts are stored in our brain, from a time when someone whom we looked up to, such as a parent, said them to us. Examples are:

- "You're a *big* girl." / "You're a *big* boy."
- "Eat up all your food."
- "You're fat."
- "You can't do anything right."
- "Don't do that."

Because these thoughts, which act like commands, may be stored in a part of the brain called the Wernicke's area, we call these thoughts "Wernicke's commands".

Research has shown that words are stored in a specific area on the left side of the brain. There is a similar area in the *right* half of the brain which is also involved with language. Both these areas are called the Wernicke's area.

According to Professor Julian Jaynes, lecturer in Psychology at Princeton University, up until around 3,000 years ago, mankind was basically not conscious as he is today. He did not think in terms of concepts, and he was not introspective. That is, he did not 'turn inwards' and think about himself. Instead he operated with what is called a "bicameral mind". The bicameral mind was man's mind before he developed self consciousness. Early man did not make any decisions on his own. The concept of "self", of being independent and self-reliant, did not exist.

Whenever a decision had to be made, early man looked for a "sign" from an outside authority, such as a king or a god, to tell him what to do. For example, if he went along a road which divided into two roads, he might throw some stones into the air to see which way they fell, to tell him which road to take.

Other signs that early man used to determine what action he should take when he was faced with a decision were often "voices" which he heard in his head and which brought immediate obedience.

Experiments have shown that if the Wernicke's area in the left half of the brain is electrically stimulated during speech, it will interfere with the ability to talk properly, almost halting speech. That is how we know that words are stored in the left half of the brain.

The same type of stimulation to the Wernicke's area in the *right* brain, causes a person to hear "voices" or "commands". These are usually of an authoritarian or dictatorial nature, and can be identified as the voice of one who was feared, admired or "looked up to" by the person being stimulated. We call these commands "Wernicke's commands", because they are commands stored in the Wernicke's area of the brain.

The two Wernicke's areas are connected to each other by a thin bridge of tissue. This is where the term "bicameral mind" comes from. It seems that the "voices of the gods" were in fact internal dialogue coming from the right half of the brain.

If mankind was to become civilized, this simple mind had to greatly improve and consciousness had to develop. However, the bicameral tendency is still present today! It is the bicameral mind, the right side of the Wernicke's area, which we "hear" when we hear those little words of self-invalidation and sabotage.

The 'authorities' who might have put commands into this mind are no longer "gods" - they are anyone that we might have looked up to at some time. These can include parents, teachers, peers, politicians, and doctors.

Have you ever been told to:

- "Grow up."
- "Shut up."
- "Eat up."
- "Forget that."
- "Give up."

Has anyone ever said to you:

- "You're mad."
- "You're bad."
- "You're fat."
- "You're stupid."
- "You'll never make it."

If somebody you thought was important or powerful said, "You're too fat", "You'll never change", "You'll forget", "You're a slow learner", "Eat *all* your food", You're not good enough", "strong enough", "pretty enough", "clever enough" "You'll go to Hell" etc. then they may have made an 'entry' in your right Wernicke's area, an implanted command, which is still influencing you to this day!

Wernicke's commands are not all powerful, but they do affect people, sometimes quite a lot. They particularly affect people during times of stress, or when they set a goal to do something that goes against the commands.

When people do any kind of work or therapy to get rid of negative beliefs, the beliefs they try to get rid of are usually worded as "I (etc. etc.) " For example, "I don't love myself", "I'm not pretty enough" or "I'm too fat". But these beliefs are not filed in the brain under an "I" point of view. The commands are entered as said by another person, as if the person is right there, talking to you! For example, the subconscious belief may be "I'm no good" but the original command (which is stored in the brain) was "You're no good".

In 1996 my Australian Naturopath & Kinesiology Teacher David Bridgman combined this knowledge with his knowledge of kinesiology, to create a powerful technique which removes these commands from the brain, called the Wernicke's correction. Sometimes, people who have this technique done to them have reported remarkable successes afterwards. I teach this technique in my DVD training system *Perfect Health with Kinesiology & Muscle Testing*, which was designed for lay people as well as health practitioners. Additional information on the Wernicke's correction is available at www.PerfectHealthSystem. com/wernickes.htm.

If you have been eating healthily, avoiding toxins and doing exercise, but are still not getting the results you want, this may be the missing key you have been looking for. Plus, it has applications in all areas of life, including relationships, money and success.

CHAPTER 45

CLEANSE YOUR ORGANS

There are a number of natural herbal cleanses which have helped people to get healthier and more energetic, and which therefore help with fat loss as a 'side-effect'.

The main cleanses that have helped people are:

- Intestinal.
- Gallbladder.
- Liver.
- Kidneys.
- Parasite (this was discussed in the chapter on parasites).

There are many different recipes for these, and you can find some of them on the internet. I have some recipes on my "Health, Wealth & Happiness" website at www.Relfe.com. Here is a brief summary of two of these, an intestinal cleanse and a gall bladder cleanse.

INTESTINAL CLEANSE

It's a dirty subject, but what if no one talks about it? More people have problems with their intestines than most people realize. How can you lose fat if you are constipated or have a dirty bowel?

Intestinal cleansing is often called colon cleansing, but it likely helps more than just the colon. Intestinal cleansing uses herbs to help your body to heal health problems which are often related to intestines that are not functioning as well as well as they were designed to function.

The most important organ cleanse to do is *intestinal* cleansing, because if you have dirty intestines with impacted fecal matter, this will create extra toxins which the other organs then have to continually detox.

The Merck Manual, the medical industry's standard text for the diagnosis and treatment of disease, tells us that colon degeneration is increasing at an alarming rate. Here are its figures for diverticulosis for people over 45 years old:

1950   10%
1955   15%
1972   30%
1987   Almost 50%

Modern natural healers prefer to talk about nice, clean things like vitamins. These are important, but are often money down the toilet because many people are rotting from the inside out because of all the toxins they ingest combined with lack of nutrition from plants.

Believe it or not, some healers have had people in their clinic who had only had one bowel movement a month! Where did all that food go? These people must have their bowels frozen solid. Their other organs were being squashed by all the extra material down there.

HOW OFTEN SHOULD ONE HAVE A BOWEL MOVEMENT?

People in less developed countries living simple, natural lives have two or three bowel movements a day, without straining. Once you go on a wholefoods, plant based diet with no wheat or soy and few grains, and a lot of raw food, you will likely find that this becomes normal for you as well.

A client of mine in Dallas told me that many of her friends had a bowel movement only once every five days. Unbelievably, when they told doctors this, the doctors said that this is normal! It may be common, which just shows how far we have come from where we are meant to be, but it's sure not meant to be that way.

I used to believe that doing a few colonic irrigations might be helpful to some clients for their intestinal health. However now, with the prevalence of prion disease and morgellon's disease, I no longer recommend colonics. The infectious agents that cause prion disease and morgellon's disease cannot be killed with standard sterilization equipment, and so I believe that colonic procedures are too dangerous to perform.

Ultimately, you need to get your bowels working by themselves. A herbal intestinal cleanse, can work wonders, especially if you also do a herbal parasite cleanse before it, and also do kinesiology and improve your diet.

Herbs can not only clean and scrub, but also draw out old fecal matter and toxins, stop bleeding, disinfect, kill and expel parasites, destroy and remove cancer, kill *Candida albicans* overgrowth (which is a major contributor towards Irritable Bowel Syndrome and Crohns disease), regulate and balance intestinal flora, remove toxic metals (such as lead, mercury and radioactive metals) and strengthen the muscles of the colon to promote normal bowel movements (and therefore heal spastic colon).

Good bacteria (probiotics) can also make a huge difference as they are an essential part of digestion. Many of us don't have all the good bacteria we should, because of antibiotics and because farming practices are so far removed from nature. I like iFlora probiotics by Sedona Labs.

Many people believe that problems that don't appear to be directly related to the colon, often improve with colon cleansing. All parts of the body, affect all parts of the body. Excess fat, pain and disease are caused by toxins, and a dirty bowel is full of toxins.

IMPORTANT: No one should rely on any herbs all their life. They act like drugs, just not with so many bad side effects. Many old people who have used laxatives all their life can no longer have a bowel movement - they evacuate only by enemas. You want to eat foods that support, rather than control, the body.

TIP FOR EASIER EVACUATING: SQUAT DON'T SIT

Believe it or not, the current toilet seat is a comparatively new invention. It was developed in the Industrial Revolution by people who thought it was more 'dignified' to sit on a 'throne' than the way the natives did. However, many doctors at the time were worried that this would cause health problems, because it went against nature. But in Victorian England where even table legs were covered with long tablecloths, because they suggested 'legs' (which were called only 'limbs'), it was considered very improper to discuss such things.

If you have ever felt, as many, many people do, that after you have evacuated, there is still something left, here is the reason: The anal canal is *unstraightened* when seated. This causes an obstruction.[1] Adopt a relaxed, full squat position and the anal canal *straightens*.

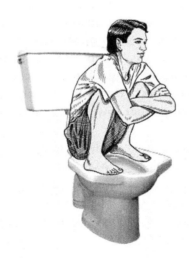

Picture courtesy of NaturesPlatform.com

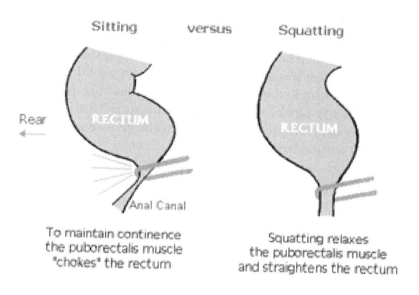

Picture courtesy of NaturesPlatform.com

Squatting rather than sitting can therefore help greatly with constipation. Later, other health improvements can also occur, because your body has been freed of more toxins.

Oncologists have observed that 80% of colon cancers occur in the cecum and the sigmoid colon, the two areas that are not fully evacuated in the sitting posture. This causes fecal stagnation and is probably a major reason why colon cancer is one of the leading cause of cancer deaths in the United States. In traditional Asian and African cultures where squatting is the norm, colon cancer is virtually unknown.

Many sufferers usually notice significant improvement within seven days of making this simple change of habit to the squat posture, because body wastes pass through the straightened anal canal.

I began to learn about this when I visited India, where I learned to use an Asian toilet ("Eastern toilet"). The first one I saw was in an airport. I went into the cubicle. It was very clean and there was no smell. It all seemed quite strange, but I had been warned. The cubicle was fully lined with tiles. In the middle is a gutter. You squat either side of the gutter.

A story told by my mother made me realize that this may be more important than we think. Mum said how one day she was out somewhere in Australia and went into a public toilet. Accidentally she walked into a toilet where there was another woman. The strange thing was, she saw that the woman in there was balanced up, squatting on the toilet seat! Now, that is a lot of trouble to go to. I assume that if you have been used to squat all your life, then you really know how unnatural and difficult our modern toilets really are.

After discussing this subject with a woman I met, she told me that she once dated a man from a South American country. He said that he was very angry at the Catholic Church because before they came everybody squatted. And after they came in, people changed to western style toilets, and a high percentage of the population developed all kinds of health problems which they did not have before.

One problem we in the west have with squatting is that most of us have lost the ability that we had as children to squat with our feet flat on the floor. I didn't even realize this until I visited India. Two ladies came and cleaned the tiled floor of a room I was staying in. I was amazed to see them clean the floor while squatting, and walk around while squatting, with their feet flat on the floor the whole time.

If you have children, encourage them to squat fully every day to maintain this ability. And have them squat on the toilet lid, while they still have the muscles to enable them to do so! (Note: Adults should not do this as the toilet seat will break under the excess weight).

USE A FOOT STOOL

Maybe one day people will build houses with eastern toilets. You can buy some products which help to make squatting possible on a western toilet, such as "nature's platform". In the meantime, it is important to use a *foot stool* every time you use the toilet.

GALLBLADDER CLEANSE

The following information on gall stones and the gall bladder is from the very good book *Are you Stoned?* by chiropractor Claude M.

Lewis, Edith Hiett and Leon Hiett.

The gall bladder stores bile, and releases it in optimum quantities when it is needed. Without your gall bladder, the liver will *still* produce bile, but the bile will leak inside you because it will not have a proper place to go.

What is bile? The spleen breaks down worn-out red blood cells into bile salts and other substances. What a wonderful system is our body! Even worn out blood cells get used. Bile salts are normal in the body when in normal amounts.

The liver removes excess bile salts and wastes and sends them to the gall bladder for storage. The liver is the body's principal chemical plant. If a man built a plant to perform all the chemical functions one mans' liver could perform, the plant would cover *500 acres.*

While the products are in the gall bladder, water is reabsorbed and so the waste products get more and more concentrated and form bile. Bile is needed for 3 things:

1. It neutralizes the acid from the stomach, because bile is very alkaline.
2. It breaks down fats so that they can be digested.
3. It is a natural laxative for the colon.

Bile is essential for the *digestion of fats.* When you eat a meal with fats, the gall bladder releases a large amount of bile to digest the fats. One big problem when a person has gall bladder surgery is that the body has nowhere to store bile until it is needed. Therefore, it just drips continually. And when a large amount is needed to digest a meal with a lot of fat, there is not anywhere enough bile added to digest it properly.

GALL STONES

Stones can form anywhere in the body where there is a liquid containing mineral salts that can be crystallized, and where the fluid is held for a while in a hollow organ, such as the gall bladder.

The stones may be large or small, and sometimes grow together causing extra large stones. Small stones are often excreted along with the bile and eliminated with no problem. Larger ones, however, can become lodged in the ducts, causing gall stone colic, one of the most painful illnesses known. At other times, gall stones may be silent. In autopsies, examiners often find gall bladders full of gall stones, although the deceased had no complaints about them.

A gall stone is not a true stone. They are rather rubbery and soft. Most gall stones float. They are mostly green. The size varies from rice grains to golf balls.

There are numerous recipes for gallstone cleanses, mostly involving lemon juice and a large amount of oil. On my website Relfe.com I have a summary of a cleanse from the book *Are you stoned*. Here are a few success stories from the book, to encourage you to do research on gallstone cleanses:

"I had my gall bladder removed three years ago, but now I seem to have the same symptoms as I had before the operation: Nausea, gas, poor digestion, pain and general run-down condition. After taking your gallstone removal treatment, I got rid of two cups of stones!" (This woman began to feel better immediately after, and went to work the next day). Mrs. N. Richardson, Texas

"I feel fine, but to encourage my wife to take the treatment (since she needed it so badly) I decided to go ahead and do it myself. I didn't realize just how good I could feel." Mr. C.N. Texas

"In the past eight months, I've done the gall bladder flush four times, each time passing progressively larger stones. I was really packed! ... The pain in my stomach and esophagus is gone."

"About two weeks after taking the gall bladder treatment I noticed that my skin condition had greatly improved. This is the first time in thirty years that my skin has not looked like a teenager with acne. The acne and skin blemishes are gone and my digestion had improved so much that I no longer have to take digestive aids." Mr. C.K. Texas

"I passed a cupful of stones - four stones were the size of prunes... The next day I had so much energy, I felt like a new person". Mrs. M.C. Texas

"Ten of the stones that I passed were the size of a penny. My energy level is easier to maintain and now I get by on 6 hours sleep without fatigue". Mr. J.F. Texas

"For more years than I care to remember, I have had trouble with constipation. I could not have a bowel movement without taking something....In a 25 year period, I had 66 rectal operations. At one point, my digestion became so difficult with gas attacks and sour bile creating much distress that I relied heavily on antacids to relieve the problem.... I passed approximately 100 gall stones ranging from pea size to quarter size ... The stones ranged in color from the red and tan ... to green and quite a number of black gall stones. I have carefully adhered to the follow-up treatment. My overall health has greatly improved thanks to this gall bladder treatment and my strict adherence to these guidelines. Most amazingly, my bowels are functioning in a normal manner now!" J.B.R. Texas

LIVER CLEANSE & KIDNEY CLEANSE

Again, there are herbs that can help you with these. Please do some research on the internet and ask your health practitioner and at your health food store.

CANDIDA

Many people who are overweight have what naturopaths call a Candida imbalance. This means that there is an excess of the yeast *Candida albicans* in the body. Many doctors do not believe that this is a problem, because Candida occurs naturally in the body, as an aid in digestion. But the problem is not that Candida exists, the problem is with balance.

Maybe another reason why doctors don't want to acknowledge

that Candida plays a major role in weight gain and health problems is because they are a major cause of Candida imbalances, by prescribing antibiotics. Candida is normally kept under control by the good bacteria in the gut. When the good bacteria are killed off, for example, by antibiotics, the Candida goes wild. It also grows out of control with certain foods, especially sugar.

My training DVD series *Perfect Health with Kinesiology & Muscle Testing* teaches a technique called the Candida Balance. I have had women come to me with Candida problems, who were feeling itchy between their legs from Candida overgrowth, who literally had the feeling stop by the end of the session! Having a good balance of Candida is important for weight loss. Taking good probiotics, such as iFlora by Sedona Labs (which has more species in it than just *Acidophilus*) can help with weight gain and digestive problems.

CHAPTER 46

KEEP YOUR ORGANS

I have had clients come to me who have had various parts of their body cut out of them. Often after doing this, they put on quite a lot of weight. That's no wonder, because it's then harder for the body to do what it was designed to do, because it doesn't have all the parts it should have. Before you take the drastic and permanent step of cutting out part of a body organ, please consider what would happen if a part of your car was not working, and you just tore it out and threw it away?

Every part of your body is necessary for something. The fact that science has not fully understood the body yet, is not enough reason to rip out something that we can't understand. For example, we have only very recently discovered that fat cells produce the most important hormone in the body (leptin)!

A lot of people have problems after surgery, but it's too late to be sorry then. Before you consider surgery, you might like to read books such as the excellent *Confessions of a Medical Heretic*, by Dr. Mendelsohn. You can't heal something once it has been removed. Doctors have never managed to make a human body, so chances are that if God gave you a body part, that body part is there for a reason.

Our body is designed to repair itself. It can't repair anything that has been cut out. Even with cancer, realize that every human being has cancer cells in their body[1]. Most people don't even know they have cancer cells because their immune system safely and easily kills their cancer cells as they form. As long as there is a balance between the number of new cancer cells in the body, and the strength of the immune system, they will never "get cancer," meaning the cancer cells will never grow out of control. Did you know that, according to the excellent website, CancerTutor.com, there are *four hundred* 'cures' for cancer? However, modern medicine, that makes about $300,000-$1.3 million[2] from each cancer patient, generally offers only the three toxic choices of radiation, chemotherapy and surgery.

If anyone recommends that you get any part of your body cut out, as long as you are not in a life-threatening situation, please get several other recommendations first. Find out exactly what that particular part of the body is used for. Make sure you *ask for a printed, full list of side effects*. Better yet, ask the person who will do the operation to sign a document saying that they will be *financially responsible* for any negative side effects that occur as a result of the operation. They will never do this, so that should tell you something.

Note that if you go to a butcher, he will not suggest that you buy lettuce. Please realize that an operation is a *product*, like a toaster or a car. It is not a "favor" someone is doing for you. Have a look around and see what other products are offered as well. If necessary, even look outside your country.

REFERENCES

1. www.anewdayanewme.com/dr-oz-cancer-truths-all-of-us-has-cancer-cells-growing-inside-and-more/
2. www.beating-cancer-gently.com/index.html

CHAPTER 47

ELECTROMAGNETIC
CAUSES OF FAT GAIN

Our bodies are *electrical* instruments. They don't like to be in electrical fields. I have found from working with my kinesiology clients that a lot of people are *much* more affected by electromagnetic stress than most people realize, including the scientific community. This electromagnetic stress puts our brains and bodies out of balance, which makes our bodies less efficient, which makes it harder for us to reduce fat, in addition to adding to pain and health problems.

The Bioinitiative Report 2012[1] supports much of what I am going to say in this chapter. The Bioinitiative Report 2012 was prepared by 29 authors from ten countries, ten holding medical degrees (M.D.s), 21 Ph.D.s, and three Ms.C., M.A. or M.P.Hs. Among the authors are three former presidents and five full members of the Bioelectromagnetics Society.

In my early days, clients would come to me with health problems and I would put them in balance with kinesiology. Once a person's body is in balance, it should stay in balance. But in many cases when I saw them a week later, their health problems were no better, because once again, they were out of balance. When I muscle tested for the cause of why the balances did not hold for longer than a week or two, the cause was very often found to be from electromagnetic stress, rather than from emotional or nutritional stress. The particular stress was then identified, and was nearly always one of the things listed further in this chapter.

Once this was dealt with, generally the person would stay in balance, and their health symptoms would heal. This is probably a major reason why some of my clients happily reduced weight, even when they weren't trying to.

More and more of us are under stress from electromagnetic radiation and ionizing radiation. Just because you can't see it doesn't mean it's not doing anything! The following list of the main causes of electromagnetic stress was created by myself, from research on my clients in my kinesiology practice, and by observation of what it took to heal them.

ELECTRIC BLANKET

This is possibly the very worst thing you can do as far as electromagnetic stress is concerned. It creates a very high electromagnetic field, which causes electromagnetic interference with your body, for a long period of time. This greatly harms your body. Keep it off the bed at all times.

I would say to throw the blanket out, but I have heard of one use for an electric blanket. A woman had bronchitis. She left her electric blanket going on her bed night and day for 3 days. After that, her bronchitis went away and didn't return. I believe that the electric blanket killed whatever organisms were living in her bed, and contributing to her bronchitis. It would be interesting to try this for asthma sufferers. If you do this, don't sleep in the bed while it's on.

Instead of an electric blanket, use comforters which are warmer than blankets, flannelette sheets and put a blanket under your bottom sheet.

I am sorry for hotel staff, but when we stay in a hotel, if there is an electric blanket on the bed, we remove it. Just unplugging it is not enough, because a lot of coiled metal creates enough charge to interfere with your body.

EATING MICROWAVED FOOD

Muscle testing has shown me that this is one of the few things that is almost always guaranteed to make sure that a body goes out of balance. I have had clients come to me for their second visit who were out of balance, and the body told me that they had eaten microwaved food since the last session, *even though* I did not know this, and had told them to not eat it. After I found this out, the person then verified that this was the case. Please see the chapter on microwaved food for more information.

MOBILE AND CORDLESS PHONES

Few people want to hear that something that they now regard as "indispensable" might cause serious harm to their health. But since cell phones *kill brain cells*[2], they can be a major contributing factor to any health problem, apart from brain cancer. Since they kill brain cells, I believe that suggesting that they are contributing to obesity is not a wild idea.

Your cell phone is a microwave transmitter and it should bear a strong cancer warning. The Journal of Cellular Biochemistry reports microwaves promotes rapid cell aging[3].

Cordless phones marked 900 megahertz or 2.4 gigahertz emit the same dangerous microwave radiation as cell phones.

In 1993 the telecom industry committed $25 million dollars for a series of research projects designed to prove that cell phones are safe. The studies proved just the opposite! They proved that federal microwave exposure standards are dangerously inadequate. Cell damage and tumors can be easily induced in the lab at about one third of the FCC's exposure. How can you expect your body to work properly if you are giving your brain cancer?

Spanish researchers have shown that cell phones can alter electrical activity of a child's brain for hours, causing drastic mood changes and possible behavior and learning disabilities. Because of this, and the fact that cell phones will give millions, if not billions, of people brain cancer, children should never, ever talk on a cell phone.

Insurance studies in England showed that an average driver talking on a cell phone is actually more impaired in function and reaction time than a drunk!

Finland's Radiation and Nuclear Safety Authority reports that one hour of exposure to mobile phone radiation can cause human cells to shrink.

The Interphone Study Group eventually acknowledged that so-called *"heavy users" of cell phones* had an approximately *doubled* risk of a life threatening and often-fatal brain tumor called glioma, after only 10 years of cell phone use. But their definition of a "heavy user" was someone using a cell phone for about *two hours per month*[4]! What would happen if someone used a cell phone for two hours a day?

People are addicted to mobile phones for some as yet unknown reason. There is a new psychological disease called "nomophobia", where people suffer stress or even panic attacks if they can't find their phone or it is out of range. This 'disease' affects a massive two thirds of people! That shows you that cell phones are affecting people's brains in ways that no one has yet even discovered[5]. They are actually addictive. You know this is not natural when a shocking one in five people suffer as much stress, when their cell phone is out of range or lost, as if they are moving or getting divorced![6]

Please, give up the cell phone and cordless phone. Please use only these alternatives:

- Landline.
- Voicemail.
- Hands-free kits.

If you think this idea is just too "radical", please do research on the internet to verify this information. Even many multi-millionaire celebrities are starting to do without cell phones because of the radiation danger. Don't put that transmitter next to your brain!

RADIO CLOCK NEXT TO THE BED

Having a radio clock near the head of the bed seems to affect a surprisingly large number of people. Presumably the radio clock puts out an electromagnetic field which interferes with the brain's electrical field. The fact that you are in the bed for so many hours every night gives the effect extra strength, at the time when you most need to be unaffected by anything, and the main time when you burn fat.

Move the radio clock as far from the head of your bed as possible. Ordinary alarm clocks are okay, but don't get one with luminous lights, because any light can interfere with the quality of your sleep.

USING A COMPUTER FOR TOO LONG

Before I found kinesiology, I had an office job where I was on a computer all day. By the end of the day I was totally exhausted. How can one exercise or feel like eating right when one is exhausted? Muscle testing showed me that my body went into stress after just one hour on the computer. Then a kinesiology technique was done which rebalanced my brain around computers, to increase my body's resistance to computers. Since the brain is a living super-computer, this is a bit like adding more memory to it.

Muscle testing then showed that I could be on a computer for eight hours before my body went into stress, an improvement of seven hours. Sure enough, from then on, I had plenty of energy at the end of the day! I have used this technique on many clients, with similar success. This technique is taught in my DVD training system, *Perfect Health with Kinesiology & Muscle Testing.*

Here are some solutions for reducing electromagnetic stress from computers:

- Turn off the monitor whenever practicable.
- Keep any computers or printers you are not using turned off as long as possible.
- The worst effects come off the sides and the back. Don't ever place a computer so that its back is pointing at someone.
- Drink water frequently whenever you are using the computer, or anytime you are in an area with a strong electromagnetic field.

X-RAYS & MAMMOGRAMS

Maybe this has nothing to do with obesity, but I thought I would include x-rays for completeness, as they are so harmful to the human body. X-rays cause cellular damage that is cumulative. Therefore, x-ray breast examinations cause breast cancer[7]. If you must have an x-ray, take extra fresh juices, vitamin C & other antioxidants before and after exposure.

STANDING IN FRONT OF A MICROWAVE

Hopefully, by now you have thrown out your own microwave. But if you are around other people who do this toxic activity, do not ever be near it when it is turned on.

WIFI & WIMAX

My husband Michael was warning people about the great dangers of WiFi and WiMax, five years before scientific studies started to show that he was correct. From my husband Michael;

"My experience includes 6 years in the military as a radar technician in the United States Navy's Advanced Electronics program. In addition, I am a graduate of the United States Naval Nuclear Power School and so I have experience with non-ionizing and ionizing radiation safety protocols. WiMax is so very dangerous because of the high signal strength, but WiFi is also dangerous. High speed broadband in the gigahertz range requires a higher signal strength than cell phones.

While it is true that we live in this electronic microwave "soup" (from the tower to you) the problem comes from your WiMax transmitter. If your transmitter is on your roof, then it is not so much of a problem. If the transmitter is on the desk next to you then it IS a problem because you are so very close to it and you are being beamed with the signal full strength. Same thing with a WiMax transmitter on a laptop. The operator is way too close to the transmitter.

Another new danger is from the home internet routers that contain both a WiFi transmitter and a 4G "smart phone" transmitter in the same box. These 4G transmitters allow "smart phones" to connect to an office network and are like having a mini cell phone tower in your office. They are extremely dangerous to a persons long term health."

My husband Michael came home one day after visiting the mall and he looked terrible, which was unusual for him. It turned out he had been inquiring about WiMax. I used kinesiology on him and he was way out of balance. Muscle testing indicated that the cause was electromagnetic radiation from WiMax. Just walking past these little black boxes can affect you.

However, WiFi is bad as well, as more studies are starting to find. For example:

"Mr Bevington "had never had any problems before the WiFi. When it was put into his classroom he suffered nausea, blinding headaches and a lack of concentration. When the school removed the WiFi, his condition improved"[8].

For your health and weight, the best blueprint is to totally boycott *all* wireless devices. That includes cell phones, smart phones, tablet pcs, WiFi in your home and WiMax as well. And if you have to use a laptop or tablet PC, always deactivate the WiFi transmitter and 4G broadband transmitter and never put them on your lap, as they constantly radiate RFI (radio frequency interference) through the case, into you, when they are turned on. The only safe alternatives are to use Ethernet cables in your home for connectivity and to avoid mobile devices that transmit any form of radiation.

BEING IN A CAR OR AIRPLANE FOR A LONG TIME

Just like with computers, muscle testing will show that a lot of people go out of balance after a certain number of hours in a car or airplane. It's harder to lose fat when you are out of balance.

Again, kinesiology can help with this. Other suggestions are: If you're driving, stop every 2 hours and walk around the car a few times. Drink water frequently. If on an airplane take your own water with you.

WALKING THROUGH A METAL DETECTOR

I have had clients come to me who were very out of balance, and suffering various unpleasant symptoms. When I muscle tested them, their bodies indicated that the cause was a metal detector at the airport, even though sometimes they had not been to an airport for a number of weeks. Unfortunately, the only solution that I know for this is the same kinesiology technique that I described in the paragraph on computers.

WEARING A WATCH

Believe it or not, and I apologize for the inconvenience of this information, I have found that wearing an electric watch affects a lot of people considerably. When people who are negatively affected by wearing a watch are muscle tested, the arm with the watch will test weak and the arm without the watch will test strong. When the watch is removed, both arms test strong.

You may remember that I discussed how we have rivers of energy called meridians flowing through our body. There are images for this in the chapter on kinesiology. We have 14 main meridians, or rivers of energy in the body. Six of these go through the wrist. The pulse given off by the watch interferes with the meridians, putting the body off balance. Even worse, one of these meridians is the meridian for the Central Nervous System. Having the Central Nervous System out of balance can cause many kinds of negative symptoms, and make fat loss a lot tougher.

I personally now, no longer wear a watch. I have had clients who gave up wearing watches who made remarkable improvements. For example, one woman was very worried and upset. She had pains and a lump under her arm. She had been to the doctor for a test, and while they didn't tell her what was wrong with her, they looked very worried and told her to come back next week for more tests. She came straight to me. I gave her a kinesiology balance, made some changes to her diet and told her to stop wearing her watch. When she went back for more tests the doctors looked very surprised - they could find nothing wrong with her.

If I need to know the time, I carry a small fold up clock in my bag or pocket, and hang clocks up in the house.

ULTRASOUND SCANS ON UNBORN BABIES

A new study in the Lancet and Canadian Association Medical Journal says that this Ultrasound is one of the most dangerous things you can do for a baby[9].

Babies are so fragile. They should only ever be in the purest electromagnetic environments possible. Please consult your Holistic M.D. to determine if you really need these procedures. And, for the same reason, please do not fly when pregnant. Seven hours in an airplane exposes you to about as much cosmic radiation as one chest x-ray[10], in addition to what the metal detector does to you.

WEARING FLASHING LIGHTS

I was at a conference when a woman told me her stomach hurt. I used muscle testing and found that one of her arm muscles was out of balance, the muscle that relates to the stomach meridian. That muscle was right underneath a badge with a flashing light that she was wearing. After I corrected the imbalance, and she removed the badge, her stomach stopped hurting.

Do not wear any flashing lights, or other electrical gadgets. I cringe at the shoes they now make for children with flashing lights on them, plus jewelry with flashing lights. A woman I know asked me why her three-year-old son had constipation. Her son had shoes with flashing lights on them. When I told her how bad these are, she realized that his constipation started around the same time that he got those shoes.

LIVING OR WORKING NEAR HIGH TENSION POWER LINES

The closer your home, office or school is to high tension power lines, the more damage it is causing. Please see the Bioinitiative Report 2012[11] for more information.

For more information on electromagnetic health dangers, please see: www.microwavenews.com and www.emrnetwork.org.

You're not fat, you're suffering from the toxic effects of electromagnetic stress. Get it out of your life and note what improvements you experience.

REFERENCES
1. www.bioinitiative.org
2. www.relfe.com/cell_phones_brain_cancer.html
3. www.relfe.com/cell_phones_brain_cancer.html
4. articles.mercola.com/sites/articles/archive/2011/08/27/do-cell-phones-cause-brain-cancer.aspx
5. news.bbc.co.uk/1/hi/education/6583213.stm
6. jag.cami.jccbi.gov/cariprofile.asp
7. www.naturalnews.com/010886_breast_cancer_mammograms.html
8. www.bioinitiative.org
9. www.telegraph.co.uk/technology/news/9084075/Rise-in-nomophobia-fear-of-being-without-a-phone.html
10. www.independent.co.uk/news/uk/home-news/phonereliant-britons-in-the-grip-of-nomophobia-802722.html
11. www.wakingtimes.com/2013/05/07/ultrasound-one-of-the-worst-things-you-can-do-to-a-developing-fetus

CHAPTER 48

THIN IS CHEAPER THAN FAT

Are you thinking that you can't afford this new way of eating? Please think again. Surprisingly, you can save a lot of money on this plan, even if you are juicing. Going to the furthest extreme, if money is really an issue, consider that millions of incredibly poor people in the world live off less than $1 a day, and are slim and healthier than many Americans, by living off lentils or stir fried vegetables. You can go one better and eat your lentils raw and sprouted, with raw sunflower seeds and apples, all of which are cheap.

WHY IT'S PROCESSED FOOD THAT IS EXPENSIVE

How do you get rich? You *add value* to something. For example, you take five cents worth of wheat, and make it into breakfast cereal, and sell it for $4.85. Or get some cucumbers and vinegar and make them into pickles for $5.00. (Better yet, add some MSG or aspartame to the product, to make it addictive). Therefore, to save yourself a ton of money, you need to do the opposite of that. Don't buy anything that anyone has "added value" to.

I continually look in people's shopping carts when I am at the supermarket. When you do this, and you know that it's toxins that make people fat, and that processed food has many more toxins than unprocessed food, you will know why people are getting bigger every year. For example, many shopping trolleys seem to be filled with about twelve different ways to turn 5 cents worth of toxic wheat into a 'different' kind of food.

All of that processed food is a whole lot more expensive than the ingredients that it's made of. Have you noticed how nearly everything seems to cost $4.00 or $5.00 now? That is where your money is going. It gets worse, because you have to pay taxes on what you earn. You might have to earn $8.00 to pay for that $5.00 item. But what's really infuriating is that a $4-$5 item has only a tiny fraction of *real food* value in it. For example, a box of cereal, whether it costs $3 or $5, has only about 5 cents of real food in it. Maybe less.

Work out how much you pay for drinks and bottled water. Know that you don't need to do this anymore once you have your own reverse osmosis water filter, plus water cooler and five gallon bottles (although you do have to get replacement filters about every six months).

You can save more money by replacing a lot of your supplements, if not all, with fresh-squeezed juices, because all the vitamins and minerals and thousands of other nutrients will be in much better proportions, and much better absorbed from your fresh juice than they are from most supplements.

In addition, once you have food that your body really wants, and give up the addiction to the toxic foods you eat because they cause addictions, not because they help your body, you will start *eating less* without even trying.

Therefore, please work out at least a rough estimate of how much you spend each year on the following toxic items:

- Alcohol, including wine.
- Beef jerky and other embalmed meat snacks.
- Breakfast cereal.
- Caffeine in any form (tea, coffee, 'energy' drinks, guarana etc).
- Cake & cheesecake.
- Candy.
- Canned soups.
- Cheese and "American Cheese".

- Chewing gum.
- Chips, pringles, similar snacks.
- Chocolate.
- Cookies.
- Crackers.
- Diet drinks.
- Fast food meals.
- Fruit juice, bottled.
- Ice cream.
- Margarine.
- Meat in any form.
- Milk.
- Olive oil (since most olive oil is lampant oil or made from non-olive oils).
- Pizza.
- Popcorn.
- Restaurant meals (top class restaurants are okay if they know where their olive oil came from, and do not use anything that is genetically modified, or that was fed GMO food. But they are still expensive).
- Sea food (animal protein is bad for you. Plus it has mercury and other toxins, such as GMO food if it's farm raised.) Plus it is poisoned with oil and corexit if it comes from the Gulf of Mexico.
- Soft drinks.
- Toxic oils (Soy, Canola, Cottonseed, Vegetable, etc).
- TV dinners.
- "Weight-loss" products.

Then add to the total:

- Prescription drugs needed now, and *in the future* if you continue your current life style. Many are not covered by insurance.

- Other medical costs such as dialysis, insulin, hospital costs not covered by insurance, etc. if you continue your current life style.

- Then include to the total the amount that you spend on vitamin supplements that are going to be replaced by foods that give much better support to health, such as fresh-squeezed juice.

- Then remember that you have to pay tax on top of the total. If you make your own food, you don't have to pay tax on your labor.

AVOID 'WEIGHT LOSS' PRODUCTS – THE $60 BILLION A YEAR' SCAM

I added "weigh loss" products to the list (unless it really has been working for you in the long run). Don't fall for those ads that tell you that all you have to do is take one bottle a month of their product (always plus exercise and water, of course!) to get the body you want. These may help a tiny bit, but only if you give up the toxins that made you the way you are now in the first place. Many of them are just diuretics. That is, they force the body to get rid of water. But if your body is holding onto water, there is a reason for that, which is probably linked to protecting it from toxins. So there will be a price to pay later on for ingesting diuretics. Go and spend the money the weight-loss merchants want you to give them, on more nuts, fruit and vegetables.

LACK OF MONEY FOR FOOD IS MOSTLY CAUSED BY LACK OF KNOWLEDGE

I once saw a story on TV about a woman who believed that she did not have enough money for food. Poor woman! It was obvious that it was not lack of money that was keeping her hungry, but lack of knowledge. For example, she showed the interviewer her cupboard, which contained a few *small boxes* of some kind of processed food. Hundreds of millions of people feed themselves every day off practically no money at all, and they don't have a box in the house. As I said, anything in a box has added value, which is super expensive. And usually, the smaller the box, the high the price per pound of food.

What that woman should have been showing was things such as big bags of rice, beans and lentils, plus piles of cheap vegetables. Things that can be cooked into vegetable stews.

Even more shockingly, this woman's house was surrounded by a big grassy area. Hundreds of millions of people would just love to have all that fertile soil, because you can use it to grow food on, much more food than you can imagine. I strongly urge you to read two books: *Secrets of the soil* by Peter Tompkins is a classic that every farmer should read, if not every person on earth. It shows how you can greatly increase the amount of topsoil you have, no matter where you live. So too does *Back from the Brink*, by Peter Andrews. *How to grow more vegetables than you ever thought possible, on less land than you can imagine* by John Jeavons, is also highly recommended. It teaches how Biointensive farming can produce on just 800 square feet (the size of an ordinary front lawn) enough vegetables for a family of four for a whole year. *Four-Season Harvest*, by Eliot Coleman, shows how to grow organic vegetables from your home garden all year long.

Please plant at least one fruit, nut or olive tree. Imagine how much extra food there would be if everyone did this!

JUICING

Never think, as someone I talked with recently told me, that you can't juice because "you can't afford it". It doesn't matter so much what you are juicing, just how cheap it is. Don't worry about organic or not (except for beets, because they are bound to be genetically modified). All you need to juice is, for example, some carrots, apples and some kale leaves. That won't cost a fortune. Ask around for cheap sources of fruits and vegetables, and search on the internet for farmers markets and Asian stores. Even supermarkets can have decently priced produce if you buy in bulk or on sale. It doesn't matter too much what you juice, so long as you don't use too much sugary fruit, and I highly recommend always including at least some leafy greens.

As for raw seeds for smoothies, nut butter and salads, raw sunflower seeds are very inexpensive and super nutritious.

FOOD THAT WILL REGROW FROM SCRAPS

To save you even more money, because plants are *living*, many of them can be grown again and again from scraps! This includes;

- Fennel.
- Leeks.
- Green onions.
- Celery.
- Romaine Lettuce.
- Cabbage.
- Bok Choy.
- Lemongrass.

Place the root in a glass jar with a little water in a sunny position. It will then grow. You can cut off what you need. As soon as you can, transplant into soil for better growth and nutrition. Other plants you can regrow are:

- Ginger: Place a spare piece in potting soil with the smallest buds facing upwards. It makes an attractive house plant as well.

- Potatoes: Cut it into pieces. Plant in soil with the eye facing upwards.

- Onions: Cut off the root end and plant in soil. You can reuse the roots forever.

- Sweet potatoes: Plant in soil. You have to give them about 4 months to produce a new sweet potato.

- Beets: Cut off the top. Put in water until it sprouts. Then plant in soil.

Break your addiction to foods that are harming not just your body, but also your pocket book. Learn to appreciate quality ingredients rather than addictive chemicals. Turn off the television and the computer, and spend some time preparing real food. Eventually, you will find that you are not just thinner, but a whole lot happier and healthier, and that the rewards for changing your lifestyle benefit you in numerous ways right now, which will become only more important as you get older.

REFERENCES

1. www.prweb.com/releases/2011/5/prweb8393658.htm

CHAPTER 49

HOW TO LOSE PREGNANCY FAT EASILY

It is quite shocking that many women are given ridiculous advice on reducing their 30 or so pounds of pregnancy weight, such as the advice on www.medicinenet.com, they said:

"Weight loss after pregnancy can take a very long time, sometimes a few years¹".

Nothing could be further from the truth. Because nothing is easier than losing pregnancy fat, so long as you do what *you were designed to do*.

And what is that? I will give you a clue, the same clue that first made me realize the truth about losing pregnancy fat. Since I had clients with this problem, I had often wondered why pregnant woman often put on an extra 20-30 pounds after having a baby, that they never lost. I was in Sydney Australia and saw my mother's neighbor's dog give birth to a litter of puppies. The mother looked nice and plump at the time, and stayed that way for weeks, while the puppies were *small*. But eventually those puppies were *really big*, and still nursing, and the mother then became skin-and-bones skinny.

That made me realize: Like everything else to do with your body, that extra 20 or 30 pounds of fat has a purpose. It's to feed your baby with. You will lose a little weight faster in the early months if you are breastfeeding than if you don't[2], and your belly will suck in a whole lot faster, but if you really want to get thin, and lose *all* the weight you put on during pregnancy, you must nurse your baby when he/she is a lot older than most women breastfeed. Obviously, you do this **in addition** to solid food, which you introduce slowly at first, when the time is right, adding one new kind of food every several days or more. Dr. Sears *The Baby Book* recommends starting solid food around 6 months or when your baby starts showing you signs that they want to eat what you are eating.

I have never been as slim as when I was breastfeeding! It was wonderful to not have to worry about how much I ate, so long as it was healthy. But the weight did not start to pour off until after my son was one year old. All you have to do to lose that baby fat permanently is to do what will also help your child to stay slim for the rest of his/her life, and that is to breastfeed for a lot longer than society has told us to. I will explain how this will benefit you, as well as your baby, in many other ways, but first I will give some evidence to show you this is true.

Babies are not meant to be weaned until they can live totally off solid food. If you think about it, doesn't that make sense? And they can't do that until they have their full digestive system developed. And a major part of the digestive system is the *teeth*, particularly the back teeth (molars), because you must have the back teeth for chewing. Therefore, babies should not be weaned at least until they have all their teeth, which may not be until they are at least three years old.

That will be shocking news to many people. But, please, consider research done by Dr. Katherine Dettwyler, Ph.D., Dept. of Anthropology at A & M University[3], which you can read in her wonderful book which I super highly recommend, *Breastfeeding, Biocultural Perspectives*. No other breastfeeding book compares to this one.

Dr. Dettwyler compared different variables such as length of gestation, birth weight and life span in apes and monkeys with age of weaning. Our bodies are similar biologically, if not spiritually, with apes.

For example, gorillas and chimpanzees share more than 98% of their genes with humans. Dr. Dettwyler did this to decide at what age humans would "naturally" wean their children if they didn't have cultural rules about it. Some of her results are:

1. In 21 species of monkeys and apes the offspring were weaned at the same time they were getting their first permanent molars. In humans, that would be at 5.5-6.0 years.

2. Pediatricians like to claim that length of gestation is approximately equal to length of nursing in many species, which suggests that one should wean at 9 months. However, the larger the adults, the longer the length of breastfeeding relative to gestation. That makes sense, since breast milk is so important to the development of the brain, which is not as important for small animals. Chimpanzees and gorillas, the two primates closest in size to us, nurse their offspring for over *six* times the length of gestation. In humans, that would be 4.5 years of nursing.

3. Pediatricians claim that most mammals wean their offspring when they have tripled their birth weight, but we are not rodents. Again, larger mammals nurse their offspring until they have quadrupled their birth weight. In humans, this occurs between 2.5 and 3.5 years.

4. One study of primates showed that the offspring were weaned when they had reached about 1/3 their adult weight. This happens in humans at about 5-7 years.

5. A comparison of weaning age and sexual maturity in non-human primates suggests a weaning age of 6-7 for humans.

6. Studies have shown that a child's immune system doesn't completely mature until about 6 years of age (so why do we vaccinate when they are babies?). Breast milk helps develop the immune system, and also helps protect the baby with your antibodies.

Therefore, the *minimum* natural age of weaning in humans is 2.5 years, with a maximum of 7.0 years! That's definitely a whole lot longer than six months. It is likely that humans should wean at 4-5 years, because only babies have the ability to digest lactose, the main carbohydrate in milk, and they lose this ability around 4-5 years old[4].

If you are worried about getting bitten, don't worry, it will only happen once. If when your baby has teeth, he/she bites you, immediately put the baby down and leave the room. They won't repeat the experience.

Each generation of women is getting fatter and fatter, with babies who are fatter each generation. A major reason for this is that women are feeding formula instead of perfect breast milk. One study found that nearly 70% of women in New York were using only formula. The poorer people were more likely to use formula. Once again, poor people are poor in their *choices*, not just in their wallets.

Compared to perfect breast milk (when a woman eats and drinks toxic-free food), formula is very toxic. It's not just a little difference. The difference is massive. Formula should only be for emergencies. Fat babies grow up to be fat men and women with health problems, who are not as smart, who make even fatter babies, and so the cycle goes on and on, as we are seeing now. It is time for this cycle to stop, and go the other way, in a direction that *improves* the human species.

Remember this statistic that I quoted earlier: In 2006, scientists at the Harvard School of Public Health found that rates of obesity, in infants less than 6 months old, have risen 73% since 1980.[5] While vaccine toxins will be contributing to this, formula has to be a major cause also.

I have been looking at babies for years and I notice that these days a lot of American babies look 'different'. If you look into their eyes, it is as if nobody is home. Their poor little bodies are struggling to deal with all that they are being treated with, especially vaccines and formula, plus excitotoxins which their mothers ingest during pregnancy. And yet, when we went to France and Switzerland in 2006, most of the babies there looked more like babies used to look decades ago – bright and alert, as well as slimmer. Please breastfeed your baby for as long as you were designed to, while you avoid toxins, and you will have a more beautiful, smarter, happier child who can easily be slim for life.

It's not as bad as that may sound. Realize that after about two years your baby will not want milk all the time. After around 2 1/2 years you might be down to just two feeds a day, one in the morning, and one in the evening when you are private and it is easier on you. You will find that your night feed will make it very easy to get your baby to go to sleep.

In fact, once you see how the weight starts to drop off you when you are breastfeeding past one year old, and how good you feel from the hormones your body is producing, you may not want to stop! But eventually your baby's body will change and weaning will be easy rather than a drama, because their body will no longer want milk. You just 'forget' to nurse and so do they.

WHY BREASTFEEDING IS THE ONLY OPTION

Normally, I would first list all the reasons why it's good for your baby, like the fact that just three months of feeding only breast milk boosts baby's brain by a massive 30%[6]. But, unfortunately, I have met, unbelievably, selfish mothers who really did not care what was good for their baby as much as they cared for themselves. So I will first list reasons why breastfeeding will benefit *you:*

HOW BREASTFEEDING IS REALLY GOOD FOR YOU

1. You will easily lose all the pregnancy fat you want, plus extra, so long as you breastfeed until your baby has all their teeth.

2. Sucking stimulates oxytocin which contracts the uterus[7]. Your tummy will go back to pre-pregnancy levels in record time.

3. Oxytoxin is also a 'feel good hormone', which is why women who breastfeed are much more happy and contented than women who don't.

4. The one thing that most mothers of babies want is more *sleep*! I believe from personal experience that breastfeeding gives your body hormones that replace quite a lot of the need for sleep. I came to this realization by watching my husband while we were raising our son. While normally it was I who needed more sleep, and I was getting a whole lot less sleep than normal, plus lots of very broken sleep, I noticed that it was Michael – not me – who looked totally haggard and sleep deprived, even though he was getting much more sleep

than me. I am not going to say that I felt fantastic, but I did feel as though I could manage it. But for Michael, it was quite otherwise.

That was when I realized that my body was doing something different. I got a clue to this when I read *The Promise of Sleep.* Everyone, both men and women, release the hormone prolactin during sleep[8]. Prolactin levels increase when women produce milk. I theorize that part of what the prolactin is doing is replacing the need for sleep. Women who use formula are deprived of these high levels of prolactin, and other hormones, that make them feel a whole lot better.

5. There is no preparing food or cleaning up! That means less work and *more sleep*!

6. Because there are no bottles to heat up, no cleaning up, and your baby is right beside you, you can feed throughout the night without getting out of bed, while you are still barely awake, and get back to sleep instantly.

7. Your baby will get to sleep a whole lot faster, which will mean *more sleep* for you.

8. Your baby is being given your antibodies, which saves you all the anxiety, time wasted and sleepless nights that happen when babies get sick.

9. You develop a super *extra* bond with your baby which you won't develop if you use formula. This bond is most rewarding.

10. This bond will also help you now and years later when discipline become an issue, when you will 'know' what is going on with your child.

11. While breastfeeding, all your other hormones will be working better. For example, estrogen levels will be lower[9], and high estrogen makes you fat.

12. Hormones released during breastfeeding make you very relaxed, maybe more relaxed than you have ever been in your life. Stress makes fat, while breastfeeding un-stresses[10].

13. Your baby will learn to love and trust *you* more, rather than an inert, cold, physical bottle.

14. You won't have to go to the doctor nearly so often, if at all. Formula fed babies visit the doctor much more often.[11]

15. Dr. Sears in *The Breastfeeding Book* said that you will save about $1,200 a year, plus not have to visit the doctor as often. But even if formula is free, you do not want it.

16. Giving your baby the very best basis for growth will save you tons of stress, drama and upset later on when they grow up to be more beautiful, smarter, healthier and happier, and greatly add to your own happiness and sense of achievement.

17. Baby will not throw up nearly as often.

18. Your baby will cry a whole lot less. There are few things more heart-breaking for a mother than a crying baby.

19. Baby's stools will not smell nearly as much.

20. Your baby will grow up looking more attractive, with a better-looking face, and much more beautiful smile.

HOW BREASTFEEDING IS SUPER GOOD FOR YOUR BABY

It's impossible to list all of the reasons why breastfeeding is good for baby, and scientists will probably find thousands more reasons in the future. Our bodies are infinitely complicated, with thousands of chemical reactions. Only God can figure out how to create the perfect food. It's a continuation of the miracle of life. A formula factory cannot come even close, and will be giving toxins that breastmilk does not.

Much of the following information is from the book, *The Breast-feeding Book*, by Dr. Sears. This is a good book to have, if you keep in mind the following error: Dr. Sears seems to believe that it is okay to have caffeine while breastfeeding because "very little is transferred"! Please, realize that caffeine is a drug, and a baby should have absolutely *zero* drugs. The same goes for excitotoxins such as MSG and aspartame. Also, while Dr. Sears' book *The Baby Book* is very useful, I believe that his information on vaccines is highly dangerous, as you can see in my chapter on "Other toxins".

Make your diet as super healthy and toxic free as possible to give your baby the full benefits of the following from breastfeeding -

- Raises IQ by at least 10 points. The longer you nurse, the higher the IQ.

- Only three months of feeding only breast milk makes your baby's brain 30% smarter[12]. What would three years do to their intelligence?

- Makes his / her eyes work better.

- Makes him / her hear better.

- Makes all body organs work better.

- Greatly reduces all kind of health problems such as ear infections, tummy upsets, even diaper rash.

- One million white blood cells in each drop of milk protect your baby from disease.

- Good fats and other nutrients keep your baby's body at a desirable size.

- The sucking in breastfeeding, and improved nutrients, make a better-shaped jaw, which ends up producing a more attractive face.

- Baby will not require a pacifier, which is aptly called a 'dumby' in Australia, since they make children look less intelligent.

- Makes a better heart, which will end up meaning improved health and athletic abilities.

- Baby will grow a whole lot faster.

- Breastfeeding protects against allergies[13], which make people fat.

- Breast milk improves everything so much that some pediatricians can even tell which babies are breastfed by their skin. Breastfed babies have beautiful skin.

- Your baby must have breastmilk, especially the colostrum in the first six hours after birth, to set correct levels of leptin. This is most important for correct appetite regulation for the rest of their life[14].

By the way, if you have a little baby and did not breastfeed, so you don't have any milk currently, do not despair. Start now! While your baby is sucking, imagine milk flowing to your breast. If the baby won't suck, have someone leak some formula down onto the nipple at the same time to encourage sucking. Keep this up for a few weeks, and it is likely that your body will start to produce milk again, possibly within a week!

If you or your baby have never been breastfed, I suggest you get some organic cow's colostrum from the health food store. I have seen people benefit from this.

To learn how to breastfeed, there are many very good books available from Amazon. I recommend *The Breastfeeding Book* by Dr. William Sears. You can also find a Lactation Consultant, which is a recognized profession, in your area. Hospitals may be able to help you to locate one.

Please, stop the growth of obesity and health problems that are becoming rampant, due to formula feeding. Increase love and beauty within your life by working with nature. Breastfeed your baby at least until all their teeth are grown. The time will fly by much faster than you ever dreamed of, and you will have the rest of your life to thank yourself that you did so, because the benefits will pay off for the rest of your life, and on into future generations of your family.

REFERENCES

1. www.medicinenet.com/script/main/art.asp?articlekey=20244

2. *The Breastfeeding Book*, by Dr. Sears, 2000, page 10

3. www.kathydettwyler.org/detwean.html

4. THE MILK LETTER : A MESSAGE TO MY PATIENTS Robert M. Kradjian, M.D., Breast Surgery Chief Division of General Surgery, www.not-milk.com/kradjian.html

5. Kim J, Peterson KE, Scanlon KS, et al. Trends in overweight from 1980 through 2001 among preschool-aged children enrolled in a health maintenance organization. *Obesity (Silver Spring)*. 2006;14(7):1107-1112.

6. www.dailymail.co.uk/health/article-2337374/Breast-really-best-want-brainy-baby-Just-THREE-months-breastfeeding-boosts-development-30.html

7. *The Breastfeeding Book*, by Dr. Sears, 2000, page 10

8. *The Promise of Sleep*, by Dr. Dement, 1999, Pages 21 and 260

9. *The Breastfeeding Book*, by Dr. Sears, 2000, page 11

10. *The Breastfeeding Book*, by Dr. Sears, 2000, page 11

11. *The Breastfeeding Book*, by Dr. Sears, 2000, page 12

12. www.dailymail.co.uk/health/article-2337374/Breast-really-best-want-brainy-baby-Just-THREE-months-breastfeeding-boosts-development-30.html

13. *Diet Wise*, Dr. Keith Scott-Mumby, 1984

14. *Mastering Leptin*, by Byron Richards CCN, 2002, third edition 2009, page 76

CHAPTER 50

SUPPLEMENTS FOR FAT LOSS

- Chamomile tea.
- Chromium picolinate.
- Iodine from kelp drops.
- Juice, fresh-squeezed.
- Magnesium.
- Minerals.
- MSM.
- Probiotics.
- Pumpkin seeds.
- Raw spirulina & chlorella.
- Vitamin D.
- Zinc.

MALNUTRITION BEGINS WITH THE SOIL

Nearly everyone today is suffering from malnutrition to some extent, even if they are eating only healthy foods. This is because today soils are overworked and poisoned by synthetic chemicals & GMOs. We continually take organic material and minerals from the soil, but don't put them back, as would happen in a forest. Therefore, the quality of food has suffered, and so has health.

Excellent human health & slim populations depend on wholesome food, and this can only come from fertile soils. Minerals & microorganisms in the soil control the metabolism of plants, animals, and people. Diseases are created chiefly by destroying microorganisms in the soil, and depleting minerals. Because of modern farming practices, that use chemical fertilizers, pesticides & GMOs, and don't add organic matter such as humus, or natural minerals such as rock dust, to the soil to replace what we take out of the soil, most of us need supplements.

However, while we need supplements of minerals and vitamins, most supplements are not worth anything, and can even cause harm. This is because inorganic minerals and synthetic vitamins are not what the body recognizes. Your body needs nutrients in their natural, organic forms, which means *whole foods* surrounded by all of the other nutrients in complex combinations. The special combinations which nature provides, and that most supplements do not, is synergy.

WHAT IS SYNERGY?

Synergy is when the sum of two or more things together is greater than the sum of the things when considered individually.

In other words, if you have synergy, 1+1 does not equal 2. Synergy is where 1+1=3, or 4, or 5, or 6… and on and on.

I'll give you an example. Take some tin, which is a soft metal. Mix it with copper, which is also a soft metal. Do you get another soft metal? No, you get bronze, which is a hard metal[1]. When there is synergy, an extra 'magic' appears from the mixing of two or more things.

Another example of synergy is when the Australian sailing team won the America's Cup, the first time that it had been won outside of America for 100 years. It was said that the America's team was a "team of champions" but the Australian team was a "champion team". Because of synergy, a chain is not as weak as its weakest link, and a team can be better than its best player.

God gives synergy in whole foods, which is why juicing and eating raw plant foods does so much more than taking most supplements.

SYNTHETIC VITAMINS FLUSH DOWN THE TOILET

Synthetic vitamins are often wasted. They literally flush down the toilet because the body can't absorb them. Certain synthetics can actually poison the body as they may be too concentrated or they are isolated from other substances which should be present to balance them out. Some even contain GMOs!

Therefore, the supplements that I recommend are generally made from whole raw foods which contain vitamins, minerals and enzymes in balanced quantities and in forms that the body can easily assimilate, such as green or raw food products that are just pure, dried food. Many of these foods are called "superfoods" or whole food concentrates. These are generally available only from healthfood stores or the internet.

CHAMOMILE TEA

Take this to fight excess estrogen. Keep to the 'no-snacking' rule and have this only at meal times (with a little almond milk and raw honey if desired, if this does not interfere with your weight reduction).

CHROMIUM

A deficiency in chromium is causing an epidemic of weight gain and fatigue, according to a study at Weill Medical College of Cornell University[2]. A lack of chromium can cause fat gain, super fatigue and excess need for sleep, overeating and depression. A chromium supplement is good to add to any fat loss and health program. Chromium picolinate may be the best form to take. It is best absorbed when there is a good intake of Vitamin C. Author Dr. John P. Docherty M.D. found that people who took 600 mcg. of chromium a day for two months experienced more energy and drop in carb cravings. He recommends up to 1,000 mcg. of chromium daily[3].

IODINE FROM KELP DROPS

Why do young people stay thin no matter what they eat? The answer is hormones. Your body needs many different minerals and vitamins to keep its hormones working properly. An essential substance needed for

hormones is iodine, and it is something that is almost completely missing from our diets. In fact, lack of iodine contributes to many health
problems including breast cancer and mental retardation[5].

The little bit of iodine that is added to salt and milk is not nearly
enough. However, there is a problem with supplementation, in that
overdosing on iodine supplements is very dangerous.

The answer is to have iodine in a safe, natural, organic form. That
form is kelp. Why are the Japanese thin and healthy, apart from not
eating wheat and dairy? The answer is that they eat a lot of kelp sea-
weed, which has plenty of natural iodine. The Japanese consume more
than 12,000 micrograms, *fifty times* what Americans eat[6]. (Symbols for
micrograms are ug. or mcg.). You can get your iodine by taking liquid
kelp drops. I take them daily.

JUICE, FRESH-SQUEEZED VEGETABLE

This is your ultimate supplement, full of vitamins, minerals, enzymes and thousands of nutrients that scientists don't even know about
yet. Please see the chapter on raw food for more information.

Most people eat a lot of food, because the food they eat is addictive, plus they are hungry because they are suffering from malnutrition,
from lack of the many different vitamins, minerals and many other
nutrients the body must have to work properly. That is why supplementation should help people lose weight. But often, it doesn't. This is
partly because our bodies are so complex, and really want a huge variety of nutrients. It is also because many of the products sold for high
dollar amounts in health food stores are designed to make money for
the manufacturer, not to get you as healthy as possible for the smallest amount of money.

You may be able to juice fruit as well, but watch yourself. If you get
hungry afterwards, or bloated, or don't reduce as much as you want,
reduce or cut out the fruit in your juice.

WHAT'S IN A VITAMIN TABLET?

As an example, a co-called "complete" multi-vitamin may contain:

- Vitamin A (Vitamin A Acetate, 29% Beta Carotene)
- Vitamin C (Ascorbic Acid)
- Vitamin D (DL-Alpha Tocopherol, Ergocolciferol)
- Vitamin E (DL-Alpha Tocopheryl Acetate)
- Vitamin K (Phytonadione)
- Thiamin (Thiamine Mononitrate)
- Riboflavin
- Niacin
- Vitamin B6 (Pyridoxine Hydrochloride)
- Folic Acid
- Vitamin B12 (Cyanocobalamin)
- Biotin
- Pantothenic Acid
- Calcium
- Iron
- Phosphorus
- Iodine
- Magnesium
- Zinc (Zinc oxide)
- Selenium
- Copper
- Manganese
- Chromium (Chromium Chloride)
- Molybdenum
- Potassium
- Boron
- Nickel
- Silicon
- Tin
- Vanadium
- Lutein
- Lycopene

WHAT'S IN A CARROT?

But what's in vegetable juice? Let's take a carrot for example. A carrot contains[7]:

- 2-Methoxy-3-Sec-Butyl-Pyrazine
- 3,4-Dimethoxy-Allyl-Benzene
- 3-Methoxy-4,5-Methylenedioxy-Propyl-Benzene
- 5,7-dihydroxy-2-Methyl-chromone
- 6-Hydroxy-Mellein
- 6-Methoxy-Mellen
- Acetaldehyde
- Acetone
- Acetylcholine
- Alanine
- Alpha-Amyrin
- Alpha-Bergamotene
- Alpha-Carotene
- Alpha-Caryophyllene
- Alpha-Humulene
- Alpha-Ionone
- Alpha-Ketoglutaric-Acid
- Alpha-Phellandrene
- Alpha-Pinene
- Alpha-Terpinene
- Alpha-Terpineol
- Alpha-Tocopherol
- Aniline
- Arabinoside
- Arginine
- Ascorbic-Acid
- Ash
- Aspartic-Acid
- Barium
- Benzoic-Acid-4-0-Beta-D-Glucoside
- Benzylamine

- Bergapte
- Beta-Amyrin
- Beta-Bsabolene
- Beta-Carotene
- Beta-Cryptoxanthin
- Beta-Farnesene
- Beta-Pinene
- Beta-Stitosterol
- Betaine
- Biphenyl
- Borneol
- Bornyl-Acetate
- Boron
- Bromine
- Butyric-Acid
- Cadmium
- Caffeic-Acid
- Caffeoylquinic-Acid
- Calcium
- Campesterol
- Carbohydrates
- Carotatoxin
- Carotol
- Carypohyllene
- Caryophyllene-Oxide
- Chlorogenic-Acid
- Choline
- Chromium
- Cis-Beta-Bergamotene
- Cis-Gamma-Bisabolene
- Citric-Acid
- Cobalt
- Copper
- Courmarin
- Cyanidin-Diglycoside
- Cystine

- D-Glucose
- Daucic-Acid
- Daucosterol
- Dec-2-En-1-Al
- Deca-Trans-2,Trans-4-Dien-1-Al
- Dehydroascorbic-Acid
- Giosgenin
- Dipentene
- Dodecan-1-Al
- Eo
- Epsilon-Carotene
- Ethanol
- Ethylamine
- Ethyl-Methyl-Amine
- Falcarindiol
- Falcarinol
- Fat
- Ferulic-Acid
- Fiber
- Fluorine
- Folacin
- Folate
- Fructose
- Fumaric-Acid
- Galactose
- Gamma-Bisabolene
- Gamma-Carotene
- Gamma-Decanolactone
- Gamma-Muurolene
- Gamma-Terpinene
- Geraniol
- Glutamic Acid
- Glutamine
- Glycine
- HCN
- Heptan-1-Al

- Heraclenin
- Histidine
- Ionene
- Iron
- Isocitric-Acid
- Isoleucine
- Isopimpinellin
- Isoprene
- Kaempferol-3-)-Beta-D-Glucoside
- Lauric-Acid
- Lecithin
- Leucine
- Limonene
- Linalool
- Linoleic-Acid
- Linolenic-Acid
- Lithium
- Lupeol
- Lutein
- Luteolin-7-o-Beta-glucoside
- Lycopene
- Lysine
- Magnesium
- Malic-Acid
- Maltose
- Malvidin-3,5-Giglucoside
- Manganese
- Mannose
- Methionine
- Methylamine
- Mevalonic-Acid
- Molybenum
- Mufa
- Myristic-Acid
- Myristicin
- N-Methyl-Aniline

- N-Methyl-Benzylamine
- N-Methyl-Phenethylamine
- Neurosporene
- Niacin (B)
- Nickel
- Nitrogen
- Non-2-En-1-Al
- Nonon-1-Al
- Nopol
- Octan-1-Al
- Oleic-Acid
- Osthole
- Oxalic-Acid
- Oxypeucedanin
- P-Coumaric-Acid
- p-Cymene
- P-Hydroxybenzoic-Acid
- Palmitic-Acid
- Palmitoleic-Acid
- Pantothenic-Acid
- Pectin
- Pectinesterase
- Peroxidase
- Phjylanlanine
- Phosphofructokinase
- Phosphorus
- Phytin
- Phytofluene
- Phytosterols
- Potassium
- Proline
- Protein
- Psoralen
- Pufa
- Quinic-Acid
- Rhamnose

- Riboflavin (b)
- Rubidium
- Sabinene
- Scopoletin
- Selenium
- Serine
- SFA
- Shikmic-Acid
- Silicon Sodium
- Starch
- Stearic-Acid
- Stigmasterol
- Strontium
- Suberin
- Succinic-Acid
- Sucrose
- Sulfur
- Syringic-Acid
- Tartaric-Acid
- Terpinen-4-Ol
- Terpinolene
- Tetradecenoic-Acid
- Thiamin (b)
- Threonine
- Tin
- Titanium
- Toluidene
- Trans-Gamma-Bisabolene
- Tryptophan
- Tyrosine
- Uronic-Acid
- Valine
- Vitamin A
- Vitamin C
- Vitamin B6
- Vitamin E

- Vitamin K
- Water
- Xanthophylls
- Xanthotoxin
- Xylitol
- Xylose
- Zinc
- Zirconium

ARE YOU STARTING TO SEE THE "BIG PICTURE"?

All of those nutrients work together to produce massive synergy (where 1+1 can equal 3 or 4 or more). The carrot was created by God, and therefore everything in it is in the correct *balance*. The multivitamin was processed in a factory which does all kinds of strange things to the ingredients. Raw, whole foods are the best for you. Juicing them makes you absorb super concentrated nutrients quickly and easily.

Once you start having food that your body really wants, and give up the toxic foods that you want because they cause addictions, you will start eating a lot less, and you will reduce that unwanted weight, for life.

MAGNESIUM

This is so important that it has its own section. Please see the chapter on magnesium.

MINERALS

I have mentioned a number of times how minerals, such as iron, calcium, magnesium, copper and zinc help with fat loss. Many people believe that minerals are more important than vitamins for being slim and healthy, because the body can make vitamins, but it can't make minerals, and because every chemical reaction depends on minerals. Currently the levels of minerals in our food are much lower than they were in prehistoric times. Ultimately, the best way to raise your level of minerals is to eat plant food from farmers who add minerals, such as rock dust, and organic matter back to the soil.

In the meantime, a good mineral supplement is important. Your mineral supplement should be in plant derived form to be effective, and preferably liquid. Also, many people report that edible clays have helped them.

MSM FOR ORGANIC SULFUR

Please see the chapter on MSM.

PROBIOTICS ("GOOD BACTERIA")

Your digestive system has a complicated system of good bacteria that help keep you alive and healthy. These good bacteria perform many vital functions within the body. Here are just a few:

- Help digest food.
- Guard your body against *harmful* bacteria, yeast and viruses.
- Produce essential vitamins.
- Maintain your body's chemical and hormone balance.
- Perform a vast number of necessary tasks to maintain high energy levels.

Antibiotics, chlorinated water, food preservatives and drugs damage and unbalance this delicate ecosystem. Naturally, antibiotics are the worst, as they are *anti*-bacteria, and affect good bacteria as well as bad bacteria. This causes:

- Inability to digest or absorb food.
- Build-up of toxic sludge in the intestines.
- Deficiencies in vitamins.
- Other problems that can lead to weight gain, cancer, heart disease, diabetes, low energy, chronic fatigue, depression, sleeplessness and many other health challenges.

Bear in mind that both "good" and "bad" microorganisms live in the human intestines at the same time. Often, each contributes to the overall function and health of the intestinal tract, while keeping the other in "check."

To enjoy true health, you must restore balance in your body's eco-system. To do this, it is good, at least for a while, until your intestines are working properly again, to take a supplement called probiotics. Be aware that some probiotic supplements are useless because the bacteria in them are dead.

Just taking acidophilus is not enough. There are many species of good bacteria which do different things. That is why we like to take, occasionally, iFlora made by Sedona labs, because it contains sixteen strains of the most powerful, beneficial microorganisms needed by the human body.

PUMPKIN SEEDS, RAW

Also called "pepitas", they are super high in magnesium, as well as containing good oils and much other nutrition. Eat some of these frequently, raw. They taste a bit like butter.

SPIRULINA & CHLORELLA FOR B12, IRON AND ENERGY

Both of these plants are algae that are called superfoods, because they contain so many nutrients and massive synergy. That is, the combination of everything in these algae provides massive health benefits. It's good to have both at different times, as each has different benefits. Some people who can't take spirulina can still have chlorella.

While meat eaters are often short of many vitamins, just about the only vitamin that a plant eater may be short of is vitamin B12. Neither plants nor animals make vitamin B12, which is made by bacteria. Although recommendations for vitamin B12 are very small, a vitamin B12 deficiency is a very serious problem leading ultimately to anemia and irreversible nerve damage.

Both spirulina & chlorella, contain a large amount of Vitamin B12, which is difficult to find in other plant foods. Both spirulina and chlorella are also very rich in iron, which is the most common mineral deficiency. Some nutritional yeast products & organic free-range egg yolks also contain B12.

Anytime you feel that you just have to have something sweet, and can't avoid it, take instead 6 or more spirulina or chlorella tablets. You may be surprised to see how this stops the craving. Both are fantastic brain food to have when you are doing mental work. If you can, it is best to chew the tablets, if no one is around who will mind you looking like a green-mouthed monster!

Women who are pregnant or breastfeeding should first consult with their health care practitioner before adding spirulina or chlorella to their diet.

Prices vary a lot. Try iHerb.com or VitaCost.com. Work out how many grams you are getting for each dollar. However, it is also important to verify that products are harvested from a pure source, and not mass-produced in contaminated waters. I recommend Earthrise products.

VITAMIN D

Please see the chapter on Vitamin D.

ZINC

Our soil is so deficient in zinc that a number of us are deficient as well. The trouble is, it can be dangerous to take too much as a supplement. I take "zinc tally" by Metagenics sometimes. They say that if it tastes like water, then you could be zinc deficient. If it tastes nasty, you don't need to take any more.

REFERENCES
1. *Critical Path*, by Buckminster Fuller
2. *First* magazine, 4/3/06
3. *First* magazine, 4/3/06
4. *Woman's World* 5/30/11
5. www.lewrockwell.com/miller/miller20.html
6. www.lewrockwell.com/miller/miller20.html

7. naturalhealthtechniques.com/carrots-and-glycemic-index.htm

CHAPTER 51

SECRET TIPS TO GET THIN

1. KEEP YOUR PLANS TO YOURSELF

When Ricki Lake lost 62 pounds, she said that one of her secrets to success was to keep what she was doing totally to herself[1]. Ricki must have accidentally found a key to achieving any goal: Do not tell *anyone* your plans. Although many people believe that it is good to make a public declaration of your plans, tests done since 1933 show that people who talk about their intentions are less likely to make them happen![2]

Announcing your plans to others, satisfies your self-identity just enough so that you are less motivated to do the hard work that is needed to make it happen.

In 1933, W. Mahler found that if a person announced the solution to a problem, and was acknowledged by others, it was registered in the brain as a "social reality", even if the solution hadn't actually been achieved. NYU psychology professor Peter Gollwitzer found that **those who kept their intentions private were more likely to achieve them,** than those who made them public and were acknowledged by others. This is one of the secrets of the ultra rich.

Once you've told people of your intentions, it gives you a "premature sense of completeness." So, keep that energy within you, for any goal. I have found that when I set a goal, if I don't tell anyone about it, the energy just builds and builds inside me so that I just *have* to do something about it and manifest it. But if I tell someone anything about what I am going to do, the energy goes out. It feels much like the air going out of a balloon.

When you feel that you just *have* to tell someone – just *don't*. Take that energy instead and use it to make the goal *come true*!

2. GROW SOME HERBS

Fresh herbs are easy to grow, and make ordinary meals very tasty & satisfying, especially if you are having a raw meal. Best of all, when you grow herbs, or lettuce, you don't have to wait for them to actually produce something, like you have to do if you grow something like to-matoes. Just snip off what leaves you want, and let it keep on growing. This way, you can have fresh, tasty, truly organic food frequently. You might be amazed at the difference that fresh herbs and greens make, compared to even an organic salad bought from the store. Your own plants are so much more satisfying. Somehow, something is missing from the store-bought organic salads, probably because a lot are grown hydroponically and not in living soil, with all of its microbes, which are part of what we need.

If you have an outdoor area, make a raised garden bed. Concrete blocks are easy, cheap, don't rot and you can fill the holes in the blocks with soil, and plant herbs in them. If you don't have a yard, you can still grow herbs. Just get a few containers. Even just one will do wonders for you. Just get started.

Suggested plants to start with are:

- Basil (grows like a weed).
- Lettuce (coz is healthier than iceberg).
- Italian parsley.
- Mesclun.

A good place to look for cheap seeds is online. Try Ebay.com and AmericanMeadows.com. If you get into this in a big way, then you can get supplies from GrowersSupply.com.

3. HOW DO YOU KNOW YOU ARE HUNGRY?

I used to think I was hungry because my belly did not have food in it, so it was a shock for me to learn from my kinesiologist/ naturopathic teacher David Bridgman that this is not how to tell when you are hungry. You see, your belly is not meant to be constantly processing food. It's quite exhausting for it to do so. It's good for it to have a rest now and again. You will remember in the chapter on leptin that one of the rules is to have three meals a day, but no snacks.

The real way to tell if you are hungry is: If you think of something raw and nutritious, do you start salivating in your mouth? If not, then you are not hungry. Whatever you are feeling is something else, such as an urge from some addictive substance, or simply a new feeling that you are not used to yet, such as a stomach that does not have its walls pushed out.

Therefore, before you reach for some food, see if you are salivating at the thought of raw, healthy food, to give you more feedback. If not, maybe you are just dehydrated and need a glass of reverse osmosis water instead. Remember from the chapter on water how most of us have bodies that do not distinguish between thirst and hunger.

If you are still hungry, how long has it been since you had some parasite-killing herbs, or food grade diatomaceous earth, or used the Hulda Clark zapper? Anytime I start getting hungry, I believe it's usually from parasites, because using one of these usually fixes it. Although sometimes it's because I've had too much high-sugar fruit.

If you are still hungry after drinking water, have some brazil nuts, or spirulina or chlorella. Massively good nutrition will also get rid of those hunger pangs.

4. EAT OFF A SMALLER PLATE AT DINNERTIME

Studies have shown that if you eat off a smaller plate, you will eat less and still feel as full as if you had eaten off a bigger plate.

5. EAT ONLY WHEN SITTING

Never eat when standing, and preferably not when in the car. Also, don't eat when you are doing something else. Focus on your food so that you know that you ate something.

6. THINK THIN

You are not fat. And you are not a victim of your genetics. You just have some toxins to remove from your body and your habits. Think and act like a thin person. Tell your body that you love it. Write a goodbye letter to your fat self. Look at thin clothes and know they are coming to you.

7. BREATHE DEEP

Unfortunately, sucking in our bellies is yet another reason why we are getting fatter, because it helps to prevent intake of more oxygen[3]. Breathe deep into your belly to get more oxygen to your cells. This is extra important as the amount of oxygen in the atmosphere goes down every year, from destruction of trees and plankton in the ocean.

Instead of sucking in your belly, rotate your pelvis forward, so that it is directly underneath your neck. This will rock your belly back onto the pelvis, so that is it not so visible. Good posture can do wonders for improving appearance. Another posture tip from "Alexander technique" is to focus on the back of the top of your head, and lift it up and back as far as possible.

8. DON'T EAT LESS FOOD EVERYDAY

Studies conducted by Dr. Krista Varady Ph.D., an assistant professor of kinesiology and nutrition at the University of Illinois, reveal that reducing calories on alternating days, and eating as much as you want in between, can trigger weight loss of up to 80 pounds in 8 to 10 weeks[4]. If you want to get thinner, have less food, but do not do it every day, or your body will figure out that you have a pattern of starving, and adapt to your reduced level of calories, without making you thinner.

9. BLOATED BELLY? SUSPECT CANDIDA

If you have a bloated belly, part of the problem could be an over-growth of *Candida albicans*. Candida is a fungus that occurs naturally in our bodies and is needed for digestion. Normally it is kept under control by "good bacteria". However, antibiotics kill 'good' as well as 'bad' bacteria, and other things make it grow like crazy, particularly sugar, caffeine and yeast, which is in many foods including bread and vinegar. Besides bloated belly, it can cause a whole host of other symptoms, including fatigue and acne.

My experience is that the best way to heal an overgrowth of Candida is to take some quality probiotics (good bacteria, available from a health food store) and give up all sugar, caffeine and yeast (which is in many foods including vinegar, bread and cheese) for at least 3 weeks. In addition if you can manage it, it works great to do the kinesiology Candida correction which I teach in *Perfect Health with Kinesiology and Muscle Testing*. I have even had women clients come in who were feeling itchy between their legs, have the itch totally stop by the end of a session when I have done this correction!

One other common cause of a bloated belly is gas from fermenting sugars, often from fruit. Reduce the amount of high sugar foods you eat.

10. DON'T COOK HOTTER THAN 350°F

The higher the temperature, and the longer the food is cooked, the more toxins it will have, and the less nutrition. When I was growing up, food was cooked at 350°F. But over the years I have seen people recommending hotter and hotter ovens, so that now even 425°F is recommended. Don't do this. If you are going to use the oven, keep the temperature no higher than 350°F.

11. NO CHEWING GUM

Firstly, you should not have chewing gum because it has either sugar or artificial sweeteners, and both are toxic. But, in addition, chewing gum messes up your digestive system. When you chew, you are telling your body that food is on its way, and so the stomach starts pumping out acids to digest what food that it thinks is coming, but never arrives. Your body does not like you doing that. Besides, even a very beautiful woman who chews gum, looks like a cow chewing the cud.

12. WORDS HAVE POWER

Words have power. They speak to your subconscious mind, which controls your body. So don't talk about "losing" weight. If you do, you very well might find it again one day. Instead use the words "reducing" weight or fat.

13. DON'T FALL FOR "INSTANT WEIGHT LOSS" PRODUCT SCAMS

There's a new one out all the time. There is no one product which is going to give you the body you want, but that doesn't stop criminals from making up a great story, fake pictures and even bribing people to promote their product, because they know that most people want a magic pill and something easy. They are promoting a fantasy, a lie. You need a wholistic approach and good habits instead.

14. EAT SLOWER AND EAT LESS

It takes time for your brain to let you know that you have had enough. Give your body time to get those signals. This is especially important for people who are overweight, because they very likely have leptin resistance, and until this is healed, they usually don't feel satisfied eating a normal amount. Slow down, chew more and work out ahead how much you will have. Be strong for 20 minutes, because it could take your body 10-20 minutes after the meal is over before your brain tells you that you have had enough[5]. This is particularly important to do at dinner time.

Remember that studies of animals which had their caloric intake reduced by one third, lived 30-80% longer. That is the equivalent of a human living 160-220 years old[6]. That may sound crazy, but there have been numerous studies that suggest that people should be able to live to 140 years old[7,8,9] at least.

15. CONSIDER THE TOXINS ON YOUR SKIN

Your skin absorbs what you put on it. You know that because a number of drugs these days are given in the form of patches[10]. Ultimately, you should not put anything on your skin that you would not want in your mouth. So:

1. Get some hypoallergenic gloves for washing dishes, such as Kimberley-Clark nitrile gloves (I got a rash from the normal rubber gloves being sold).

2. Try shea soap or African black soap.

3. Wear a respirator when cleaning the shower or mowing the lawn.

4. Read the ingredients of your shampoo, and try washing your hair less often.

5. Consider omitting conditioner.

6. Reduce the amount of makeup you use, and look for healthier options.

7. Rinse thoroughly all surfaces cleaned with detergent or chemicals, including benches, floors and toys.

16. DO DRY SKIN BRUSHING

There is nothing more important than having good eating, drinking and exercise habits. But once you have done that, an extra habit that is said by many to beautify and energize you, and to remove cellulite, is dry skin brushing, for at least one minute a day. The skin is an important organ for detoxing. Skin brushing helps clean toxins out of the lymphatic system. Remember how toxins collect in the lymph system but can only move out of the lymph if the muscles around them move. If you think about belly fat, that is going to be harder to do than in the legs. So give your lymphatic system a boost with regular skin brushing. People have reported that skin brushing made their skin soft and glowing, that cellulite disappeared and that they felt noticeably more alive. You need a stiff, almost scratchy skinbrush which costs around $8. Do skin brushing daily before a bath or shower. The brush must be dry. Start at the feet and brush the feet and legs towards the heart, at a steady speed. Brush your belly, hips and buttocks towards the heart. Brush the hands and arms towards the heart. Especially work on problem areas.

SKIN BRUSHING BEAUTY TIP

For your face, I read of two women who looked years younger using a soft toothbrush on the face, in circular movements. Brush up the neck. When doing around the eyes, start at the bridge of the nose, go up and around to the outside of the eyes and then come down and into the nose.

This comment was posted on the internet:

"I lost 20 pounds in 3 months with dry skin brushing alone. I'm 52 years old and my husband noticed my skin felt so much softer after a few weeks of skin brushing".[11]

17. KEEP A FOOD DIARY

People who write down everything they eat and drink reduce twice as much weight as those who do not[12]. It's possible that one reason this works is because it gives you feedback as to what is toxic and allergic for you.

REFERENCES

1. *Woman's World*, 9/14/99

2. sivers.org/zipit

3. *First* magazine, 4/3/06

4. *First for Women* magazine, 10/31/11

5. *Mastering Leptin*, by Byron Richards CCN, 2002, 3rd edition '09, pg 144

6. *The Rosedale Diet*, by Dr Ron Rosedale M.D., page 43

7. www.dailymail.co.uk/sciencetech/article-1290993/Found-natures-freezer-secret-living-140.html

8. newyork.cbslocal.com/2012/02/14/could-the-next-generation-live-to-be-150/

9. www.chinadaily.com.cn/life/2013-03/11/content_16298196.htm

10. en.wikipedia.org/wiki/Transdermal_patch

11. drjessechappus.com/dry-skin-brushing-benefits-and-technique/

12. www.webmd.com/diet/news/20080708/keeping-food-diary-helps-lose-weight

CHAPTER 52

YOUR NEW SHOPPING LIST

I am going to show you how to make this new way of living easy. *The most important key* to making this plan work for you for life is to *already have* all the good food you need in your house. If you have to look up a recipe, and then shop for that recipe, then it becomes way too complicated, and you won't do enough of it to replace the processed and toxic food you have been eating.

Once you have bought plenty of food from the following list, this is all you have to do before any meal: Just look at what fresh or dried food you have, go to a search engine on the internet, put in "recipe, vegan" or "recipe, raw" and list some of the items you want to use, and see what comes up. You can also search for "recipe, vegetarian" and leave out or replace the dairy. E.g. search on "cabbage ginger recipe vegan". Print out favorite recipes and keep them in a ring binder.

Eventually you will learn to prepare food without recipes. You just throw it all together! The key is in having the right ingredients available with you in the first place. So, I am going to give you the shopping list you need.

Please make sure you read the rules at the start of the Recipe chapter. Please note: Obviously, do not buy anything that you hate or that you think you may have an allergy to. See my chapter on allergies for more information. But, please, be adventurous and try out plants you have never eaten before. You may be surprised to find that they become your favorites.

NON-FOOD ITEMS

The first things I recommend you buy are the following. If you can't get all these yet, that's okay. Just keep it in mind that you are aiming to get them.

1. **A good magnifying glass.** This is essential for reading the list of ingredients on foods, to avoid toxins, preservatives and especially anything that could contain GMOs. Do not buy anything, even trail mix or bulk food, without reading the ingredients. There is way too much toxic packaged food, even in 'health' food stores! You may be surprised at how many times things such as GMO corn, sugar, canola, GMO soy and MSG get sneaked into even so-called 'healthy' food. It doesn't matter what the label says on the front, back or sides. The only thing that matters is the list of ingredients.

2. **A good food processor.** Make sure it's a quality one. It is going to get a work out, and the cheap ones aren't powerful enough to grind up tough food like nuts and dates.

3. **A good blender.** For raw smoothies.

4. **A juicer.** A good juicer will pay for itself in the long run, because other juicers waste a lot of money and work from inefficient juicing. If you can't afford that yet, get a cheap one until you can go deluxe. There is no perfect juicer that will perform every juicing operation with equal quality. Some are messier and easier to clean than others. Search the internet for reviews and consider before purchasing:

- Can it juice all plants, such as carrots and greens?
- Ease of cleaning. How messy is it?
- Noise level (loud noises hurt your hearing long term).
- Speed of juicing.

- Length of warranty.
- Does it make ice cream from frozen fruit?
- How efficient is it, in terms of wasted juice.

4. **A wok.** Non-aluminum.

5. **Stainless steel or ceramic cookware**. Throw out all the microwave, non-stick, aluminum and plastic cookware. They are toxic.

6. **Half gallon containers** with lids. Several dozen, for all the new seeds, nuts, flour and legumes you are going to add to your pantry. You can get these in PET plastic or HDP plastic at www.Uline.com.

7. **Big Asian soup bowls.** You want a bowl that holds enough liquid for a main meal. Asian soup bowls hold over three times the amount of a normal soup bowl. You can use these for vegetable stews, Asian meals with liquid and also for giant salads.

8. **A set of scales that measures in tenths of a pound**. Yes, you can get thinner while you don't get lighter, but the more feedback you have, the better. If you find that you put on 2 pounds from the day before, chances are you ate something toxic that your body did not like. It's great to see regular reductions in weight, even if it's just 0.2 pounds, but if your scale only measures in half pounds, then you won't see this change.

9. **Ear muffs** to protect your hearing when blending. It can be noisy, and the cumulative effect of a lot of machinery damages hearing. Studies have found that hearing loss is caused by loud noises, not by aging[1].

10). **Good carving knife and Sharpener**. It's essential that you have a very sharp, large knife, and that you can keep it sharp. You will be using it a lot.

FOOD SHOPPING LIST

Do you love food? If so, then you have all that it takes to be a great cook, if you aren't already one, especially when you are preparing food this new way. See my recipe chapter for a few basic ideas on what to do for any meal.

All that you have to do to be a great cook is open containers, cut up the food that you like the taste of, mix it together and sometimes do a few extra things that a recipe will tell you about. It's easy. It's not rocket science. You just have to want to do it.

Going on a totally raw diet for a while taught me to never be afraid of a recipe. Basically, on the raw diet, you take raw plant food, chop or blend them up, mix them together and then eat them. Sometimes you might dehydrate some of them, but basically that is it. You just get some plants, mix them together, and eat them. Simple. Same thing if you want to turn it into a stew or stir fry. That is why you can do this. Anytime you want to heat something, just cook it as little as possible (I am assuming that you are not including any meat that has to be cooked properly to kill dangerous germs and parasites).

The following is a suggested shopping list only, to get you started. By all means, add to it. Suggested suppliers for these products are:

- Health food stores.
- The Internet.
- Supermarkets.
- Asian food stores.
- Indian food stores.
- Farmers' markets.

VEGETABLES, FRESH

Buy fresh produce depending on the recipe, but I suggest you keep in the fridge at all times most of the following-
- Avocado (Get at least two, even if they are expensive).
- Bean sprouts (mung beans, not soy beans).
- Cabbage (Try different sorts, such as Napa & Savoy).

- Carrots.
- Cauliflower.
- Celeriac (good replacement for potatoes).
- Celery.
- Cucumbers (very alkalizing). I like the baby/pickling cucumbers best.
- NO GARLIC (use ginger instead).
- Ginger.
- Greens (eg: kale, collard greens, choys, spinach)
- Green beans (use them soon so they are fresh).
- Kohl-Rabi (good replacement for potato).
- Leeks (much tastier than onions).
- Lettuce (Coz has more nutrition than iceberg).
- Onions (Sweet onions won't make you cry when cutting them).
- Salad mix. (I suggest, without arugula - it gives me headaches. This is a clue that it's toxic. Therefore it could do the same for others as well.
- Snow peas.
- Squash. Butternut is great. Try other varieties as well.
- Sweet potato.
- Tomatoes (Small amounts. Red plants have toxins. A lot of people are allergic to tomatoes, especially cooked tomatoes, and reduce weight when they give them up).
- Lemons & Limes. Get some plastic bottles of 100% lemon or lime juice, in addition to fresh fruit.
- Zucchinis MUST be organic or they could be GMO.

A NOTE ABOUT POTATOES:

There is one plant which I suggest you don't have until you are at your desired size, and that is potato. Potatoes seem to have a lot of toxins in them, such as lectins, which is maybe why people seem to be addicted to them. Plus they have a high glycemic index, and many people are allergic to them. A 20 year Harvard study of 120,000 people found that the most fattening foods were potato chips, potatoes, sugar-sweetened drinks, red meat and processed meat[2].

FRUIT, FRESH

- Apples*.
- Bananas. Organic only, whenever possible, so they have not been gassed with ethylene, which is used in blowtorches. Have these only as treats, as many people are allergic to them.
- Bilberries.
- Blueberries.
- Cherries*.
- Dragon fruit (from Asian stores).
- Grapes*. Red are more healthy. Use to jazz up a salad or raw soup.
- Kiwifruit.
- Nectarines*.
- Oranges.
- Passionfruit.
- Peaches, if you can find some that are juicy, which is tough to do.
- Pears*.
- Pineapple (only occasionally, as it can irritate).
- Plums*.
- Pomegranate.
- Raspberries.
- Sapotas (it is ripe when you can press your thumb gently into it).
- Strawberries* (Small amounts. Red plants have toxins).
- Watermelon (Small amounts only. Red plants have toxins).

- NO Papaya - unless it's organic, as it could be GMO.

*Preferably organic. Organic produce has about twice the nutrition as ordinary fruit. But it is far, far better to have non-organic than none at all.

HERBS, FRESH

These can be ridiculously expensive. It is best to grow these yourself, even if all you can manage is one container. You can buy cheap seeds from www.AmericanMeadows.com or ebay.com. My Asian store has very fresh herbs for about 1/4 the price of the supermarket.

- Basil, Italian (Stores seem to think of this as a herb, rather than a staple, so they price accordingly. It's best to grow this yourself or ask the Asian store to get it. It grows very easily. Fantastic in salads).
- Chervil (has high potassium).
- Chives (these enliven any savory meal).
- Cilantro (USA)/ Fresh coriander (Europe/Australia). (For heavy metal detoxing & spicing up any dish).
- Italian Parsley.
- Mint.

SEEDS - RAW

Most important, because they provide good fats, kill your hunger and help you to get thin.

- Chia seeds (for omega 3 – essential for fat loss).
- Flax seeds, ground, organic, so that they are not GMO (for omega 3 – essential for fat loss. Some people say that unground flax seeds are indigestible, and the ground ones certainly seem more filling).
- Pumpkin seeds ('pepitas').
- Sesame seeds, hulled (Purchase by the pound, not by the ounce).
- Sunflower Seeds (Very cheap).

No hemp seeds. Muscle testing indicates that there are, not surprisingly, toxins in them that we should avoid.

NUTS - RAW

Provide good fats, kill your hunger and help you to get thin. Raw nuts can be purchased from health food stores and online.

- Almonds, slivered (grind them to make almond flour for

grainfree baking).
- Almonds, whole (be aware that as of time of printing, so-called 'natural' or 'raw' almonds in the USA are not raw. They have all been killed with pasteurization).
- Brazil (Have fat burning Omega 3s).
- Cashews (Good replacement for dairy).
- Pistachios (Add great flavor to anything).
- Walnuts / Pecans.

Avoid peanuts, as they are quite toxic. Make your own nut/seeds butters with a little good oil and without peanuts instead.

FRUIT, DRIED

- Apricot.
- Cherries (pitted) (Tart cherries are best[3]).
- Dates (pitted).
- Figs.
- Goji Berries (super nutritious).
- Pomegranate (super nutritious).
- Prunes.
- Raisins, organic (go easy on these).

FLOUR

- Almond flour (It's much cheaper to grind your own blanched almonds).
- Amaranth flour.
- Brown rice flour.
- Coconut flour.
- Einkorn flour.
- Millet flour.
- Oat flour (If you can have some gluten).
- Tapioca flour (use for thickening and egg replacement).

No wheat, spelt or white flour (they are all wheat flour)

STAPLES

Important: Always soak lentils, beans, oatmeal and whole grain flours in reverse osmosis water for 8 hours before using, to break down the phytates which block absorption of minerals. You may be amazed at how much more satisfying and easily digestible they become when you do this.

Note that lentils seem to be a lot more slimming and healthier than beans for most people. Many upper class people in India have lived off a vegetarian diet based mostly on lentils, with great success, for hundreds of years.

- *Basmati rice, preferably brown (lower glycemic index than other rice).
- Brown rice noodles.
- Chickpeas (Garbanzo beans).
- Dried Beans (black, kidney, pinto, navy etc.).
- Lentils, green, red, try other sorts (lentils are better than beans).
- Millet.
- Moong dal (split mung beans, very yummy) (look online).
- Shirataki noodles. Made of pure fiber, they have zero calories! (may be cheapest online). *First* magazine had stories about women who lost 24, 55, 60 and even 121 pounds using shirataki noodles!

*Only get this if you believe that it is not GMO or being affected by radiation from the Japan Fukushima disaster or other sources. Otherwise, use millet instead.

PRODUCE, FROZEN

- Blueberries (lots of these!).
- Brussels Sprouts.
- Cherries.
- Coconut, shredded (No sugar. check other ingredients).
- Corn (ONLY if it's organic so it's GMO free).

- Mango.
- Peas.
- Raspberries (small amounts. Red plants have toxins).
- Spinach / other green plants.

HERBS / SPICES, DRIED

- Basil.
- Cinnamon.
- Coriander.
- Cumin.
- Dill.
- Fenegreek (really delicious spice for Indian recipes. Look online).
- Ginger.
- Italian herbs.
- Lemongrass (frozen or fresh from the Asian store).

EXTRA FLAVOR

- Horseradish (without preservatives). Not for people with any digestive tract problems.
- Liquid mustard (without sweeteners etc. Use only on occasion, because it is very irritating. Not for people with any digestive tract problems, hemorrhoids or pain).
- Vinegar, *only* made totally from non GMO foods, such as red wine, white wine or rice.

SWEETENERS

Go very easy on these, or omit completely when serious about getting thin.

- Coconut sugar (for very rare treats).
- Maple syrup, 100%.
- Molasses, organic, so it's not from GMOs.
- Raw honey (Not grown near GMO corn fields).

No artificial sweeteners of any kind. No Agave syrup. It is worse than high fructose corn syrup. No Stevia: It tastes and acts like artificial sweeteners.

MISCELLANEOUS

- Almond Milk (containers stored in the fridge are better than ones on the shelf, but get some long-life ones on the shelf for emergencies).
- Cans of coconut milk or coconut cream, with no preservatives.
- Celtic sea salt *(essential to get)*.
- Dried sun-dried tomatoes (with nothing else except maybe some citric acid). (Nuts.com has good prices).
- Grape vine leaves in glass jars, not canned.
- Olives, Black or Green, pitted. It's hard to find good ones because most are in bad oils (see the chapter on oils). Canned olives are heated.

OILS

Available mostly from health food stores.

- Coconut oil (virgin is a lot better and a lot tastier. Check out www.VitaCost.com for good prices and free shipping).
- Ghee (If you are not allergic to dairy. Only organic & grassfed, or from countries where cows are not fed GMO's.
- Cold-pressed sesame oil.
- Cold-pressed avocado oil.
- Extra virgin olive oil *only* if you can *guarantee* that it is 100% extra virgin. This might mean you have to visit a farm directly. Do not trust any beautiful looking label. 70% of the world's "extra virgin" olive oil is 'lampant' oil, which is so toxic it's good only for lighting lamps, and/or other toxic oils including Genetically Modified oils[4].
- Cold-pressed sunflower, safflower or flax oil. Do not cook with these. These are for mayonnaise / a little on salads / making

nut butter.

- Cold pressed almond oil. For making nut butters.

EGGS, ONLY FREE RANGE AND ORGANIC

Organic eggs are from chickens who are meant to be fed non-GMO grains. Non-organic factory eggs are toxic pills, because the chickens are fed lots of GMOs as well as toxic and gross stuff from rendering plants etc.

Hopefully you would want your eggs to be free range because you don't want to be responsible for keeping a poor chicken in a cruel wire cage which hurts her feet, and where she can't even stretch her wings, let alone enjoy life. However, there is an advantage to you in free-range over factory eggs, besides the great reduction in the lack of toxins. Free-range is full of a whole lot more nutrients, which will help to decrease your hunger and give your body the means to get rid of toxins and fat. For example, free-range eggs have 50% more folic acid and 30% more Vitamin E and B12 than factory eggs[5].

BUTTER

Salted, organic butter, preferrably cultured or butter from a country that does not grow or import GMO foods.

Only get butter if you are not allergic to it and can therefore lose weight eating it, or if you want it for the other people who don't have weight problems.

Cultured butter is most delicious, and how butter used to be when people had less weight problems. You can recognize it, even if it doesn't say 'cultured butter', because the ingredients will say it contains a culture. Plus it is very golden in color, and soft.

HERBAL TEA

- Chaga (wild mushroom that grows on birch trees. Helps grow muscle).
- Chamomile (to absorb estrogen).

- Tulsi (healing).

SUPPLEMENTS

Note: A large glass of fresh squeezed vegetable and fruit juice will give a lot more vitamins and minerals than any pill, plus hundreds of other nutrients.

- Chlorella tablets.
- Liquid kelp drops, for iodine.
- Magnesium chloride, food or aquarium grade, for foot baths.
- Magnesium chloride, oral supplement.
- MSM (methylsulfonylmethane - organic sulfur). Add to your juice.
- Probiotics, with more species than just acidophilus. I suggest iFlora by Sedona Labs. Share at least one bottle with your family, to refarm your intestines with good bacteria. There should be no need to take them all the time.
- Spirulina tablets (great for providing nutrients when your brain gets tired, or you get low blood sugar). Tablets are a lot easier to consume than powder.
- Vitamin D. I suggest 2,000 IU. Megafoods brand.
- Zinc Tally by Metagenics.

TREATS / OCCASIONAL USE IN MAINTENANCE PLAN

- Yogurt – organic only so it's not GMO.
- Cottage cheese – full cream - organic only so it's not GMO.
- Cream cheese – organic only so it's not GMO.
- Millet bread, buns, bagels, lavache (From health food store. Make sure you check the other ingredients).
- Oatmeal (soak, dilute with nuts etc.).
- Potato chips cooked in avocado oil (Use very rarely. See recipe).

A FINAL NOTE

1. Be sure to take *You're not fat, You're toxic* with you when you shop, so that you can easily find what you need.

2. Remember to take a cooler and an ice pack with you when shopping so that your cold food doesn't get warm and to prevent the melting / re-freezing cycle that ruins frozen fruit.

REFERENCES
1. well.blogs.nytimes.com/2013/03/25/what-causes-hearing-loss/
2. *Woman's World*, 1/30/12, page 18
3. www.naturalnews.com/033443_cherries_pain_remedies.html
4. *Extra Virginity* by Tom Mueller, 2011
5. *Transdermal Magnesium Therapy*, by Mark Sircus, Ac, M.D., 2007

CHAPTER 53

SUMMARY FOR
PERMANENT FAT REDUCTION

MAIN RULES:

1. Purchase the foods on the shopping list. If you can't think how to make them into a meal, go to a search engine on the internet and put in the words, for example "vegan recipe" or "raw recipe" and the ingredients that you want to use. Print favorite recipes and keep them in a ring binder.

2. Have no toxic foods. The main ones are in the table below, with alternatives. Remember that while you need never go hungry, you are breaking *real addictions,* which need some extra will power for a while.

3. Drink only water (reverse osmosis or spring water), like wild animals do. No flavored drinks at all. Drink 6-8, 8 oz. glasses a day. Two 8 oz. glasses should be drunk *before* breakfast. Children should also drink good water before eating.

4. Drink at least one 8 oz. glass of fresh-squeezed vegetable plus

occasionally a little fruit juice with a meal at least once a day. Always include some leafy greens (not lettuce). Drink within 15 minutes of juicing, before enzymes break down. A fresh-squeezed juice every day is very important because our bodies do not get energy from burning fuel like a car does, but from complicated chemical reactions that require a good supply of nutrients. Fresh juice supplies the nutrients to turn fat to energy.

5. Have three meals a day.

6. No snacks. If you must snack, it must be raw seeds and nuts, or spirulina or chlorella tablets.

7. No wheat at any time. Go easy on grains, or best of all, avoid them totally as well, until you are at your ideal body size. Whole grains and flours to be soaked for 8 hours before using, to break down toxins.

8. Lentils and beans should be soaked for 8 hours before using, to sprout them, which breaks down toxins and makes them more digestible. Lentils are more slimming than beans.

9. Have some raw plant food with every meal.

10. Have at least one totally raw plant meal every day.

11. If you are really keen to get thin, have a whole day where all meals are totally raw plants, once a week or more often.

12. Use Celtic sea salt or sun-dried sea salt that is moist. Do not use ordinary table salt or ordinary sea salt that is not moist.

13. Get at least 8-10 hours sleep a night. Get more if you owe your body sleep. You should have enough sleep so that it takes you at least 20 minutes to fall asleep (without the effect of caffeine or bright lights before bed). Get to bed as soon before midnight as possible.

14. Do not ever microwave anything, even water. Ask at restaurants to see if they microwave their food. Throw away your microwave oven.

Category	<u>DO NOT</u> eat/ drink	<u>DO</u> eat/drink	Have occasionally for treats
Grains	Wheat. White flour. Soy. Jasmine rice. White rice. Corn (Limited organic is okay, so it's not GMO).		*(Preferably soak whole grains & flours 8-24 hours first)* Amaranth. Basmati rice (preferably brown). Buckwheat. Einkorn. Millet. Oatmeal (very limited amounts). Quinoa. Teff. Try to avoid (for gluten): Rye, Barley.
Soy	Any soy that is not GMO free and is not fermented, including: Soy flour. Soy oil.	Soy lecithin MUST be organic so it's not GMO.	Some fermented organic GMO-free soy products are okay, including: Soy sauce. Tamari. Tofu (no more than, say, once in 2 weeks).

Category	DO NOT eat/drink	DO eat/drink	Have occasionally for treats
Meat	Meat. Chicken. Animals / birds.	*Have instead:* Vegetables. Fruit. Nuts. Seeds. Soaked Legumes.	
Fish and Seafood	Fish. Seafood.	*Have instead:* Vegetables. Fruit. Nuts. Seeds. Soaked Legumes.	
Dairy	Milk. Cheese. Yogurt. Whey. Ice cream.	Almond milk. Organic, salted butter, preferably cultured.	*(MUST be organic so it's not from GMO-fed cows)* Cottage Cheese. Cream Cheese. Yogurt. Raw cream.
Eggs	Normal eggs (they are GMO and full of toxins).	Organic, free range eggs.	
Legumes		Soak lentils & beans for 8 hours before using. You can also eat them raw after soaking. Lentils are more slimming than beans.	

Category	DO NOT eat/drink	DO eat/drink	Have occasionally for treats
Vegetables	Potatoes (use pumpkin, sweet potato, celeriac or kohl-rabi instead).	Most vegetables. Beets & zucchini must be organic so they are not GMO. Have raw, leafy greens every day. Work to include anti-estrogenic vegetables, namely - Broccoli (organic is best). Brussels sprouts. Cabbage. Cauliflower.	Some potatoes may be possible when you are at your ideal size.
Fruit	Cooked fruit. Canned fruit.	All raw fruit.	Go easy on: Grapes. Watermelon. Bananas (organic so they are not gassed). Dried fruit.
Nuts	Peanuts (actually a legume).	All nuts, preferably raw. Get some brazils for Omega 3s.	
Seeds		All seeds, especially sunflower and pumpkin. Flax should be ground and organic. Get chia and flax seeds for Omega 3s.	

Category	DO NOT eat/ drink	DO eat/drink	Have occa-sionally for treats
Drinks	Any bottled drinks including sodas & sports drinks. Alcohol.	Reverse osmosis or spring water, 6-8 eight oz glasses a day. Especially drink *2 glasses before breakfast.*	
Sweeteners	Any sweetener except for the ones in the allowed column, including: Agave nectar. Aspartame. AminoSweet. NutraSweet. Corn syrup. Fructose. High fructose corn syrup. Maltitol. Saccharin. Sorbitol. Splenda. Stevia. Sucralose. Sugar. "Sugar-free" products. Xylitol.	*Tiny* amounts of : Raw honey. Maple syrup (100%). Organic molasses (so they are not GMO).	Coconut sugar
Juice	Processed, bottled juice.	Fresh squeezed juice. Mostly vegetable with leafy greens. Limit the amount of fruit.	

Category	DO NOT eat/drink	DO eat/drink	Have occasionally for treats
Genetically Modified Food	Up to date of printing, this list includes in the USA: Alfalfa. Canola. Chicken. Corn. Cottonseed. Dairy. Eggs. Meat. Papaya. Salmon. Soy. Zucchini. (Rice & potato in other countries).		
Restaurant Food	Virtually all restaurants.	Bring your own. Eat a ton of food before you go. If you are travelling, do things like go to a supermarket and make a giant fruit and nut salad.	Restaurants that tell you what is in the food, don't use GMOs, bad oils, or any of the foods listed in the "Do not eat" column.
Microwaved Foods	Microwaved food and water. Ask first as restaurants, microwave a lot of food.	To heat or defrost, use a stainless steel saucepan, with a lid, and add a little water.	

Category	DO NOT eat/drink	DO eat/drink	Have occasionally for treats
Cooked Foods	Steam rather than boil. Bake rather than fry. Stir fry for only a minute, just enough to heat the food up a little. Add what ever you can think of raw just before serving, including the seed mix.	Eat more raw food. See the recipes chapter. Make raw soups. Blend fruit and/or vegetables and nuts or seeds in a blender. Add hot water to make them seem like cooked food. Learn a new raw recipe every few days.	
Processed Foods	Processed foods.	Don't pay for "value added" food. Make your own.	
Fast Food	Fast foods.	Pack food in a container.	
Flavor Enhancers	All of them, including: MSG. Glutamate. Hydrolyzed vegetable protein.	Never use them.	
Food Colorings	All of them.	Something that is purely part of a plant (that's non-GMO).	
"Natural" Flavorings.	Best to avoid. There is no saying what these are.		
Preservatives	All of them.		

Category	DO NOT eat/ drink	DO eat/drink	Have occasionally for treats
Caffeine.	All caffeine including: Tea-black, green, puerh, oolong. Coffee. Chocolate. Cocoa. Energy drinks. Guarana. Sodas. Ask your doctor about medications. De-caf. Kola nuts. Yerba mate. Ma huang (ephedra).	Chamomile tea. Tulsi tea. Herbal teas. Chaga.	
Salt	Table salt Any salt that is not moist.	Celtic sea salt. Sun-dried whole sea salt, that is moist.	

FATS AND OILS

Eat lots of these RAW, to promote fat loss & health.	Eat a little of these if desired, RAW ONLY	Use only these for COOKING, and that in moderation	DON'T EAT, EVER
Raw seeds, e.g. pumpkin, sunflower, sesame. **Raw nuts**, e.g. walnuts, almonds, cashews, brazil nuts. Especially use raw **chia** and **flax** seeds on different meals. **Coconut oil.** **Extra virgin olive oil**, but only if you can *totally trust* the source (which outlaws most olive oil). **Avocado.**	Flax oil. MUST have been kept in the fridge. **Safflower oil**, expeller or cold-pressed only. **Sunflower oil**, expeller or cold-pressed only. **Organic or non-gmo salted butter**, if you can eat it and still lose weight. Preferably cultured butter.	**Coconut oil.** **Sesame oil**, unrefined, cold-pressed or expeller pressed. **Peanut, almond or cashew oil**, unrefined, cold-pressed or expeller pressed. **Avocado oil.** **Extra virgin olive oil**, but only if you can *totally trust* the source. **Organic or non-gmo salted butter**, if you can eat it and still lose weight. Preferably cultured butter. **Ghee**, non-GMO	Anything deep fried. Margarine. Trans fats. Hydrogenated fats. Corn oil (It's gmo). Soy oil (it's toxic and gmo). Canola (it's toxic and gmo). Cottonseed oil (it's super toxic and gmo). Vegetable oil.

DAILY TIMETABLE

Wake up:

- Weigh yourself. And feel yourself to see if you feel thinner. Record it.

- Once a week, try on a smaller pair of pants than you normally wear.

- Spend 1-8 minutes doing the Five Tibetan Rites if you can do them without producing any pain. Remember, no pain, real gain.

- If you need something to get you going, have a shower, get your head wet, and before getting out of the shower, have a few seconds of water that is as cold as you can bear.

Before breakfast:

- Drink 2, 8 oz. glasses of reverse osmosis water. This is one of the most important things to do. Your brain needs water for energy. If you don't give it enough, it will tell you to drink more, and most of us interpret thirst signals for hunger signals.

At one meal in the day:

- Drink a glass of fresh-squeeze vegetable juice, possibly with a little fruit. Omit the fruit if you are extra serious about getting thin.

Breakfast:

- See breakfast recipes in the recipe chapter.

Lunch:

- Have a salad with leafy greens in it, along with whatever else you want. Make lunch bigger, and dinner smaller. If you are going to have anything fattening, make sure you do it at *lunch* time. See recipes.

Dinner:

- See recipes.

Exercise:

1. Walk for 20-30 minutes, at least 5 times a week. After a five minute warm up period at your normal rate, speed up as fast as you can for 8 seconds and then walk at your normal speed for 12 seconds. The best times to walk are the times that are easiest for you to fit in a schedule. Walk to:

- Lower your set point.
- Clean out your toxins.
- Replace fat with muscle, that uses up to 25 times more energy.
- Restore leptin sensitivity, which gives your body a healthy shape.

2. If you sit down a lot, stand up and walk for a few minutes every hour.

3. Lift some light weights, and spend 1-8 minutes doing Five Tibetan Rites every day, if you can do so without creating pain, in order to:

- Signal to the body that you want to have more muscle, without damaging any muscle.
- "Use it or lose it".
- Open up and energize your energy centers and chakras, to stay young and energized.

One hour before bedtime:

- Turn off the computer. (The bright screen will keep you awake).

Bedtime:

- Get 8-10 hours of sleep a night (not just lying in bed). If you fall asleep before 20 minutes is up, get more sleep next time.

- Especially, get to bed as soon before midnight as possible.

Extra Rules for helping Thinness

1. Learn kinesiology and muscle testing. Get in balance so your body can work more efficiently.

2. Avoid the electromagnetic stress described in the chapter on electromagnetic stress.

3. Take a Vitamin D supplement and get at least one hour a week of direct sun over most of the body, including belly, when it's warm enough.

4. Have a magnesium footbath occasionally.

5. Consider parasite and organ cleanses.

6. Do the best you can to work out if there is a food that you are sensitive/allergic to. Accurate muscle testing can help greatly with this. It will be something that you eat or drink most days and probably do not want to go without. Give it up for at least 3 weeks to see what happens.

7. If there is a chance of you ever having a baby, read the chapter on pregnancy fat.

8. Watch the excellent documentaries *Super Size Me, Forks Over Knives, Food Inc.* & *The World According to Monsanto.*

9. Some psychologists believe that people generally have only a 90 day attention span, which means that they don't think much about things that happened over three months ago. Therefore, I ask you please to immediately write a note in your calendar to reread this book in three months time. If you do this, you will find that a lot of what I have said, then makes more sense to you. This will also help you to fine-tune your habits, so that you can get the beautiful, healthy body you deserve.

10. If you have benefited from this book, please help others by recommending it to a friend, and write a review on www.amazon.com.

CHAPTER 54

RECIPES
FOR FAT LOSS

RULE #1:

Buy most of the foods in the "Shopping List" Chapter.

RULE #2:

Anytime you need a recipe, see what plant food you have, go to a search engine on the internet, put in "recipe, vegan", "recipe, raw" or "recipe, vegetarian" and list some of the foods you want to use, and see what comes up. (For example, put in "recipe vegan cabbage lentils"). Print the recipe and store in a ring-binder with an alphabet divider. If it's a vegetarian recipe, just substitute or leave out the dairy.

RULE #3:

Here's a basic rule that I use for most dishes, including salads, soups, stews and stir-fry. You will note that almost all packaged goods use this formula. It's not necessary to do this, but you will find it makes food more interesting. Add something of each of these categories:

<u>SOUR</u>: Add a dash of something sour – fresh **lemon or lime juice** is best, but sometimes for variety you could add a **gourmet vinegar** such as red wine vinegar with raspberry (not made from any GMO foods).

<u>SWEET</u>: Add ¼ tsp. of a healthy sweetener. That is, **maple syrup, raw honey** or **cane molasses**. No agave nectar or stevia (see chapter on sugars).

<u>SALT</u>: **Celtic sea salt** to taste.

<u>SOMETHING TASTY</u>: Fresh herbs is best – **basil, dill, mint, cilantro** etc. For Asian dishes, also **ginger, lemongrass, spices**.

RULE #4:

Always soak all grains, flours and legumes for 8 or more hours first. Where possible, also soak nuts and seeds before use. Soaking sprouts the plant, and breaks down toxins, such as:

- Lectins which damage the intestine.

- Phytates which stop the absorption of minerals, including magnesium.

Soaking also breaks down complex compounds into simpler compounds, so that your body can use the nutrition more easily. After soaking, you can *store in the fridge* for several days. Just *rinse* whole plants (not flour) once a day, as they will be growing and producing waste products.

RULE #5:

No recipe is ever sacred. You are not cooking complicated French dishes. You can add or omit whatever you want to any recipe. Any plant food is food – you just have to put it in your mouth, just like a gorilla would.

RULE #6:

It would be beneficial to read all the recipes in this chapter. But if you are not going to do that, please at least read the recipes for "Juice", "Seed & Nut mix", "Breakfast" and "Salad, Stephanie's Sumptuous".

Note #1: Tablespoons are American size. An American tablespoon (Tbsp.) is half an Australian tablespoon. An American tablespoon equals 3 teaspoons.

Note #2: A lot of raw 'uncook' books require a dehydrator for many recipes. I recommend that you get a dehydrator eventually, because then you can make delicious thinning food, such as raw kale chips. For now, none of the following recipes needs a dehydrator.

RECIPES - Contents

Juice, Fresh-Squeezed	- Raw	590
Millet, rice replacement	- Cooked	591
Muffins, Grain-free	- Cooked	592
Muffins, Non-Wheat	- Cooked	593
Nut Butter	- Cooked & raw	594
Olive & Spinach Tapenade	- Partly raw	595
Olive Pate	- Raw	596
Pad Thai	- Raw	597
Pistachio Delight	- Raw	598
Power Balls, Goji & Chia	- Raw	599
Quesadilla Filling	- Cooked	600
Salad, Estrogen Sponge	- Raw	601
Salad, Israeli	- Raw	602
Salad, Super Slimming Lentil	- Raw	603
Salad, Stephanie's Sumptuous	- Raw	604
Salad, Tabouli	- Raw	607
Sauce, Lemon Tahini	- Raw	608
Sauce, Tomato	- Raw	609
Seed & Nut Mix, Stephanie's	- Raw	610
Soup, Cabbage	- Cooked	612
Soup, Gourmet Fennel & Grape	- Raw	613
Soup, Pumpkin & Carrot	- Cooked & raw	614
Soup, Tomato, Creamy Warm	- Raw	615
Spaghetti	- Raw	616
Spinach flavor plus	- Raw	617
Sprouted Lentils to Fill You Up	- Raw	618
Squash / Sweet Potato	- Cooked	619
Stir-Fry	- Cooked	620
Tahini	- Raw	622
Toast	- Cooked	623
Tunaless Pate	- Raw	624
Walnut Meatless Balls	- Raw	625

ASPARAGUS GOURMET ROLLS   - Cooked

- Wheat-free lavache or flat bread (from health food store). (If you are super keen to get thin, use lettuce leaves instead).
- Asparagus.
- 1/2 Tbsp. Healthy mayonnaise (e.g. egg & soy free, with healthy cold pressed oils). Home made is best.
- 1 tsp. Coconut oil.
- Dash Lemon juice.
- ½-1 tsp. Liquid mustard (sweetened only with non-gmo cane sugar. Not for people with irritated digestive tracts).

Vegetables for Filler e.g.:

- Mushrooms.
- Green onion.
- Salad mix.
- Cucumber.

Steam asparagus lightly. Lightly boil mushrooms & green onions in minimal water. Mix a little lemon juice & mustard in the mayonnaise. Add a little boiling water to heat it up if desired. Lightly sauté lavache in a tiny bit of coconut oil. Put asparagus on lavache. Add all other veges, then mayo mix. Superb!

BABY FOOD   - Cooked & Raw

Baby food should not be different from anything *you* would want to eat. If you taste most processed baby food, it tastes awful. To make matters even worse, many of them are filled with fillers like cornstarch, which has no nutrition, as well as GMOs. All this despite the high price! Making your own baby food is very easy. Just make them into 'ice cubes" and store in the freezer. For very young babies, use only one ingredient for a number of days, until their digestive system gets used to it.

All you do is peel and puree raw fruit, or boil vegetables gently in a little water, or steam them. Add maybe one grain of Celtic sea salt every now and again, because non breast-fed toddlers need salt too - it's in their blood. Then blend the food, with the water you used, to keep all the minerals. Then strain the food through a non-aluminum sieve.

Use what you need now, once it's cooled. Then put the rest in an ice cube tray. Freeze them. After they are frozen, get them out of the trays and store them in the freezer in containers marked with the ingredients and date. To defrost, get them out earlier or put in a warm saucepan with a little water. Do not *ever* microwave food or water, *especially* baby food.

Suggestions: Organic raw apples or pears (peel first and use fresh), cooked carrots, sweet potato, squash, peas, spinach. For brown rice, lentils and beans, you must soak them first for 8 hours before cooking to sprout them and make them safer and easier to digest. Please research this further. Dr. Sears in *The Baby Book*, goes into this in far more detail than I can cover here.

As they get older, you can add a drop of other things they need, like essential fatty acids (cold pressed avocado or flaxseed oil).

BEANS, TASTY   - Cooked

- 1 onion.
- 1 green pepper (capsicum).
- 2 cup dried beans (black, kidney etc.).
- ¼ cabbage, chopped finely (to absorb extra estrogen).
- Fresh coriander /cilantro.
- 1 tsp. cumin.
- 1/2 tsp. honey.
- 1 Tbsp. coconut oil.
- ½ tsp. Celtic sea salt.
- Organic tamari to taste.

Soak the beans in reverse osmosis water for 8 hours. Drain. If you are not ready to cook right then, store them in the fridge. Add plenty of water and some salt, bring to boil, cover and then simmer for 4 hours. Halve the beans and store the other half in fridge or freezer for another meal at another time. Sauté on medium heat the onion and pepper in coconut oil until lightly cooked. Reduce heat to low. Add the cumin and stir well for a minute. Add all of the rest of the ingredients except for the fresh cilantro. Raise the heat. Wait until cabbage is heated up/ cooked a little. Add the cilantro just before serving.

Suggestions to serve with are baked squash/sweet potato, salad, fresh sprouts, rice etc.

BREAD, Walnut & Grain-free   - Cooked

Delicious and very filling.

- 2 cups almond flour (look online, or grind up blanched almonds, which is much cheaper).
- 2 Tbsp. ground flaxseeds.
- 2 eggs, organic and free range (so they are not GMO or toxic).
- ½ cup coconut oil, lightly melted.
- 1 cup almond milk, unsweetened.
- 2 tsp. baking powder, aluminum free.
- ½ tsp. Celtic sea salt.
- 1 tsp. cinnamon.
- 2 tsp. maple syrup.
- 1 cup walnuts, chopped.

Mix everything, except for the walnuts. Stir walnuts in after mixing. Put in a baking pan greased with coconut oil. Cook at 350° F for about 45 minutes, until a toothpick comes out clean.

BREAKFAST

- Raw

First drink two 8 oz glasses of reverse osmosis water, before you eat anything. Then, choose from one or more of the following:

1. Breakfast "Cereal":

Mix all together. This tastes as good as commercial breakfast cereal:

- Ground flaxseeds (organic, so they are not GMO).
- Seed and nut mix (see recipe).
- Fresh fruit, chopped e.g. apple / pear.
- Something sweet – e.g. trickle of raw honey. Add some raisins and it will taste like raisin bran.
- Almond milk (unsweetened).
- (Treats & maintenance only) A few raw rolled oats, soaked in water for eight hours.

2. Blueberries, frozen or fresh. Allow frozen ones to thaw. Sprinkle with Stephanie's seed & nut mix.

3. Power Balls (see recipe) / **Bowl of raw nuts and seeds**. With a little dried fruit (e.g. goji berries). Add a spoon to the bowl. If you try to pick them up in your fingers, you won't consume enough.

4. Fresh-squeezed vegetable & fruit juice (with greens added). You could add this to your smoothie, to keep the volume down, so as not to stretch your tummy.

5. Smoothie:

- 4 Tbsp. seed & nut mix, ground.
- Extra chia seeds.
- 1 Tbsp. or more of green superfoods, such as spirulina (ask at your health food store or check online). You can skip this if you are adding fresh juice with greens, such as kale/spinach.

- Handful of fruit, such as frozen blueberries and/or mango.
- 1-2 cups water (reverse osmosis filtered of course) – but, even better, use fresh-squeezed vegetable & fruit juice.
- Small amount goji berries (optional).
- Crushed ice or ice cubes to taste (optional).
- ¼ tsp. raw honey (optional). If you add fresh juice, you won't need this.

Plus, consider the following supplements:

- 3-6 spirulina tablets.
- Vitamin D tablet/s.
- MSM powder (in juice or smoothie).
- Kelp drops for iodine.

If not satisfied, or having a treat or on a maintenance plan, you may be able to have some toast, see under "toast".

BURGER, EGG – HOLD THE BURGER   - Cooked

All Australian hamburgers come with pickled beetroot, even Burger King. It makes a big difference to the taste.

- 1 beet (organic so it's not GMO).
- 1 onion.
- 2 organic, free-range eggs.
- mushrooms.
- 1 tomato.
- lettuce.
- wheat-free toast, e.g. millet bread (optional).
- 2 tsp. coconut oil.

Steam the beet. Sauté onions & mushrooms in oil. Fry eggs in oil, then turn over. Lay eggs on toast. Lay beet on eggs, then mushrooms & onions on eggs, then tomato & lettuce. For extra weight reduction, omit the toast.

BURGER, lentil   - Cooked

Delicious hot or cold. Great to take to go to a barbeque.

- 2/3 cup red lentils, soaked 8 hours.
- 2/3 cup green lentils, soaked 8 hours.
- 1/4 cup oatmeal, soaked 8 hours.
- 2 eggs, organic & free range (so they are not GMO or toxic).
- 1 carrot, grated.
- 1 potato / sweet potato, grated.
- 1 onion, grated.
- 1/2 cup sesame seeds.
- 1 tsp. maple syrup.
- 1 tsp. Italian herbs.
- coconut oil/ghee for greasing pan.
- 1 Tbsp. miso (optional).
- 2 cups water.

Add water to lentils. Bring to boil and cover. Simmer lentils until soft, about 15 minutes. Scrape the bottom occasionally so they don't burn. Mix all ingredients. Grease a baking pan with a little oil. Shape into patties and put on pan. Bake 25-30 minutes at 350° F. Turn and bake another 20 minutes or so. Alternatively, sauté on medium heat in coconut oil, about 12 minutes each side.

CARROT CAKE   - Raw

Eat as much as you want for breakfast, lunch and dinner with no guilt, while you get thin & healthy! Stores for a few days in the fridge.

- 7 medium sized carrots.
- 1 cup walnuts, preferably soaked overnight.
- 1 cup pitted dates, soaked one hour.
- 3/4 cup raisins (sultanas), soaked one hour.
- Optional: 1/2 teaspoon cinnamon.
- Optional: 1/2 teaspoon natural vanilla essence (Note: If you eat a lot of this, or to be extra healthy, omit the cinnamon and vanilla).

FROSTING:

- 1 cup raw cashews, preferably soaked overnight.
- 3 Tbsp. raw honey (creamed is tastiest).
- 2 Tbsp. fresh squeezed orange juice.

Preferably soak the walnuts and cashews overnight, to sprout. In any case, soak in good water, in separate containers, for one hour, the dates, raisins and cashews.

Peel the carrots. Blend them in a blender until super fine. Then add walnuts, dates, cinnamon & vanilla. Blend the lot really well. Take out and mix in the raisins by hand. Place the cake in a glass / ceramic dish. Make it level. Blend the icing ingredients. Place them on the cake. This is best to eat immediately. But you can also store in the freezer or fridge. I prefer it when it's been partly defrosted.

CHIPS, POTATO & COCONUT   - Cooked

Even though I suggest that you don't have potato because it's toxic to so many people, if you just have to have some chips, this should satisfy you enough without doing too much harm.

- 1 large potato per person.
- 1 dessertspoon of virgin coconut oil per person.

Slice the potatoes fairly thin. Put in a bowl of ice cold water, and keep in the fridge, for one hour. Dry them well by shaking in a clean towel.

Place the oil on a baking tray. Melt the oil in an oven at 350°F. Remove and cover the chips with the oil. Place in oven at 350°F for 20 minutes, turn and cook another 20 minutes.

Add Celtic sea salt to taste.

COCONUT DHAL   - Cooked

Dhal is a dish made from lentils, like lentil stew. This is a staple in our family. Lentils seem to be healthier than beans, and have been a staple of many upper class people in India for hundreds of years. The lemongrass gives this a great taste.

- 7 oz red lentils or Moong Dhal (soaked 8 hours).
- 2 cans coconut milk.
- 4 green onions / shallots, chopped.
- ½ leek, chopped.
- 2 Tbsp. or more lemon grass, chopped (fresh or frozen – ask at your Asian store).
- 2 tsp. chives.
- 1 Tbsp. basil, chopped (fresh or dry).
- 1-2 Tbsp. cilantro, fresh chopped.
- 1 tsp. raw honey.
- 1 Tbsp. lemon juice.
- Celtic sea salt to taste.
- 2 tsp. coconut oil / ghee (organic or from a non-GMO country).
- 1 cup water.

Lightly sauté green onions and leeks in oil/ghee, on low-medium heat until soft. Add everything else. Bring to boil, then lower heat to simmer until dhal is cooked and like thin porridge. Stir the bottom frequently so nothing sticks to the bottom and burns. Add more water if necessary.

Garnish with chopped cilantro. People not working to get thin can have some millet soaked for 8 hours or Basmati rice. Serve with chopped tomato, banana & cucumber, and for a treat, pappadums (pappads) cooked in coconut oil.

CURRY   - Cooked

- 1 cup (7 oz) red lentils or moong dhal (mung beans), soaked 8 hours.
- 1 can coconut milk (no preservatives).
- 1/4 cup grated carrot.
- 1/4 cup diced celery.
- 3 green onions.
- 1 Tbsp. chives.
- 1/2 leek.
- 1 Tbsp. organic oil / ghee (organic or from a non-GMO country).
- 1 Tbsp. fenugreek.
- 1 tsp. cumin, ground.
- 1 tsp. garam masala, ground.
- ½ tsp. coriander.
- 1 tsp. dried ginger or more of shredded fresh ginger.
- 1 tsp. tamari or soy sauce (organic so it's gmo free).
- 1 tsp. lemon juice or rice vinegar.
- 1 tsp. dried basil.
- 1/2 tsp. maple syrup.
- 1/2 tsp. Celtic sea salt.
- 2 cups or more of water.

Lightly sauté green onions and leeks in oil/ghee, on low-medium heat until soft. Reduce heat. On low heat, stir in cumin, garam masala and coriander. Stir for one minute. Add everything else. Simmer until dhal is cooked and like thin porridge. Add more water if necessary. Stir the bottom frequently so it doesn't burn.

Garnish with chopped cilantro. Serve with millet or brown basmati rice. Also maybe add pappadums (pappads), chopped tomato, banana & cucumber.

EGGS STEPHANYA   - Cooked

Fast, Low Carb Dinner.

- 1 onion.
- mushrooms.
- 2 eggs (organic & free range so they are not fed GMOs or toxic).
- fresh basil, chopped.
- Just a little cream cheese, (organic so the cows were not fed GMOs) (Optional).
- 1 tomato.
- lettuce / greens / sprouts.
- ½ Tbsp. coconut oil
- organic salted butter.

Fry eggs in a little oil & butter. Turn them over. At the same time, sauté the onion and mushrooms in a little oil & butter. Add the cream cheese and basil. Cover the eggs with the mushroom mixture, then add slices of tomato. Serve with greens, sprouts or salad. (Always have some raw food with every meal, for the enzymes.

HUMMUS, SUN-DRIED TOMATO   - Raw

- 1 cup dried chickpeas, soaked 8 hours.
- ½ cup almonds, soaked 8 hours.
- ½ cup sesame seeds.
- ½ cup sun-dried tomatoes.
- 2 pitted dates.
- ¼ cup lemon juice.
- ¼ cup parsley.
- ¼ cup cilantro.
- 1 Tbsp. fresh chives (optional).
- 1 tsp. Celtic sea salt.

Soak dried chickpeas & almonds for 8 hours. (You can store them in the fridge for a day or two if you aren't ready to cook immediately afterwards. Just rinse them once a day). Soak sun-dried tomatoes and dates for one hour or more. Blend all ingredients.

Serve with celery, carrots, brazil nuts, in avocados, on lettuce etc.

ICE CREAM   - Raw

- Bananas.
- Frozen blueberries.
- Frozen mango.
- Nut mix.
- Raw honey (optional).

Peel bananas. Freeze them. Mince frozen fruit with your juicer, if it is able to do this. Important Tip – dismantle the juicer *immediately after* making this. Sometimes it can freeze shut, and can only be pulled apart with a hammer. Add nut mix and raw honey.

JUICE, FRESH-SQUEEZED   - Raw

I was shocked when a friend of mine told me that she owned a top quality juicer, but had not used it because "she did not have a recipe". Here's the only recipe you need: Whatever is in the fridge - juice it, either on its own or mixed with other plants. Suggestions are:

- Green leaves are the *most important ingredient* because they contain chlorophyll & magnesium. Try parsley, spinach, collard greens, kale, turnip greens, different choys from the Asian store.
- Beetroot* (*only* organic so it's not GMO). Juice the greens as well.
- Carrots.
- Celery*.
- Cucumber (peeling first will make it taste better).

Add a little fruit for taste and greater range of nutrients. Note: If you are super serious about getting slim, use only lemon from this list.

- Apples*.
- Pears* (I read of one scientific research where women who ate one pear a day lost more weight because of a certain substance in the pear).
- Oranges (peel them first).
- Lemon (halve it) (has special healing abilities).
- Pineapple (peel it first. Only occasionally, as it can irritate).
- Red grapes* (have these only occasionally, and not very many when you do).

Those marked * are best to have organic, if you can afford it, as they use more pesticide on these. And pesticides work by robbing insects (and you) of minerals and damaging nerves. But it's far better to have non-organic fruit than not at all. The more leafy greens, the better. Add some leafy greens to almost every juice.

MILLET   - Cooked

Healthy replacement for rice.

- 1 cup hulled millet, soaked 8 hours.
- 1-2 Tbsp. organic, salted butter (so it's not GMO).
- ½ tsp. Celtic sea salt.
- 2 cups reverse osmosis water.

Soak millet in water for 8 hours. (Drain and store in fridge if you aren't ready to cook it then. Rinse once a day). Bring to a boil, skim, reduce heat, add salt and butter, cover tightly. Simmer on low for 15 minutes.

MUFFINS– Grainfree   - Cooked

- 2 cups almond flour (made from grinding blanched almonds).
- ¼ cup ground flaxseeds.
- 1 egg, organic & free range (so they aren't GMO).
- 1 ripe banana (organic so it's not gassed) (or add another egg).
- ½ cup almond milk.
- ¼ cup coconut oil.
- ½ cup raw honey / maple syrup / organic molasses (so it's not GMO).
- 1 tsp. cinnamon (optional).
- 1 tsp. vanilla (optional).
- Pinch Celtic sea salt.
- 1 tsp. baking powder, aluminum free.
- 1 cup flavoring – blueberries (fresh or frozen)/chopped walnuts/pecans/prunes/figs/cherries.

Mix all ingredients in the first section. Then stir in the flavorings. Grease muffin pans (non-aluminum) with coconut oil. Bake at 350° F for 22-25 minutes or until a toothpick comes out clean.

MUFFINS, Wheat-free   - Cooked

These are best to have when you are on a maintenance plan. If you want to reduce weight, the grain-free muffins are much better. It is important to soak flour because whole grains contain phytic acid, which is harmful to health because it stops the absorption of minerals. This also makes them easier to digest. I like to double this recipe and freeze the extra.

- 3 cups whole grain flour, like amaranth and/or millet, soaked 12-24 hours. It's best to use grainfree almond flour.
- 2 eggs, organic free-range.
- 5 Tbsp. coconut oil (or half coconut/half organic salted butter if you can lose fat while eating dairy).
- ¼ tsp. sun-dried sea salt.
- ¼ cup maple syrup / cane juice / molasses / raw honey.
- 2 tsp. baking soda.
- 1 tsp. pure vanilla extract (not imitation).
- ½ tsp. cinnamon.
- ½-1 cup flavorings – walnuts / pistachios / dried cherries / sultanas / blueberries.
- 1 ¼ cup water (reverse osmosis).

Soak the flour in water for 12-24 hours. Blend all other ingredients except for the flavorings. Then stir in the flavorings. Pour into muffin trays greased with coconut oil (non-aluminum, non-Teflon). Bake at 350°F for 18 minutes, or until a toothpick comes out clean.

NUT BUTTER   - Cooked & Raw

Making your own nut butters is much healthier and cheaper than buying them. These make a great replacement for peanut butter, as peanuts are toxic and should be avoided. Use as much or as little of each nut or seed as you wish.

- Almonds, raw.
- Cashews, raw (less of these).
- Pistachios, raw.
- Sunflower seeds.
- Pumpkin seeds.
- 2 pitted dates to sweeten it (optional).
- Some Chia seeds (great way to eat Omega 3s, which are great for weight loss).
- Pinch of Celtic sea salt if desired.
- Cold-pressed almond / sunflower / sesame / avocado / safflower / sesame oil.

Blend. Add just enough oil to make it stick.

OLIVE PATE   – Raw

- 1 cup black olives (Canned olives are cooked. Get raw if you can).
- 1 carrot.
- 2 Tbsp. seed mix.
- 1 Tbsp. lemon juice.
- Fresh basil to taste.
- Almond milk as needed to process.

Blend.

OLIVE & SPINACH TAPENADE   – Partly raw

- Spinach.
- Fresh basil.
- Black olives (canned olives are cooked).
- Raw pistachios / walnuts.
- Lemon Juice.

Blend the above. Serve with any vegetables such as:
- Asparagus, steamed.
- Tomatoes.
- Cucumber.
- Celery.
- Sliced Carrots.

PAD THAI   – Raw

Noodles:
- Super thin slices of Napa cabbage / carrots / organic zucchini (so it's not gmo).

Sauce:

- ¼ cup chopped cashews.
- 1 avocado.
- ½ cup coconut pulp (this can be frozen).
- 1 Tbsp. raw honey.
- 1 Tbsp. fresh ginger juice.
- 2 Tbsp. lime juice.

Blend the sauce. Put on noodles.

PISTACHIO DELIGHT   - Raw

- 3 Plum/Roma tomatoes.
- 2 avocados.
- ½ zucchini (organic so it's not GMO).
- 1 green onion.
- 2-3 Tbsp. raw pistachios.
- 2 Tbsp. raw almonds.
- 2-3 Tbsp. fresh basil.
- 1 Tbsp. fresh cilantro/coriander.
- ½ Tbsp. fresh mint (if available).
- Juice of ½-1 lemon.

Blend. Serve on it's own, wrapped in lettuce, with carrot/celery sticks etc.

POWER BALLS
                                                    - Raw

Super nutritious, with tons of magnesium, omega 3s and coconut oil. No need to pay high health food store prices when you can make your own so easily.

- • 1 cup raw sunflower seeds.
- • 1/3 cup goji berries.
- • ¼ cup chia seeds.
- • ¼ cup raw cashews.
- • 2 Tbsp. raw sesame seeds.
- • 1-2 pitted dates.
- • ¼ tsp. Celtic sea salt.
- • 1/3 cup raw pistachios.
- • 4 Tbsp. virgin coconut oil, melted.
- • 1/2 Tbsp. raw honey.
- • 3 Tbsp. water.

Grind up the first 7 ingredients in the blender until fine. Then add the honey, water, and coconut oil. When blended, add some of the pistachios and mix a little, but allow some of them to retain their shape. Shape into balls. Refrigerate until hard. Store in the refrigerator.

QUESADILLA FILLING   - Cooked

- Quesadillas, wheat-free (from health food store).
- Napa cabbage.
- Mushrooms.
- Onions.
- Roma Tomatoes, chopped finely.
- Avocado, chopped.
- Chives, chopped.
- Butter, organic salted, 1/2 Tbsp. Or use coconut oil.

Sauté the onions lightly in butter/oil. Add the mushrooms and cabbage for two minutes or so. Add all remaining ingredients and serve immediately.

SALAD, ESTROGEN SPONGE   - Raw

- Carrots, shredded.
- Cabbage, shredded.
- Apple, diced.
- Raisins, a few.
- Lemon juice, a dash.
- Celtic sea salt, to taste.
- Maple syrup, ¼ tsp.
- Sunflower seeds, as many as you can bare to eat.

SALAD, ISRAELI   - Raw

Try this. It's much tastier than it looks.

Equal parts finely chopped:

- Tomatoes.
- Green peppers.
- Green onions / shallots.
- Lebanese/pickling cucumbers, peeled.
- 2 Tbsp. lemon juice.
- 1 tsp. good oil, e.g. avocado / cold pressed sesame oil.
- Celtic sea salt to taste.

Chop equal proportions of the vegetables into very small pieces, the smaller the better. Mix in the rest.

SALAD, SUPER SLIMMING LENTIL - Raw

Surprisingly filling and satisfying.

- 1/3 lentils soaked for 8 hours.
- 1/3 apple, chopped.
- 1/3 carrot, chopped.
- Fresh squeezed lemon juice.
- Tiny bit maple syrup.

SALAD, STEPHANIE'S SUMPTUOUS   - Raw

Many women who've eaten at my house have raved about my salads. I'm going to teach you how to do the same thing. It's easy. There are thousands of recipes out there for salads, but you don't need a recipe. You just need a method to incorporate lots of different raw nutrients into your body. Plus free yourself from the need to have a recipe every time. We're not baking a cake where it's important to have the correct quantities of each ingredient. If it's a raw fruit, vegetable, nut or seed, you can eat it!

Leafy Greens

Half fill, or more, the bowl with one or more greens such as:

- Lettuce, Romaine or coz have more nutrition than iceberg.
- Mezuna.
- Spinach.
- Italian parsley, chop really well.
- Kale.
- No arugula – it's toxic for me, and therefore I suspect for others as well.

Extra Flavor

Add one or more of one the following:

- Basil, fresh(super easy to grow).
- Dill, fresh.
- Fennel, fresh (cut up part of one – delicious mild licorice taste).
- Cilantro.
- Mint.

Other Green Vegetables

Add one or more of what you feel like of:

- Celery.
- Cucumber.

Other Vegetables

Add one or more of what you feel like of:
- Olives.
- Carrots – grated or sliced super thin.
- Green onions /shallots (a little goes a long way to giving taste).
- Avocado.
- Tomatoes (less often since people get allergic to these).
- Sprouted lentils (see recipe).
- Broccoli / Cauliflower, raw (to absorb estrogen).

Fruit

I love to add some fruit to most of my salads. Just go easy on them:

- Apples, chopped.
- Pear, chopped.
- Grapes or Raisins.
- Oranges, chopped in the middle of the segments, so the juice shows.

Seeds - raw

Raw seeds are more important than nuts. They have all they need to grow a plant in them. Nuts do also, but nuts sometimes muscle test as negative for people, probably because the oils in them have deteriorated.

- Chia (super high in Omega 3).
- Sunflower.

- Pumpkin (pepitas).
- Sesame (buy these by the pound or they are too expensive).
- Stephanie's Seed mix.

Nuts

Make them raw as often as possible. Variety is a key to nutrition. Different plant types will give your body different molecules that it needs.

- Almonds, chopped.
- Walnuts, chopped.
- Pecans, chopped.
- Pistachios.
- Cashews.

Oil

Your body would prefer zero processed oil. It is unnatural. If you absolutely must have oil, make it a tiny amount of one of the following:

- Coconut oil (this one you can be generous with).
- Cold-pressed flax, sesame, sunflower, safflower.
- If you use olive oil, you absolutely need to be totally certain that it really is extra virgin olive oil, and not lampante oil or diluted with other oils, which 70% of Extra virgin olive oil is.

Vinegar or vinegar substitute

Your body does not like vinegar. It's acidic, and very unnatural. The best substitute is lemon or lime juice, preferably raw. If you want vinegar for a treat, try balsamic raspberry vinegar (delicious). Make sure it is made from a non-GMO source.

SALAD, TABOULI   - Raw

Fantastic way to eat leafy greens, that are super good for you. Eat this often and add to sandwiches and wraps.

- 2-3 cups of raw Italian parsley.
- 1-2 tomatoes, chopped finely.
- 1-2 green onions /shallots.
- 3 Tablespoons (or more) raw sunflower seeds
- Juice of 2 lemons.
- 1 Tbsp. good oil e.g. expeller pressed safflower / sunflower / sesame oil (optional).
- ½ tsp. 100% maple syrup.
- Celtic sea salt to taste.

Chop up the parsley as fine as possible. Chop the tomato and green onions into very small pieces. Mix everything together thoroughly.

SAUCE – LEMON TAHINI   - Raw

This makes anything taste good.

- 1/4 cup raw, hulled sesame seeds.
- 3 Tbsp. lemon juice.
- 1/4 cup of fresh herbs, such as basil, dill, mint, cilantro.
- 1 Tbsp. cold pressed sesame or avocado oil (to help blend the sesame seeds).
- Water / almond milk.
- Pinch Celtic sea salt.

Grind up well. Add water / almond milk to desired consistency. Add to salads or steamed, baked or raw vegetables.

SAUCE, TOMATO   – Raw

Tastes as good as cooked tomato sauce.

- 2 tomatoes.
- 10 sun-dried tomatoes, soaked one hour.
- Celtic Salt to taste.
- Something sweet – e.g. 1 date, plum, raisins.

Soak sun-dried tomatoes for one hour. Blend until smooth.

SEED & NUT MIX, STEPHANIE'S   - Raw

Seeds have everything in them for a plant to grow, which means they have everything that your body needs also. They are pure nutrition. Plus they have ingredients that hasten fat loss, such as Omega 3's and magnesium. Interestingly, seeds seem to muscle test as positive for people more often than nuts do. Add as much of this seed and nut mix as you can to smoothies, juice, salads and sandwiches. Eat them raw only, as cooking creates toxins. Sneak some onto cooked food before serving, so you get the family to eat some. Make this up ahead of time, and store in an airtight container. The fridge would be best but is not necessary. There's nothing special about this recipe. Feel free to make any changes at all to this.

Keep two containers of this:

- **Whole** seeds and nuts.
- **Ground** seeds and nuts that are ground up into small pieces in a blender, so it's easier to digest and to sneak onto meals without noticing that it's there.

Everything is RAW.

- 1 cup sunflower seeds.
- 1 cup pepitas (pumpkin seeds).
- ½ cup pistachio nuts.
- ½ cup cashews.
- ½ cup walnuts.

Add to **Whole seeds and nuts** mixture:

- ¼ cup goji berries.
- ½ cup Brazil nuts (they have omega 3s).

Add to **<u>Ground Up</u>** mixture:

- ¼ cup pitted dates, to sweeten things up.
- 1 cup chia seeds (these are a bit too messy to eat with the whole seed mixture).
- ½ cup ground Flax seeds.

Almonds: I would add a lot of these, but only if you can get them raw. The trouble is, currently all U.S. so-called 'raw' almonds are actually pasteurized. They have been cooked and won't grow. Therefore they are dead, have added toxins and some of their nutrition has been destroyed. They are not raw - they just look as though they are. This is very sad because almonds are the most nutritious and least toxic nut to have, and never hurt anyone. Once again, we see that someone has made a decision that is not for our higher good. Hopefully, this situation will change.

SOUP, CABBAGE   – Cooked

Woman's World had several articles talking about all the weight that people lost from eating cabbage soup. The articles spoke of this being because it was high volume for low calories, but it may be because cabbage is one of the best anti-estrogenic foods. People are fat these days partly from too many toxins, such as soy and pesticides, in our food, that act as though they are estrogen.

- ½ head cabbage, chopped.
- 1 cup carrots, shredded.
- 1 can diced tomatoes with liquid / fresh tomatoes.
- 1 stick celery, chopped finely.
- 1 tsp. coconut oil / salted organic butter.
- 1 large onion.
- Dash of lemon juice.
- ¼ tsp. maple syrup.
- Celtic sea salt.
- Optional: ½ cup brown rice pasta, cooked first (best for maintenance only).

If using pasta, cook it in water as per instructions. Sauté onion lightly in oil/butter, add everything else, simmer until cabbage is tender. Add pasta.

SOUP, GOURMET FENNEL & GRAPE   - Raw

This delicious recipe was inspired by Iron Chef Geoffrey Zakarian.

- ½ cup fennel.
- 1 cup red grapes.
- ½ cup almonds.
- 2 large cucumber, (pickling cucumbers are tastiest – use more of them).
- Celtic sea salt, to taste.
- 1 cup reverse osmosis water.

Heat up the water separately if desired. Blend all ingredients. Add water.

SOUP, PUMPKIN & CARROT   - Cooked & Raw

Super filling, & cheap.

- 2 cups pumpkin / butternut squash, steamed.
- 8 carrots.
- ½-1 cup greens (e.g. spinach/bok choy).
- 10 almonds.
- 1 Tbsp. coconut oil.
- 1-2 Tbsp. lemon juice.
- Celtic Sea salt to taste.
- Hot water.

Steam the pumpkin. Peel the carrots. Blend till smooth. Blend in boiling water just before serving.

SOUP, CREAMY WARM TOMATO   - Raw

- 3 tomatoes.
- 1 avocado.
- 3 Tbsp. Stephanie's Seed Mix.
- 1 Tbsp. cilantro.
- 1 tsp. virgin coconut oil.
- 1 tsp. lemon juice.
- 2 cups water.

Heat up the water separately if desired. Blend all ingredients. Add water.

Variations: Add carrots, shredded coconut, or one pear to sweeten it.

SPAGHETTI with TOMATO SAUCE   - Raw

Tastes as good as cooked sauce!

- 4 zucchinis (organic so they are not genetically modified).
- 1 cup of sun-dried tomatoes, soaked one hour (these make the sauce 'meaty').
- 1 cup tomatoes, cut up.
- 1 date, soaked for one hour.
- 1-1/2 cup basil, chopped.
- 5 green olives.
- ½ tsp. Celtic sea salt.
- ½ cup water, just boiled.

In a food processor or with a mandolin, shred 4-6 zucchini. This is the pasta.

Blend the rest in a blender to make the sauce. Add reverse osmosis water if necessary. Then add zucchini pasta and sauce to hot water and stir to heat it up without cooking it.

SPINACH FLAVOR PLUS - Raw

Even children may like this.

- 2 cups spinach, raw.
- 1 can olives.
- 2 roma tomatoes.
- 2-4 sun-dried tomatoes, soaked 1 hour.
- 1 apple.
- 1 avocado.
- ¼ cup sesame seeds, raw.
- ¼ cup basil, fresh.
- 2 green onions.
- 1 Tbsp. lemon juice.

Blend. Serve by itself, with veges, on lettuce, on wheatfree bread etc.

SPROUTED LENTILS to Fill You Up   – Raw

Sprouted plants are super nutritious, because they have tons of life force. Also, the complicated molecules in them have been broken down so it is easier for you to absorb them. You don't have to see a sprout to appear for a seed to be 'sprouted'. After a few hours, the plant is changing on the inside.

- 1 cup lentils.
- 2 cups water, reverse osmosis.

Soak in water for 8 hours. Drain after 8 hours. You can lay them out for a day to sprout a little more. Or you can store them in the fridge now to prevent mold. Rinse and drain once a day, as they will keep growing in the fridge, and producing waste products.

Eat some straight, or add to whatever else you are eating. Great with apples! Do this every day. You may be surprised at how filling these are, because they are so nutritious.

SQUASH / SWEET POTATO   – Cooked

- Squash / sweet potatoes.
- Cooked bean dish / organic cottage cheese / one of the sauce recipes / steamed broccoli.

Add squash/sweet potatoes to a baking pan. Add a little water to keep moist. Cover and bake at 350° F for 1½ hours or until soft. Add fillings.

STIR-FRY   - Cooked

This is one of my favorite recipes. I suggest that if you are not going fully raw, that you make this one of your staples. You will note that Asians, before they started to eat more western dairy and other foods, were slimmer than westerners, and lacking in many western diseases. This is likely at least partly because they don't eat dairy, or much wheat, and because they eat so many different plants, especially lots of leafy, green plants that most of us have never heard of, as well as a lot of coconut.

It's fast, nutritious and you can vary it as much as you want. If you are cooking for the family, they will love it if you add rice noodles (which you should omit from your plate if you are really keen to burn fat). You can also throw in leftovers.

The keys to a successful stir-fry:

- It must be cooked *hot*. You really do need a wok for this.
- Get out all you need, and cut up *everything* before you start.
- Once you get going, everything is cooked within a minute to two (unless you are using meat, which should be long enough to kill the parasites in it) Think of it as doing little more than heating up the food.
- To get as close to raw as possible, have a few ingredients that you throw on at the last second, such as mung bean sprouts

Ingredients

- Cabbage (try different varieties such as napa / savoy).
- Leafy greens, such as bok choy (have a look in your Asian store for new varieties).
- Grated carrot.
- Mung bean sprouts.
- Onions.
- Green onions.
- Chives.

- Rice noodles (small amounts. Leave these out if you are extra keen to reduce fat, but they are a great way to encourage the family to enjoy this meal. Note: There is now a danger of rice being GMO.)
- 1 Tbsp. Coconut oil / ghee from non-gmo countries / cold-pressed sesame oil.

Extra flavoring & nutrition:

- Sesame seeds.
- Slivered almonds.
- Basil, fresh.
- Cilantro, fresh

Plus:

- Tbsp. / dash tamari or soy sauce (organic so it's not gmo).
- Tbsp. / dash lemon / lime juice.
- Sun-dried sea salt to taste.
- ¼ tsp. maple syrup.

Plus at the end:

- Seed mix.

If you are using rice noodles, soak them for 15 minutes in warm water. Heat up the oil on high. When it is very hot, add the onions and green onions. Stir frequently. One minute later add the cabbage. Stir frequently. One minute or so later add everything else for a few seconds to heat them up, then serve. Then add some raw chopped seed mix on top.

TAHINI   - Raw

Super good for you. Add to salads and as a topping on anything.

- Hulled raw sesame seeds.
- Cold pressed sesame oil.

Blend thoroughly. Use just enough oil to make it sticky enough for the blender to blend it.

TOAST
                                              - Cooked

More for a maintenance plan, or when you feel super wheat-deprived. Do not eat this if you are serious about reducing weight.

- Wheat-free toast from health food store (e.g. brown rice / millet bread. Check ingredients).
- A little salted, cultured, GMO-free butter (e.g. organic or from Europe).
- *Lots* of home-made nut butter.
- Tiny bit of jam/jelly with nothing in it except fruit. No "fructose" or "natural flavorings".
- Cover with chia seeds.
- (Optional for treats): Add a gob of organic cream cheese (so it's not GMO).

TUNA-less PATE   - Raw

- 2 cups raw sunflower seeds, soaked 8 hours to sprout them.
- ½ cup raw sesame seeds.
- 2 pitted dates, soaked 1 hour, or ½ tsp. raw honey.
- 2-3 Tbsp. fresh basil or mint.
- 1 Tbsp. good oil (e.g. cold pressed sunflower oil).
- ½ cup lemon juice.
- 2 green onions / shallots.
- ½ tsp. Celtic sea salt.

Blend till smooth. Eat by itself with sticks of carrot or celery, or wrapped in kale / spinach / celery leaves.

WALNUT 'MEAT' BALLS   - Raw

- 1 1/3 cup raw walnuts, soaked for several hours.
- 1 date, soaked for one hour.
- 1 Tbsp. of nutritional yeast.
- 1 ½ Tbsp. of good oil.
- 2 tsp. of fresh lemon juice.
- 1 tsp. Celtic sea salt.
- 1 tsp. green onion / shallot, finely chopped.
- 2 Tbsp. fresh parsley, chopped finely.

Drain and rinse the walnuts. Mix the ingredients in food processor and shape into meatballs. Dip them in raw tomato sauce (let them soak in it a bit) and set aside.

A Final Word from Stephanie Relfe

Congratulations on getting to the end of this book! Well done!

I hope this book has upset you. It certainly upset me writing it. While I knew at the outset some of the information in this book, until I did all the research, I had no idea how evil and widespread were the toxins in our food supply, or how intentional some of it is, by the Food Mafia and the Medical Mafia. Get angry. Use that anger to make yourself take personal responsibility for what you feed you and your family, for the future of mankind.

If you haven't already done so, please go shopping with the "shopping list" to guide you. And then read the recipe chapter and get going.

Since the attention spans of most of us are only three months long, according to psychologists, may I please suggest that you mark in your calendar in three months time to re-read this book? You will find that there are many points which make more sense to you, especially if you have been taking advantage of this information.

Would you please do the following to help other people?

- Send us your testimonial describing your successes.

- Visit Amazon.com and share your testimonial with others, who want to improve their body like you have done.

- Send us 'before and after' pictures that we can share with others on our website.

- Please help others get thin. Share our websites. Give a book as a gift. Learn Kinesiology. And fight these bad corporations.

YOU ARE NOT ALONE

Please don't be discouraged or quit fighting. No matter where you are in your battle against weight, you are not alone. Always remember that you're not fat, you're toxic. And you **can** get thin. You are a victim of long term, laser targeted, expensively funded *projects*, whose goal is to make you a fat and sick consumer of toxic foods, drugs and diet products. Your weight is no accident. It was planned. So please get started immediately and never, ever give up the fight. Always remember:

FIGHT THE FOOD MAFIA

FIGHT THE DRUG MAFIA

FIGHT THE DIET MAFIA

And please tell as many of your friends as possible to do the same.

For more information and support on your fat loss journey, please visit our other websites:

www.YoureNotFatYoureToxic.com

Health, Wealth & Happiness
www.Relfe.com
Valuable natural health, mind, spirit, financial and other
information unifying the whole,
rather than just educating a part of the whole.
Established 1998

www.PerfectHealthDVD.com
See a trailer for our 11 hour training system:
"Perfect Health with Kinesiology & Muscle Testing"

www.PerfectHealthSystem.com
Learn more about our DVD training system:
"Perfect Health with Kinesiology & Muscle Testing"

www.SynergisticKinesiology.com
Explore the world of Kinesiology and learn this exciting system of
health and vitality.

www.Relfe.net
Direct order link for our Kinesiology books, DVDs and other
interesting things you may have never seen before.

Please see this book by Stephanie Relfe:

*Homeschool Natural Health & Biology
Comprehension Curriculum Workbook
For Grades 7 – 12*

English worksheets for reading comprehension,
at the same time that your child learns
how to be slim and healthy.

To be used in conjunction with the book
You're not fat, You're toxic

Bibliography

Books & Documentaries quoted in *You're not fat, You're toxic.*

Note: For an up-to-date listing of books, please visit
www.relfe.com/books.html

Ancient Secret of the Fountain of Youth, by Peter Kelder.
Anti-Estrogenic Diet, The, by Ori Hofmekler.
Baby Book, The, by Dr. William Sears M.D.
Body, Mind & Sport, by John Douillard.
Breastfeeding Book, The, by Dr. William Sears M.D.
Breastfeeding, Biocultural Perspectives, by Katherine Dettwyler.
Caffeine Blues, by Stephen Cherniske.
Chelation Answer, The, by Morton Walker D.P.M.
Cure for All Diseases, The, by Dr. Hulda Clark.
DASH Diet, by Mariza Snyder.
Dead Doctors Don't Lie, by Dr. Joel Wallach D.V.M., N.D.
Diet Wise, by Prof. Keith Scott-Mumby.
Don't Drink Your Milk, by Frank Oski.
Eat Fat, Lose Fat, by Dr. Mary Enig.
Emerging Viruses, by Dr. Leonard Horowitz.
Enzymes, the Fountain of Life, by Dr. D.A. Lopez.
Excitotoxins, by Dr. Russell Blaylock.
Extra Virginity, the Sublime and Scandalous World of Olive Oil, by
Tom Mueller.
Fat, Sick & Nearly Dead (DVD), directed by Joe Cross.
Fats that heal, Fats that Kill, by Udo Erasums.
Fluoride Deception, The (Book & DVD) by Christopher Bryson.
Food, Inc. (DVD), directed by Robert Kenner.
Forks Over Knives (DVD), with Drs. Campbell & Esselstyn.
Horowitz on Vaccines, by Dr. Leonard Horowitz.
Lick the Sugar Habit, by Nancy Appleton.
Lose Wheat, Lose Weight, by Antoinette Savill & Dawn Hamilton Ph.D.
Lose the Wheat, Lose the Weight, by Dr. William Davis M.D.
Magnesium Factor, The, by Mildred Seelig.

Mastering Leptin, by Byron Richards CCN.
Medical Mafia, by Guylaine Lanctôt.
Omnivore's Dilemma, The, by Michael Pollan.
One Brain, by Gordon Stokes.
Perfect Health with Kinesiology & Muscle Testing, (DVDs & Books) by Stephanie Relfe B.Sc. (Sydney).
pH Miracle for Weight Loss, The, by Shelley Redford Young.
Promise of Sleep, The, by Dr. William Dement, M.D., Ph.D.
Rainbow Green, Live Foods Cuisine, by Dr. Gabriel Cousens M.D.
Rawsome, by Brigitte Mars.
Revolutionary Way of Thinking, A, by Dr Charles Krebs.
Rosedale Diet, The, by Dr. Ron Rosedale M.D.
Running to the Top, by Arthur Lydiard.
Sea Salt's Hidden Powers, by Dr. Jacques De Langre Ph.D.
Sugar Blues, by William Dufty.
Super Size Me (DVD), Directed by & Starring Morgan Spurlock.
Transdermal Magnesium Therapy, by Mark Sircus.
Vitamin D3 Miracle, by Jeff Bowles
Wheat Belly, by Dr. William Davis, M.D.
Wheatgrass Book, The, by Ann Wigmore.
World According to Monsanto, The (DVD), Directed by Marie Robin.
Your Body's Many Cries for Water, by Dr. F. Batmanghelidj.

Index

About the author

Stephanie Relfe was born in Sydney Australia. She graduated with a Bachelor of Science degree from Sydney University, majoring in zoology and histology (the study of cells). She has been a professional kinesiologist since 1993 and is the author of the books & DVD training series *Perfect Health with Kinesiology & Muscle Testing*. (See www.PerfectHealthDVD.com & www.PerfectHealthSystem.com). She is also the webmaster of *Health, Wealth & Happiness* at www.Relfe.com, a website established in 1998 which provides valuable natural health, mind, spirit, financial and other information unifying the whole, rather than educating a part of the whole. Stephanie is married, with one son.

CPSIA information can be obtained
at www.ICGtesting.com
Printed in the USA
BVOW10s1923191017

498055BV00007B/149/P